D1573892

The Multiple Ligament Injured Knee

Springer
New York
Berlin
Heidelberg
Hong Kong
London
Milan
Paris
Tokyo

Gregory C. Fanelli, MD
Chief, Arthroscopic Surgery and Sports Medicine, Fanelli Sports Injury Clinic, Department of Orthopaedic Surgery, Geisinger Clinic Medical Center, Danville, Pennsylvania

Editor

The Multiple Ligament Injured Knee

A Practical Guide to Management

With 157 Illustrations in 217 Parts, 50 in Full Color

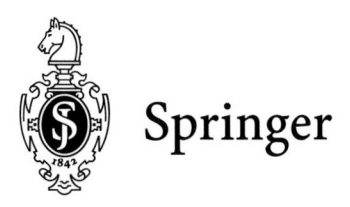

Springer

Gregory C. Fanelli, MD
Chief, Arthroscopic Surgery and Sports Medicine
Fanelli Sports Injury Clinic
Department of Orthopaedic Surgery
Geisinger Clinic Medical Center
Danville, PA 17822
USA

Cover illustration: Background photo from Getty Images, c 2003; inset photo courtesy of the authors.

Library of Congress Cataloging-in-Publication Data
The multiple ligament injured knee: a practical guide to management / [edited by] Gregory C. Fanelli.
   p. ; cm.
  Includes index.
  ISBN 0-387-40548-8 (hardcover : alk. paper)
  1. Knee—Wounds and injuries—Treatment. 2. Ligaments—Wounds and injuries—Treatment. 3. Orthopedics—Diagnosis. I. Fanelli, Gregory C.
  [DNLM: 1. Knee Injuries—therapy. 2. Ligaments, Articular—injuries. WE 870 M9605 2003]
RD561.M856 2003
617.5′82044—dc21   2003054408

ISBN 0-387-40548-8   Printed on acid-free paper.

© 2004 Springer-Verlag New York, Inc.
All rights reserved. This work may not be translated or copied in whole or in part without the written permission of the publisher (Springer-Verlag New York, Inc., 175 Fifth Avenue, New York, NY 10010, USA), except for brief excerpts in connection with reviews or scholarly analysis. Use in connection with any form of information storage and retrieval, electronic adaptation, computer software, or by similar or dissimilar methodology now known or hereafter developed is forbidden.
The use in this publication of trade names, trademarks, service marks, and similar terms, even if they are not identified as such, is not to be taken as an expression of opinion as to whether or not they are subject to proprietary rights.
While the advice and information in this book are believed to be true and accurate at the date of going to press, neither the authors nor the editors nor the publisher can accept any legal responsibility for any errors or omissions that may be made. The publisher makes no warranty, express or implied with respect to the material contained herein.

Printed in the United States of America.   (BS/MVY)

9 8 7 6 5 4 3 2 1   SPIN 10938409

Springer-Verlag is a part of *Springer Science+Business Media*

springeronline.com

*To my wife Lori, and my children,
Matthew, David, and Megan,
who are a continuous source of inspiration.*

Foreword

This is not just another book on the knee. Dr. Fanelli's book, *The Multiple Ligament Injured Knee: A Practical Guide to Management*, written with a team of experienced contributors, is about a subject that is pertinent, as well as often underestimated and underappreciated. The surgeon's thorough knowledge of this subject is essential for the care of the patient with multiple ligaments injured in the knee. Such knowledge is indispensable if the patient's well-being and future function are to be restored. Time, technique, judgment, and decisiveness are critical. These are the surgeon's responsibilities.

We have all come to be arthroscopic knee surgeons. We cannot, however, let this diminish our judgment or skill in open surgery. Often in the multiply compromised knee, open surgery is a requisite. We must return to the principles that Drs. O'Donoghue, Slocum, Hughston, Trillat, Mueller—the fathers of modern knee surgery—taught us. Open exposure may be essential in some cases; we must know when it is necessary. This textbook helps resolve the impasse that often occurs in this arena of evolving art and science. Young surgeons who were not there before the arthroscope might not appreciate the awful injury that frequently is associated with the multiligament knee injury. We all know Dr. O'Donoghue's firm dictum that early diagnosis and anatomic repair is the best and most appropriate method of treatment. Time has not invalidated this advice. Our diagnostic acumen has improved, but with this improvement there seems to be a pervasive trend to wait, to obfuscate, to substitute rehabilitation for ligament repair. For the knee with multiple ligamentous injuries and multiplanar laxity, waiting is just as much the death knell for the knee today as it was in O'Donoghue's day. Accurate diagnosis and anatomic repair have never been more needed than they are now in the era of high-speed sports, high expectations of return to play, and the stringent requirements of physical function in some industrial vocations.

How and why does *The Multiple Ligament Injured Knee* help us in our quest for knowledge? Does the knowledge help us to be ready if a patient with multiple injuries to the knee and lower extremity is thrust upon us unexpectedly, abruptly, with violence and trauma sufficient to jeopardize a limb's viability? This text is indispensable for this situation: it helps us to be prepared. Dr. Fanelli and his contributors offer solutions to these complex knee injuries that are well thought out, clearly presented, and anatomically and kinematically sound. The depth of wisdom in the chapters is apparent and useful. The chapters build upon each other, or they may stand alone. The contributing authors have been appropriately selected for their internationally recognized credibility. Dr. Fanelli's quest for excellence is apparent everywhere. The illustrations are generous, useful, and well done. The case studies are gems. Of course, I am biased—but the case study method when appropriately applied is efficient and meaningful. Dr. Fanelli has chosen appropriate and meaningful case studies to guide us in this essential learning process. The case studies will efficiently help us to focus our diagnostic and surgical skills when that inevitable day comes that one of these horrific limb-threatening injuries is thrust upon us.

This book may be approached in many ways—as a reference text for all knee surgeons; as a library addition for in-depth perusal; as a volume the mature practitioner will want to review for update, standard of practice, and result evaluation; and to other knee surgeons as an opportunity to see how the experts do it.

It is a special honor to be invited to write the foreword for this impressive work because I have lived the history, I have known the problems, I know the authors, and I know in my experience and teaching that the knowledge contained herein is exceptional for its depth, breadth, and usefulness. So many times, I have had to hunt for a key reference in the complex area of the multiligament injured knee; to wonder if my way was the best way. No more; it is all in one place, all concise and precise, readable, and usable. Dr. Fanelli and his team are to be commended on the recognition of a niche that needed filling and on a job well done. Dr. O'Donoghue would be pleased and proud of our progress in knee surgery and the principles espoused in this text. I share his pride. This text honors his memory and the memory of so many of our mentors. To the authors, we say thank you for a job well done in a subject where the information, principles, and practical advice is useful, meaningful, and comprehensively presented.

John A. Feagin, MD, FACS
Jackson, Wyoming

Preface

Our practice environment largely determines the pathways that our individual orthopaedic careers take. It has been a blessing to be in a position that enabled me to expand my surgical techniques and research interest in the evaluation and treatment of the multiple ligament injured knee. I believe the same situation exists for other contributors to this book. We all share a passion and a commitment to the treatment of complex instabilities of the knee. The purpose of this book is to provide experienced knee surgeons, general orthopaedic surgeons, fellows, residents, medical students, and other healthcare professionals having an interest in the multiple ligament injured knee with a useful tool for the management of the complex injuries.

The Multiple Ligament Injured Knee: A Practical Guide To Management is composed of four functional segments. The chapters were organized and written so that they build upon each other, and also so that they can stand alone. This will enable the reader to explore the topic of the multiple ligament injured knee at length or to use the text as a quick, practical reference when the need arises.

Chapters 1 through 4 address anatomy and biomechanics of the knee, initial assessment, classification, and nonsurgical management of the acutely dislocated knee. Chapters 5 through 9 provide multiple authors' techniques and opinions on the surgical treatment of the multiple ligament injured knee. Chapters 10 through 17 present methods to evaluate and manage associated complex conditions that occur in treating the multiple ligament injured knee. These include vascular injuries, nerve injuries, fixed posterior tibial subluxation, revision surgery, the role of osteotomy, postoperative rehabilitation, special aspects of functional bracing, and complications. The final chapter, 18, presents six case studies in the management of the multiple ligament injured knee. Each case study presents a different knee instability problem and then takes the reader through the decision-making process, the surgical treatment, and the final outcome.

The multiple ligament injured knee is an extremely complex pathological entity. I believe that through research, improved surgical techniques, the use of allograft tissue, advancement in surgical equipment, careful documentation, and experience, we are progressively improving outcomes in treating this devastating condition. It is my personal hope that this book will serve as a launch pad for new ideas to further develop treatment plans and surgical techniques for the multiple ligament injured knee.

I want to acknowledge the following people who have directly and indirectly contributed to this textbook. Rob Albano (editor) and Merry Post (developmental editor) at Springer-Verlag, New York, for their help in creating this book; the faculty and residents in the Department of Orthopaedic Surgery at Geisinger Medical Center, who have supported the multiple ligament injured knee research program; Craig J. Edson, M.S., P.T./A.T.C., friend, colleague, and research associate who is an outstanding clinician and teacher; and the Orthopaedic Surgery Team at Geisinger Medical Center, who are the best orthopaedic support staff in the world. Their dedication and drive for excellence are unequaled. My colleagues and friends have taken time out of their busy schedules to contribute chapters to this book. Mary Zubowicz and Kristin Notz Reinheimer, P.A.C., my secretary and physician assistant, are both able to keep patient care, schedules, and deadlines organized and moving forward, all with a smile.

Gregory C. Fanelli, MD
Danville, Pennsylvania

Contents

Foreword by *John A. Feagin, MD, FACS*		vii
Preface		ix
Contributors		xiii
1	Anatomy and Biomechanics of the Knee *Anikar Chhabra, C. Curtis Elliott, and Mark D. Miller*	1
2	Initial Assessment: Physical Examination and Imaging Studies *Jeff C. Brand, Jr., and Darren L. Johnson*	19
3	Classification of Knee Dislocations *Robert C. Schenck, Jr.*	37
4	Nonoperative Treatment of the Acutely Dislocated Knee *Bradley F. Giannotti*	51
5	Graft Selection *Kevin R. Willits and Walter R. Shelton*	57
6	Surgical Treatment of Acute and Chronic ACL/PCL/Medial Side Injuries of the Knee *Craig H. Bennett, Kevin E. Coates, Corey Wallach, and Ronald A. Hall*	63
7	Surgical Treatment of Acute and Chronic ACL/PCL/Lateral Side Injuries of the Knee *Daniel C. Wascher*	95
8	Combined ACL/PCL/Medial/Lateral Side Injuries of the Knee *Gregory C. Fanelli*	111
9	Open Surgical Treatment *Richard S. Richards II and Claude T. Moorman III*	133
10	Management of Arterial and Venous Injuries in the Dislocated Knee *Peter J. Armstrong and David P. Franklin*	151

11	Management of Acute and Chronic Nerve Injuries .... *Timothy J. Monahan*	167
12	The Role of Osteotomy .... *Annunziato Amendola and Michelle Wolcott*	185
13	Management of Chronic Posterior Tibial Subluxation ..... *Steven C. Chudik, Peter T. Simonian, and* *Thomas L. Wickiewicz*	193
14	Postoperative Rehabilitation .... *Craig J. Edson*	207
15	Complications Associated with Treatment .... *John C. Richmond*	217
16	Revision Surgery .... *Gregory C. Fanelli*	227
17	Brace Treatment .... *H. Jurgen Eichhorn and Daniel Pflaster*	243
18	Selected Case Studies .... *Gregory C. Fanelli*	249
	Index	261

Contributors

Annunziato Amendola, MD
Associate Professor, Department of Orthopaedics, Director, University of Iowa Sports Medicine, University of Iowa Hospitals and Clinics, Iowa City, IA 52242, USA

Peter J. Armstrong, MD
Chief of Vascular Surgery, Section of Vascular Surgery, Eisenhower Army Medical Center, Fort Gordon, GA 30905, USA

Craig H. Bennett, MD
Chief of Sports Medicine, University of Maryland, Head Orthopaedic Surgeon, Baltimore Ravens, Timonium, MD 21093, USA

Jeff C. Brand, Jr., MD
Orthopaedic Surgeon, Alexandria Orthopaedics and Sports Medicine, Alexandria, MN 56308, USA

Anikar Chhabra, MD
Chief Resident, Department of Orthopaedics, University of Virginia, Health Sciences Center, Charlottesville, VA 22908, USA

Steven C. Chudik, MD
Orthopaedic Surgeon, Hinsdale Orthopaedics Associates, Hinsdale, IL 60521, USA

Kevin E. Coates, MPT
Department of Orthopaedic Surgery, University of Pittsburgh Medical Center, Center for Sports Medicine, Pittsburgh, PA 15203, USA

Craig J. Edson, MHS, PT, ATC
Chief, Physical Therapy, Department of Orthopaedic Surgery, Geisinger Healthsouth Rehabilitation Hospital, Danville, PA 17822, USA

H. Jurgen Eichhorn, MD
Professor of Orthopaedic Surgery, Orthopadische Gemeinschaftspraxis, Straubing, 94315 Germany

C. Curtis Elliott, MD
Orthopaedic Surgery and Sports Medicine, Coastal Orthopaedic Associates, Conway, SC 29526, USA

Gregory C. Fanelli, MD
Chief, Arthroscopic Surgery and Sports Medicine, Fanelli Sports Injury Clinic, Department of Orthopaedic Surgery, Geisinger Clinic Medical Center, Danville, PA 17822, USA

David P. Franklin, MD
Chief, Vascular Surgery, Section of Vascular Surgery, Geisinger Clinic Medical Center, Danville, PA 17822, USA

Bradley F. Giannotti, MD, FACS
Chief, Department of Orthopaedic Surgery and Sports Medicine, St. Bonaventure University Team Physician, Charles Cole Memorial Hospital, Coudersport, PA 16915, USA

Ronald A. Hall, MD
Visiting Instructor of Orthopaedic Surgery, Department of Orthopaedic Surgery, University of Pittsburgh Medical Center, Center for Sports Medicine, Pittsburgh, PA 15203, USA

Darren L. Johnson, MD
Chairman, Department of Orthopaedic Surgery, University of Kentucky Sports Medicine Center, Lexington, KY 40536, USA

Mark D. Miller, MD
Associate Professor, Department of Orthopaedic Surgery, University of Virginia, Health Sciences Center, Charlottesville, VA 22908, USA

Timothy J. Monahan, MD
Orthopaedic Surgeon, Summit Orthopaedics, Bluegrass Community Hospital, Georgetown, KY 40324, USA

Claude T. Moorman III, MD
Director of Sports Medicine, Department of Orthopaedic Surgery, The Sports Medicine Center, Duke University Medical Center, Durham, NC 27710, USA

Daniel Pflaster, MS
2550 Abedul Street, Carlsbad, CA 92009, USA

Richard S. Richards II, MD
Department of Orthopaedic Surgery, University of Pittsburgh Medical Center Horizon, Greenville, PA 16125, USA

John C. Richmond, MD
Department of Orthopaedic Surgery, Tufts University School of Medicine, New England Medical Center Hospital, Boston, MA 02111, USA

Robert C. Schenck, Jr., MD
Department of Orthopaedics and Rehabilitation, Head Team Physician, University of New Mexico Lobos, University of New Mexico Health Sciences Center, University of New Mexico, Albuquerque, NM 87131, USA

Walter R. Shelton, MD
Mississippi Sports Medicine and Orthopaedic Center, Jackson, MS 39202, USA

Peter T. Simonian, MD
Associate Professor, Department of Orthopaedic Surgery, Chief of Sports Medicine, University of Washington, Seattle, WA 98195, USA

Corey Wallach, MD
Department of Orthopaedic Surgery, University of Pittsburgh Medical Center, Center for Sports Medicine, Pittsburgh, PA 15203, USA

Daniel C. Wascher, MD
Associate Professor, Department of Orthopaedics, Health Sciences Center, University of New Mexico Medical Center, Ambulatory Care Center, Albuquerque, NM 87131, USA

Thomas L. Wickiewicz, MD
Chief of Sports Medicine and Shoulder Service, Department of Orthopaedic Sports Medicine, The Hospital for Special Surgery, New York, NY 10021, USA

Kevin R. Willits, MD
Florida Orthopaedic Institute, Tampa, FL 33606, USA

Michelle Wolcott, MD
Denver Orthopedic Clinic, Denver, CO 80218, USA

Chapter One

Anatomy and Biomechanics of the Knee

Anikar Chhabra, C. Curtis Elliott, and Mark D. Miller

Multiple ligament knee injuries, although rare, are severe injuries because they result in the loss of the passive and active knee stabilizers as well as often compromising neurovascular structures. Treatment of these injuries is controversial, and results after surgery are often poor. Because of the multiple ligament disruptions, the knee is at a biomechanical disadvantage. Surgeons performing reconstructions in patients with these injuries must have a complete understanding of the normal anatomy and biomechanics of the knee to optimize the timing of surgery, the order of ligamentous reconstruction, and the anatomic placement of grafts. This chapter outlines the osteology, the ligamentous stabilizers of the knee, the menisci, and the neurovasculature of the knee. The biomechanics of the knee are detailed by describing the roles of the anatomic structures and their relationships in the uninjured knee. In addition, commonly used grafts and surgical approaches are described. This knowledge is critical to surgeons attempting reconstruction of the multiple ligament injured knee.

Anatomy of the Knee

Osteology

The bony anatomy of the knee joint consists of the articulations among the distal femur, the proximal tibia, and the patella. The height of the femoral condyles is asymmetric, and the medial condyle projects more distally than the lateral femoral condyle. The medial condyle is also larger; however, the lateral condyle projects more anteriorly. The condyles are separated by the femoral groove anteriorly and by the femoral notch at their distal aspect. The lateral condyle can be identified by its sulcus terminale and groove of the popliteus insertion[1] (Figure 1.1).

The medial and lateral menisci help to increase the conformity between the round femoral condyles and the relatively flat tibial plateaus. The entire tibial plateau slopes posteriorly approximately 10°. The tibial spine separates the medial and lateral plateaus. The anterior horn of the medial meniscus, the anterior cruciate ligament, and anterior horn of the lateral meniscus

---

A version of this chapter by the same authors was published in *Sports Medicine and Arthroscopy Review*, Volume 9 (3), 2001 pp. 166–177. Permission has been granted by Lippincott, Williams & Wilkins for use in this book.

Fig. 1.1. The relationship of the medial and lateral femoral condyles: 1, the high point of the lateral femoral sulcus; 2, the high point of the medial femoral sulcus. (From Tria AJ, Alicea JA. Embryology and anatomy of the patella. In: Scuderi GR, ed. The Patella, New York: Springer-Verlag; 1995:15.)

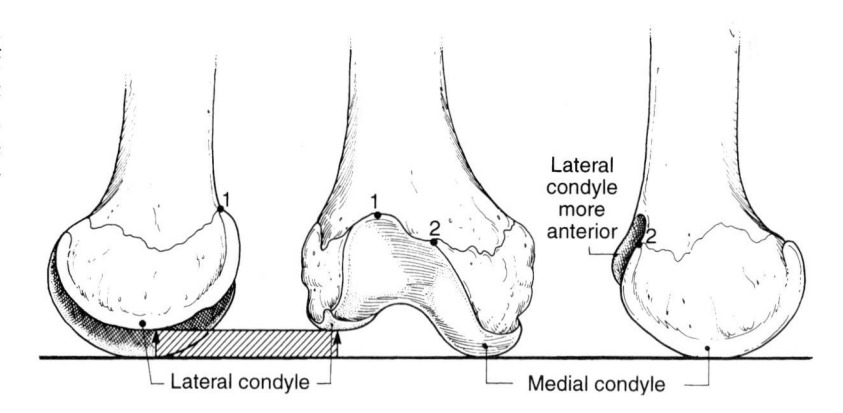

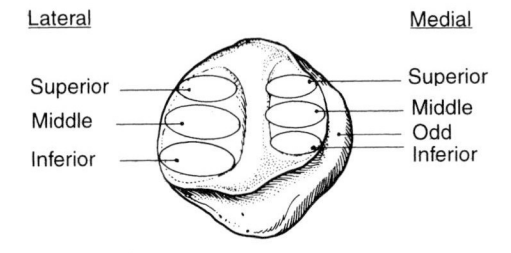

attach anterior to the tibial spine. The posterior cruciate ligament and the posterior horns of the medial and lateral menisci attach posterior to the tibial spine.[2]

The patella is the largest sesamoid bone in the body, measuring approximately 5 cm in diameter. The articular surface of the patella is the thickest in the body, owing to the normal high joint reactive forces between the femur and the patella. It consists of seven facets (Figure 1.2). The patella is triangular and serves three functions: it provides a fulcrum for the quadriceps, a protective surface for the knee joint, and an improved cosmetic appearance to the front of the knee.[3]

Cruciate Ligaments

Anterior Cruciate Ligament

The anterior cruciate ligament (ACL) extends from a broad area anterior to and between the intercondylar eminences of the tibia to a semicircular area on the posteromedial lateral femoral condyle. It not only prevents anterior translation of the tibia on the femur but also allows for normal helicoid knee action, thus preventing the chance for meniscal pathology. It is composed of two bundles: an anteromedial bundle, which is tight in flexion, and a posterolateral bundle, which is more convex and tight in extension (Figure 1.3).[4] Anatomic studies have shown that the ACL ranges from 31 to 38 mm in length and 10 to 12 mm in width.[5] The ACL is intra-articular; however, it is encased in its own synovial membrane. The vascular supply of the ACL is derived from the middle geniculate artery, as well as from diffusion through its synovial sheath.[6] The innervation of the ACL consists of mechanoreceptors derived from the tibial nerve and contributes to its proprioceptive role.[7] Pain fibers in the ACL are virtually nonexistent, which explains why there is minimal pain after an acute ACL rupture prior to development of a painful hemarthrosis.[8]

Fig. 1.2. The seven facets of the patella. (From Tria AJ, Alicea JA. Embryology and anatomy of the patella. In: Scuderi GR, ed. The Patella. New York: Springer-Verlag; 1995:16.)

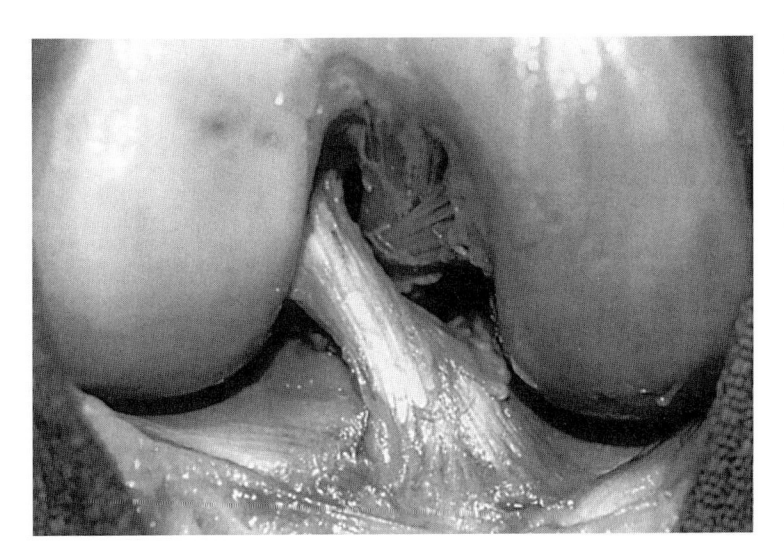

Fig. 1.3. Human anatomic specimen showing the complex helical arrangement of the ACL and its broad femoral attachment. (With permission from Brown CH, Steiner ME. Anterior cruciate ligament injuries. In: Siliski JM, ed. Traumatic Disorders of the Knee. New York: Springer-Verlag; 1994:211.)

Posterior Cruciate Ligament

The posterior cruciate ligament (PCL), like the ACL, is intra-articular and extrasynovial, with a much larger part existing extrasynovially. It extends from a broad semicircular area on the lateral aspect of the medial femoral condyle and projects to a sulcus that is posterior and inferior to the articular plateau of the tibia. The PCL consists of two bundles: a larger anterolateral bundle, which is tight in flexion, and a smaller posteromedial unit, which is tight in extension.[9,10] Its average length and width at its midportion, as reported by Girgis et al., are 38 and 13 mm, respectively.[11] The PCL cross-sectional area is 50% greater than the ACL at the femur and 20% greater at the tibia. In contrast to the ACL, the PCL is larger at its femoral insertion than at its tibial insertion.[9] Two intra-articular accessory ligaments, the meniscofemoral ligaments, extend from the posterior horn of the lateral meniscus and insert anterior and posterior to the PCL onto the medial femoral condyle. These are termed the ligaments of Humphrey and Wrisberg, respectively, and are not present in all knees. They average approximately 22% of the entire cross-sectional area of the PCL.[9] They serve as secondary stabilizers to posterior tibial translation. The vascular supply of the PCL is similar to that of the ACL, since both are derived from the middle geniculate artery. The vascular supply is mainly soft tissue based, not osseous based.[12] The innervation of the PCL is from the tibial and obturator nerves. As with the ACL, this serves primarily as a proprioceptive function.[7]

Medial Stabilizers of the Knee

The medial collateral ligament (MCL) is the primary static restraint to valgus stress placed on the knee joint. It has two portions: the superficial fibers, sometimes termed the tibial collateral ligament, and a deep portion, sometimes termed the medial capsular ligament. Both portions originate from the medial femoral epicondyle. The orientation of its fibers has implications in the valgus stability of the knee during range of motion. The superficial tibial collateral ligament has two bundles of fibers. The anterior bundle has vertically oriented fibers and inserts just posterior to the insertion of the pes anserinus, while the posterior bundle's oblique fibers insert inferior to the tibial articular surface. The medial capsular ligament also has two

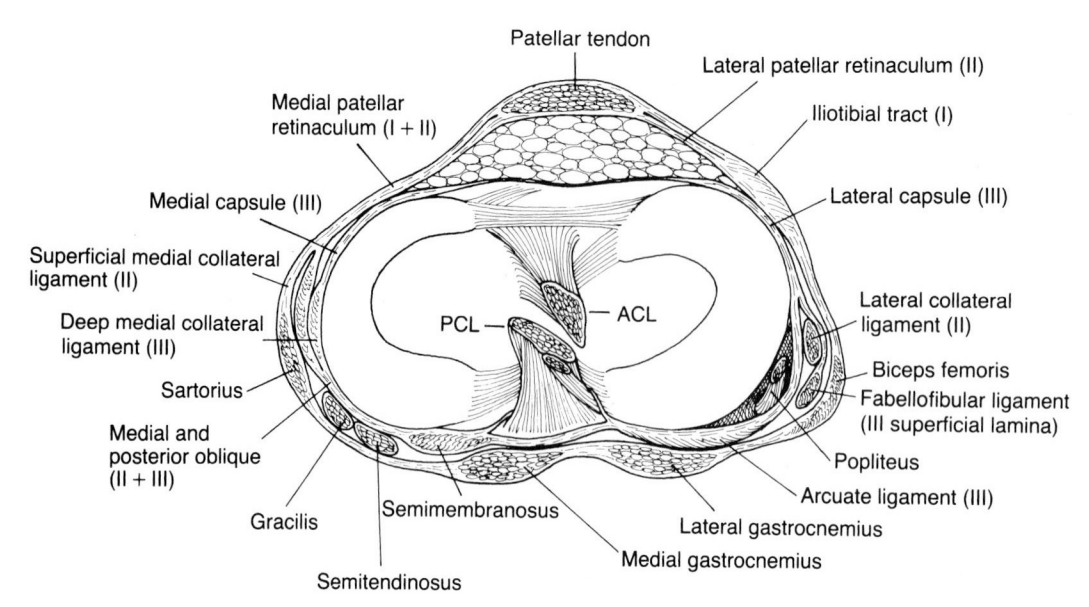

Fig. 1.4. The medial and lateral structures of the knee can be considered as three layers. (With permission from Blevins FT, Boublik M, Steadman JR. Anatomy: ligaments, tendons, and extensor mechanism. In: Siliski JM, ed. Traumatic Disorders of the Knee. New York: Springer-Verlag; 1994:10.)

bundles that differ in orientation, the meniscofemoral and meniscotibial portions, which are attached to the medial meniscus through the coronary ligaments. Three layers of medial structures provide support against a valgus stress: the superficial layer consists of the sartorius and its fascia; the middle layer contains the posterior oblique ligament and semimembranosus, in addition to the tibial collateral ligament; and the deep layer contains the joint capsule with the medial capsular ligament (Figure 1.4).[13]

Lateral and Posterolateral Stabilizers of the Knee

The posterolateral stabilizers of the knee can be grouped into three layers (Figure 1.4). Superficially, layer I consists of the iliotibial (IT) band, the biceps femoris, and the fascia. The IT band expands anteriorly, while the biceps lies more posteriorly. The peroneal nerve is just deep to the biceps at the level of the distal femoral condyle. Layer II consists of the patellar retinaculum anteriorly and the patellofemoral ligaments posteriorly. The deep layer, layer III, consists of the lateral collateral ligament (LCL), popliteus tendon, popliteofibular ligament, fabellofibular ligament, arcuate ligament, and joint capsule. The LCL is the primary static restraint to varus stress of the knee and secondarily resists external rotation of the knee. It extends between the fibular head and the lateral femoral condyle, with its femoral attachment superior and posterior to the geometric center of the lateral condyle. The popliteus originates on the posterior tibia, and its tendon inserts onto the lateral femoral condyle anterior to the LCL attachment after passing through the hiatus in the coronary ligament. It can actively internally rotate the tibia, helping to unlock the knee from a fully extended position, while also passively preventing excessive external tibial rotation. The popliteofibular ligament extends from the posterior aspect of the fibular head to the popliteus tendon, in effect connecting the posterior fibular head to the lateral femoral condyle. This rather large ligament has gained importance in posterolateral corner injuries and reconstructions. It provides static support for resisting posterior translation, external rotation, and varus angulation. Both the arcuate and fabellofibular ligaments reinforce the posterolateral capsule and are not always present.[14,15]

Menisci

The menisci are two crescent-shaped fibrocartilaginous structures that are triangular when viewed in cross section. The menisci are attached to the peripheral border of the joint capsule, lie flat on the tibia, and deepen the articular surface of the tibia plateau for articulation with the femoral condyles.[2] Only the peripheral 20 to 30% of the menisci are vascularized, supplied by the medial and lateral geniculate arteries. Historically, repaired meniscal tears in this red–red zone have a better healing potential than tears in the red–white or white–white zone, which are the middle and inner thirds, respectively.[16]

Medial Meniscus

The medial meniscus is C shaped (Figure 1.4).[13] Its stability can be attributed to its multiple attachments. Posteriorly, it is attached to the posterior intercondylar fossa of the tibia. The anterior aspect of the medial meniscus is attached to the anterior horn of the lateral meniscus through the transverse intermeniscal ligament and to the tibia at the anterior intercondylar fossa. It sometimes inserts below the tibial plateau anteriorly. Medially, the coronary ligament attaches the medial meniscus to the tibial margin distal to the articular surface. In addition, the capsule of the knee thickens at the midportion of the meniscus, giving rise to the deep medial ligament, which augments the tibial attachment and also attaches to the femur.[2,17]

Lateral Meniscus

The lateral meniscus is more circular and accommodates the narrower lateral tibial plateau. It is smaller than the medial meniscus, but it covers a larger percentage of the lateral tibial plateau. Thus, the lateral meniscus is an important weight-bearing structure, and its preservation is paramount in preventing degenerative changes in the lateral knee compartment (Figure 1.4). The anterior and posterior horns of the lateral meniscus attach to the intercondylar fossa in front of the ACL footprint and behind it, respectively. The ligaments of Humphrey and Wrisberg, when present, help to augment the posterior horn attachment.[2,17] The popliteus tendon inserts into the periphery and superior margin of the lateral meniscus posterolaterally.[18]

Musculature

The quadriceps muscle consists of the rectus femoris, the vastus lateralis, the vastus medialis (VMO), and the vastus intermedius. These four muscles are all innervated by the femoral nerve and insert onto the patella through fibrous expansions on the patellar retinaculum and the patellar tendon.

The musculature on the lateral side of the knee consists of the biceps, the IT band, and the popliteus. The long head of the biceps originates from the medial aspect of the ischial tuberosity and inserts onto the fibular head and lateral tibia, while the short head of the biceps originates from the linea aspera and inserts onto the lateral tibial condyle. They are innervated by the tibial and peroneal nerves, respectively. The IT band, which is a continuation of the tensor fasciae latae, inserts at Gerdy's tubercle on the tibia. It lies anterior to the knee axis in extension, thus providing lateral stability to the knee. It moves posterior to the knee axis at about 30° of flexion, accounting for the posterior shift of the tibia in an abnormal pivot shift exam.[14] The anatomy of the popliteus and its importance as a stabilizer of the posterolateral corner have been discussed.

The medial supporting musculature about the knee consists of the pes anserinus (sartorius, gracilis, and semitendinosus) and the semimembranosus. The insertion of the pes tendons are on the anterior/medial aspect of the tibia. The sartorius has a broad fascial insertion, with the tendons of the gracilis and semitendinosus running along its deep surface. The gracilis and the semitendinosus are oriented horizontally near their insertion on the tibia with the gracilis lying proximal to the semitendinosus. These two tendons may be used as autografts in ACL and/or posterolateral corner reconstructions. The semimembranosus originates on the lateral aspect of the ischial tuberosity and has five heads of insertion: the oblique popliteal ligament, the posterior capsule, the posterior tibia, the popliteus, and the medial meniscus.[13]

The posterior musculature consists of the medial and lateral heads of the gastrocnemius and the plantaris. The gastrocnemius inserts onto the posterior aspect calcaneal tuberosity through the Achilles tendon. It acts as a strong plantar flexor of the foot as well as a weak knee flexor. The plantaris originates from the lateral femoral condyle and also inserts onto the calcaneus. The long tendon of the plantaris is clinically significant because it is often used for tendon reconstructions or augmentations following injuries to the Achilles tendon. The posterior knee musculature is innervated by the tibial nerve.

The popliteal fossa is bordered by the two heads of the gastrocnemius, the semimembranosus, and the biceps, with the floor consisting of the popliteus muscle. The popliteal vessels course through the popliteal fossa. When the tibial inlay technique for PCL reconstructions is performed, the medial head of the gastrocnemius is mobilized and retracted laterally. The popliteal neurovascular structures are safely retracted laterally with the medial head of the gastrocnemius muscle. By partially elevating the popliteus fibers, the normal PCL attachment on the posterior/superior aspect of the tibia can be visualized.

Vasculature

Branches of the femoral and popliteal arteries supply the knee and its structures. The descending geniculate artery is a branch of femoral artery proximal to Hunter's canal and supplies the vastus medialis at the anterior border of the intermuscular septum. The medial and lateral geniculate arteries wrap around the distal femoral condyles and supply the menisci, while the middle geniculate artery supplies the cruciate ligaments.[2,19,12] The superior lateral geniculate is often injured during lateral release procedures, while the inferior lateral geniculate artery is often injured during posterolateral corner reconstructions[20] (Figure 1.5).

The geniculate arteries, the descending branch of the lateral circumflex femoral artery, and the recurrent branches of the anterior tibial artery form the anastomosis around the knee that connects the femoral, popliteal, and anterior tibial arteries.

Innervation

The innervation of the knee consists of terminal branches of the tibial, sciatic, and femoral nerves. Sensory fibers exist intra-articularly in the menisci, ligaments, and subchondral surfaces. The medial and lateral popliteal nerves arise from the sciatic nerve in the popliteal fossa and not only innervate the surrounding musculature but also have several articular branches. The common peroneal nerve, the smaller terminal division of the sciatic nerve,

1. Anatomy and Biomechanics of the Knee

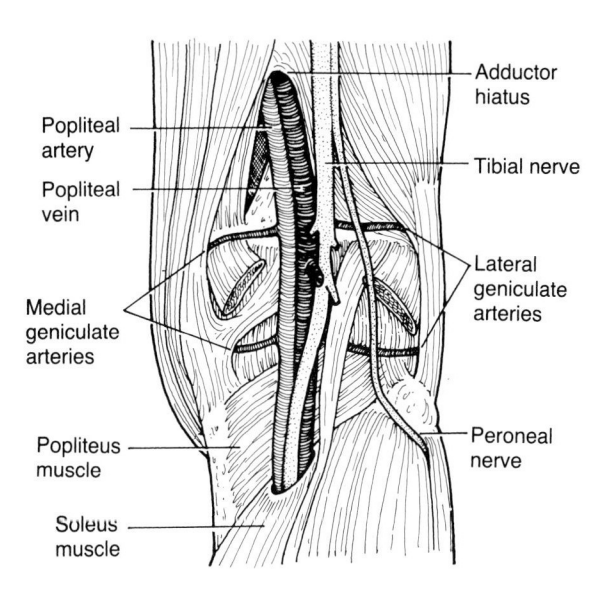

Fig. 1.5. The vasculature of the knee viewed posteriorly. (With permission from Plancher KD, Siliski JM. Dislocation of the knee. In: Siliski JM, ed. Traumatic Disorders of the Knee. New York: Springer-Verlag; 1994:316.)

courses laterally in the popliteal fossa between the medial border of the biceps and the lateral head of the gastrocnemius.[19] This nerve needs to be protected during procedures such as an inside-out meniscal repair and often has to be visualized during posterolateral corner dissections.

Cutaneous innervation about the knee is provided by the posterior and lateral femoral cutaneous, lateral sural cutaneous, saphenous, and obturator nerves (Figure 1.6). The saphenous nerve becomes subcutaneous at the medial aspect of the knee and often can be injured by medial surgical approaches, especially inside-out meniscal repairs. The patellar plexus, which supplies cutaneous innervation anterior to the patella and patellar ligament, is formed from the cutaneous nerves of the thigh and the infrapatellar branch of the saphenous nerve.[2]

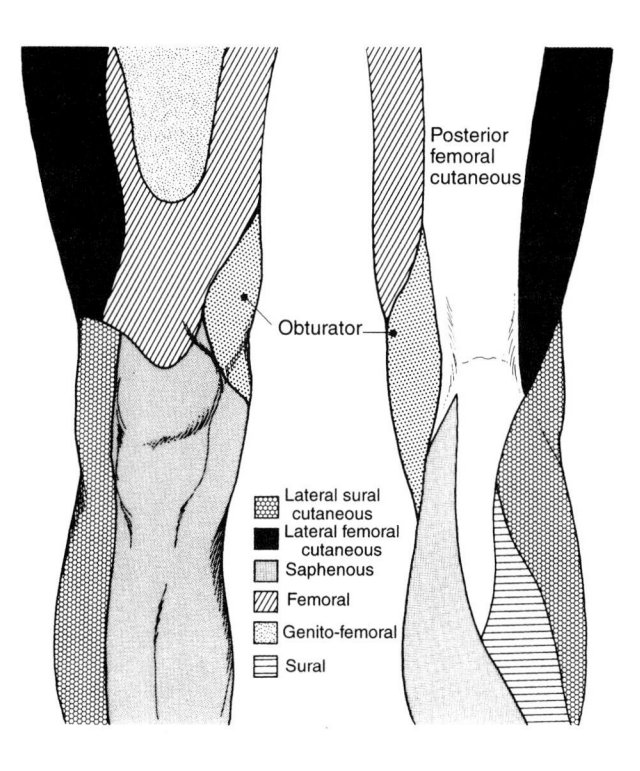

Fig. 1.6. The cutaneous innervation of the knee viewed anteriorly and posteriorly. (With permission from Tria AJ, Alicea JA. Embryology and anatomy of the patella. In: Scuderi GR, ed. The Patella. New York: Springer-Verlag; 1995:21.)

Common Surgical Approaches to the Knee with Anatomic Pearls

Medial Parapatellar Approach

The medial parapatellar approach is most commonly used for total knee arthroplasty; it utilizes a midline incision and a medial parapatellar capsular incision. The infrapatellar branch of the saphenous nerve is sometimes cut, often leading to a painful neuroma.

Medial Approach

The medial approach is used for an open repair of the medial meniscus and the repair of the medial collateral ligament and capsule. The exposure is gained by splitting the sartorius fascia to expose the deeper structures, including the superficial and deep MCL, the capsule, and the posterior oblique ligament. Throughout this exposure, the saphenous nerve and vein must be identified and protected (Figure 1.7).[13]

Lateral Approach

The lateral approach, used for repair of posterolateral corner injuries, lateral meniscal tears, and lateral collateral ligament ruptures, utilizes a plane between the IT band and the biceps femoris, and a second window between the IT band and the IT tract. Dangers include the common peroneal nerve and the superior and inferior lateral geniculate arteries (Figure 1.8).[15]

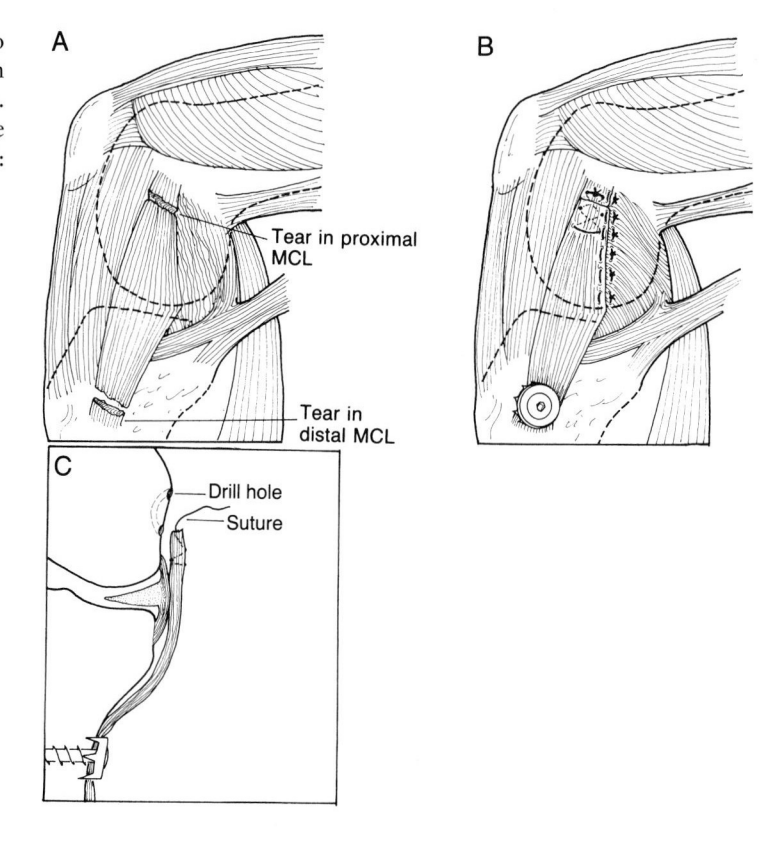

Fig. 1.7. The medial surgical approach to the knee. (With permission from McMahon MS, Boland AL. Collateral ligament injuries. In: Siliski JM, ed. Traumatic Disorders of the Knee. New York: Springer-Verlag; 1994: 307.)

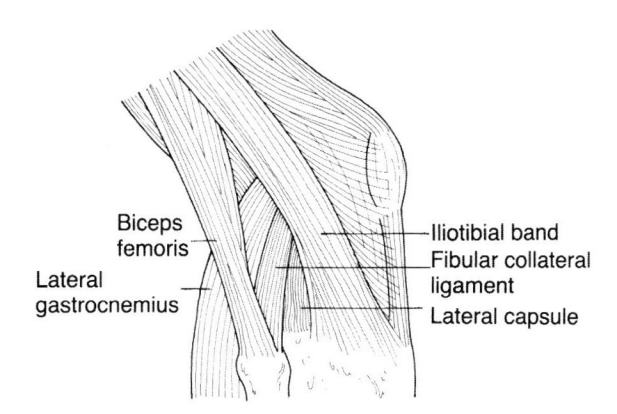

Fig. 1.8. The lateral surgical approach to the knee. (With permission from McMahon MS, Boland AL. Collateral ligament injuries. In: Siliski JM, ed. Traumatic Disorders of the Knee. New York: Springer-Verlag; 1994:302.)

Posterior Approach

The posterior approach is required to address posterior capsular pathology, for vascular repair following a knee dislocation, or for placement of a PCL graft by means of the tibial inlay technique. Classically, an S-shaped incision is made extending from proximal/lateral to distal/medial. If greater exposure is necessary, the gastrocnemius can be detached. The dangers of this approach are the popliteal vessels.[19] Alternately, a curved hockey stick incision can be made and the medial head of the gastrocnemius mobilized and retracted laterally to protect the neurovascular structures.[21]

Biomechanics and Kinematics of the Knee Joint

The goal of all joints is to allow for motion of the bony segments surrounding the joint while withstanding the loads against gravity imposed by these movements. Biomechanics is defined as the science of the action of forces on the living body. The complex interaction of femur, tibia, and patella allows the knee joint to withstand tremendous forces during normal phases of ambulation. Kinematics is defined as the study of body motion without regard for the cause of that motion.[20] Six planes of motion exist for the knee: anterior/posterior translation, medial/lateral translation, cephalad/caudad translation, flexion/extension rotation, internal/external rotation, and varus/valgus angulation.[22] The knee joint must provide a normal amount of motion without sacrificing stability during static activities such as standing to more dynamic functions such as walking, jogging, running, pivoting, and ascending or descending stairs. These goals are achieved by the interaction of the osseous anatomy, articular surface, ligaments, menisci, and surrounding musculature about the knee.[23] Changes in any of these components can alter the biomechanics of the knee joint, greatly increasing the loads and functional demands placed on the remaining structures. Understanding the normal interactions of these structures is necessary prior to attempting any reconstructive procedures.

Passive Motion of the Knee

The primary motion of the knee is flexion and extension. The knee joint averages from 0 to 135° of flexion in the sagittal plane.[23] The passive motion of the knee joint is dictated by the anatomy of the articular surfaces and the surrounding soft tissue capsule and ligaments.[24] As a result of the distal asymmetry between the medial and lateral femoral condyles, motion between full extension and 20° of flexion is accompanied by rolling of the lateral femoral condyle posteriorly more than the medial femoral condyle. This allows the femur and tibia to unlock from full extension and occurs without the assistance of any dynamic muscle involvement.[25] After 20° of flexion, passive flexion of the knee joint occurs by a sliding motion, with relative tibial movement on the femur.[23]

Function of the Menisci

The menisci are composed of collagen fibers that are arranged radially and longitudinally. Their wedge shape aids in providing conformity to the femoral and tibial articular surfaces. The primary functions of the menisci are to bear loads, to distribute the load of the knee joint medially and laterally, and to absorb shock.[26] The longitudinal fibers help to dissipate the hoop stresses in the menisci, and the combination of the fibers allows the meniscus to expand under compressive forces and increase the contact area of the joint. The tensile stiffness and strength of the menisci is approximately 10 times greater than that of articular cartilage.[27] This allows the menisci to withstand the large hoop stresses generated by the knee joint. The deformation behavior of the meniscus is more dependent on its multidirectional arrangement of the collagen fibers, rather than the type of collagen itself. The water content of the meniscus adds to its viscoelastic properties, aiding in its ability to withstand shear forces and to distribute tensile and compressive loads.

The menisci may also function as a secondary restraint to anterior translation in an ACL-deficient knee. The medial meniscus is more firmly fixed to the tibial plateau than the lateral meniscus and, consequently, has half the excursion of the lateral meniscus during knee flexion and rotation. This may account for the greater number of medial meniscal tears associated with ACL-deficient knees. The increased mobility of the lateral meniscus also aids the articular conformity in the screw home mechanism.[28]

The Functional Biomechanics of the Cruciate Ligaments

Of the knee ligaments, the cruciates are the most important in providing passive restraint to anterior/posterior knee motion. If one or both of the cruciates are disrupted, the biomechanics during ambulatory activities may be disrupted.

The primary function of the ACL is to prevent anterior translation of the tibia. In full extension, the ACL absorbs 75% of the anterior translation load, and 85% between 30 and 90° of flexion.[29] In addition, other functions of the ACL include resisting internal rotation of the tibia and varus/valgus angulation of the tibia in the presence of collateral ligament injury. Loss of the ACL leads to a decreased magnitude of this coupled rotation during flexion, and an unstable knee. Many studies have been performed to determine the biomechanical properties of the ACL. However, uniform testing with regard to strain rates and orientation is impossible. Several recent studies have demonstrated that the anterior bundles (both medial and lateral) have higher maximum stress and strain than the posterior bundles.[30] The tensile strength of the ACL is approximately 2200 N but is altered with age and repetitive loads.[20,31,32] As the magnitude of the anterior drawer force increases, the in situ force of the ACL also increases.[5]

The primary function of the posterior cruciate ligament (PCL) is to resist posterior translation of the tibia on the femur at all positions of knee flexion.[33] The anterolateral band is tight in flexion and is most important in resisting posterior displacement of the tibia in 70 to 90° of flexion. The posteromedial portion is tight in extension; thus, it resists posterior displacement of the tibia in this position. The double-bundle technique for PCL reconstruction, which attempts to restore both bands of the PCL, has recently gained some popularity.

Isolated PCL ruptures may cause a mild increase in external rotation at 90° of knee flexion; they do not greatly alter tibial rotation or varus/valgus angulation, however, because of the intact extracapsular tissues and ligaments. With both PCL and posterolateral corner injuries, there is a marked increase in tibia external rotation because of the lack of supporting restraints.[34] Harner et al. demonstrated that the anterolateral component had a greater stiffness and tensile strength than the posteromedial bundle and the meniscofemoral ligaments.[9] Furthermore, Fox et al. demonstrated that at varying degrees of knee flexion, different in situ forces existed. At 0°, the PCL had an average tensile strength of 6.1 N, while at 90° it had a tensile strength of 112.3 N. The posteromedial bundle attained a maximum force of 67.9 N at 90° of knee flexion, while the anterolateral bundle reached a maximal force of 47.8 N at 60°.[35] Understanding these relationships is critical in reconstructive surgery to ensure that the grafts are tensioned properly.

In addition to its known role in the sagittal plane, the PCL influences knee motion in the frontal plane. This occurs because the PCL inserts onto the lateral aspect of the medial femoral condyle and is oriented obliquely. This orientation of the PCL aids in the articular asymmetry between the medial and lateral femoral condyles and permits adequate tensioning of the PCL during the rolling of the lateral femoral condyle posteriorly in early flexion.

The popliteus muscle aids the PCL in resisting posterior tibial translation and enhancing stability. Harner et al. demonstated that in a PCL-deficient knee, the popliteus muscle reduced posterior translation of the tibia by 36%.[36]

The Interplay of the Cruciate Ligaments

The complex interaction between ACL and PCL at varying degrees of flexion and extension helps account for the dynamic stability of the knee joint. The length and tension of the ACL and the PCL change during flexion and extension owing to their asymmetric insertion sites. In full extension, the ACL is taut, while the PCL is relatively lax. When a person is standing with the knee in hyperextension, the joint is passively stable, with little need for muscular support. As the knee flexes, the posterolateral portion of the ACL become lax, while the PCL tightens, especially the anterolateral bundle. Stability is more tenuous between 20 and 50° of flexion, since neither cruciate ligament is very taut. The change in the orientation of the ACL and PCL fibers during knee flexion allows for dynamic stability in the sagittal plane. With increasing flexion, the ACL changes from a vertical position to a more horizontal orientation in relation to the joint line. The PCL's orientation is opposite to the ACL's during flexion and extension. Consequently, as the knee reaches higher degrees of flexion, the PCL becomes more important in preventing distraction of the joint.[25,37] This interplay between ACL and PCL is often referred to as the four-bar cruciate linkage system[38] (Figure 1.9). The intersection of these ligaments demonstrates that the center of joint rotation moves posterior with knee flexion. This allows for both sliding and rolling movements of the femur during flexion and prevents the femur from rolling off the tibial plateau at extremes of flexion.[23]

Fig. 1.9. The four-bar cruciate linkage system. (With permission from Boublik M, Blevins FT, Steadman J. Anatomy: bony architecture, biomechanics, and menisci. In: Siliski JM, ed. Traumatic Disorders of the Knee. New York: Springer-Verlag; 1994:6.)

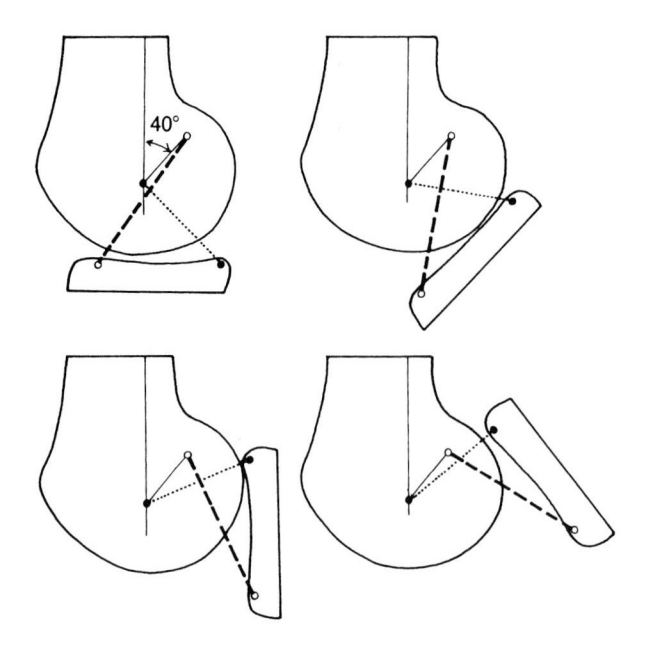

During the different phases of the gait cycle, the force vectors about the knee in the sagittal plane change. The mechanical loads across the knee joint are altered by changes in foot position as well as by the intensity and type of ambulatory activity. During normal ambulation, a joint reactive force of 2 to 5 times the body weight is produced; this force is up to 24 times the body weight during running. Dynamic muscle forces help to balance these functional loads and joint reactive forces, especially as the knee flexes and the weight-bearing axis shifts from a position anterior to the knee joint to one posterior.[39] If a ligamentous, muscular, and/or bony injury occurs that alters this delicate balance of forces, the joint is not as effective at withstanding these loads, hastening the degenerative process of the knee.[25]

The dynamic actions of the surrounding muscles are restrained by the cruciate ligaments during knee flexion and extension. The quadriceps muscles, by way of the patellar tendon, ultimately insert onto the anterior tibia, and, consequently, the tibia is translated anteriorly by the extensor mechanism and constrained by the pull of the ACL. The biomechanical advantage is maximized when the center of rotation of the knee joint is perpendicular to the joint line. If anterior translation occurs in the sagittal plane during ambulation, as with ACL deficiency, the center of rotation is altered and the resultant increase in forces across the knee joint places increased stress upon the secondary restraints. The moment arm of the knee extensor apparatus is decreased, causing an increase in the muscle forces necessary to maintain balance across the knee joint. This leads to an increase in joint reactive forces and, ultimately, stressed or injured supporting structures.[40] In an ACL-deficient knee, increased stress is placed on the secondary restraints of anterior translation, including the menisci and the surrounding soft tissue capsule. When the quadriceps become atrophied after an ACL rupture, the extensor pull on the tibia lessens, decreasing the stresses placed on the secondary stabilizers.

The screw home mechanism again demonstrates the importance of the dynamic muscles in knee motion. As the lateral femoral condyle rolls posteriorly in early flexion, the moment arm of the extensor apparatus increases. This gives a mechanical advantage to the knee in stair climbing and running, when there is maximal demand on the knee joint.[37]

The Collateral Ligaments and Varus/Valgus Motion

Medial and lateral stability of the knee joint is achieved mainly through the collateral ligaments. The cruciates provide minimal secondary stabilization to varus and valgus stresses and would not be able to withstand these forces during ambulation without the collaterals. The orientation of the two portions of the MCL is critical in providing valgus stability to the knee during normal range of motion. In extension, the anterior vertical fibers are relaxed and the posterior oblique fibers are taut, while during flexion, the anterior fibers are taut and the posterior oblique fibers are relaxed. The degree that the MCL resists a valgus load depends on other ligamentous injuries. Valgus angulation, external rotation, and anterior translation of the tibia may all be increased when the posteromedial capsule, ACL, and PCL are injured.[41]

According to Burstein and Wright,[37] the knee joint withstands the forces in the coronal plane by means of three mechanisms. First, during normal gait, there is typically a medial force acting at the foot that produces a varus moment at the knee. The flexion moment, which also occurs because of ground reaction forces, is countered by the quadriceps force. To maintain equilibrium in the coronal plane, this force must be divided asymmetrically, with the medial femoral condyle absorbing more of the load than the lateral. Thus, balancing this normally applied varus moment is accomplished by a moderate shift in joint reactive force between the condyles.

As increasing varus moments are produced, a second protective mechanism is induced. Increased voluntary force applied through the quadriceps and hamstrings can produce increased joint loads. This again will tend to be balanced by increasing the medial compartment pressure, hence, producing an internal knee valgus moment to oppose the externally applied varus moment. It has been reported that medial stability of the knee can be increased by up to 50% with concurrent contraction of the quadriceps and hamstrings.[41]

If the externally applied load exceeds these internal equilibrating forces, or if they are produced at a high rate, the contribution of the ligamentous stabilizers becomes important. The collateral ligaments, and to a much lesser degree, the cruciates, are able to provide a large counterforce to the externally applied loads. If an equilibrium cannot be established because of the magnitude or rate of the externally applied load, ligamentous disruption will occur.

Patellofemoral Biomechanics

Although the emphasis of this chapter is on multiple ligament injuries, no discussion of knee joint biomechanics is complete without mention of the patellofemoral joint. The patella is functionally important because it increases the strength of the extensor mechanism by increasing the center of rotation away from the knee, creating a larger moment arm. This has been reported to increase extensile strength by up to 50%.[42] Joint reactive forces change during knee range of motion. As the knee flexes from 0° to 120°, the summation of the quadriceps and patella tendon vectors creates gradually increasing forces on the patella. However, the contact area on the patella increases as well, moving from its distal pole to the proximal pole. Also, at extremes of flexion, the quadriceps tendon makes substantial contact with the femur. Thus, the increasing contact area helps to compen-

Fig. 1.10. The patellar stabilizers. (From Tria AJ, Alicea JA. Embryology and anatomy of the patella. In: Scuderi GR, ed. The Patella. New York: Springer-Verlag; 1995: 17.)

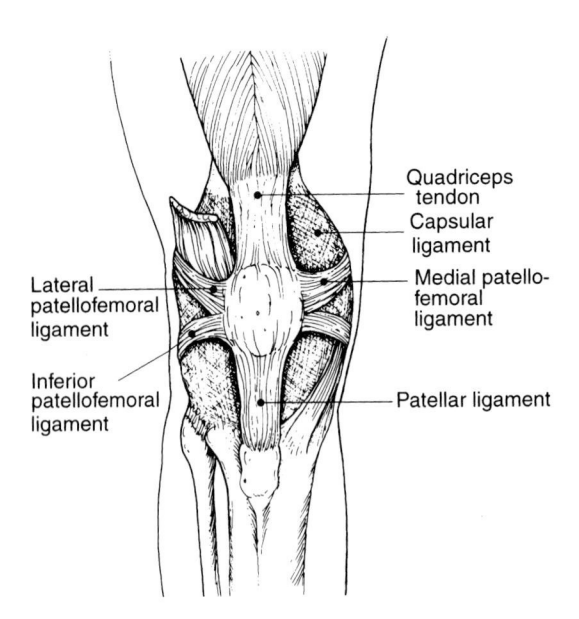

sate for the increasing joint reactive forces. This helps to keep the joint contact pressure, which is the ratio of the joint reactive force to the contact area, in a safe physiologic range.[43]

Owing to the normal valgus alignment of the lower extremity, the resultant quadriceps vector tends to pull the patella laterally. The amount of valgus is measured by the Q angle, which is the angle portended by a line from the anterior superior iliac spine to the patella and a line from the patella to the tibial tubercle. This angle averages 12° in males and 15° in females. The lateral pull on the patella is resisted by static and dynamic restraints. Static restraints include the patellofemoral articulation and the medial capsular structures.[44] These include the medial patellofemoral ligament (MPFL), lateral patellofemoral ligament, inferior patellofemoral ligament, patellar ligament, patellameniscal ligament, and quadriceps tendon (Figure 1.10). The MPFL is the primary static restraint to lateral translation of the patella, contributing 60% of the force, while the medial patellameniscal ligament and medial retinaculum contributed 13 and 10%, respectively.[45] The dynamic restraint against lateral patellar motion is produced primarily by the oblique pull of the VMO muscle. Poor tracking of the patella may cause lateral instability and pain while also decreasing the mechanical advantage supplied by the patella for flexion/extension of the knee joint.

The Biomechanics of Ligament Reconstruction

As the incidence of multiple ligament knee injuries increases, the order and necessity of the reconstruction of the ACL, PCL, and the posterolateral corner in combined injuries have become controversial. Harner et al. have demonstrated that in isolated PCL injuries, reconstruction led to an average posterior tibial translation of 1.5 and 2.4 mm at 30 and 90°, respectively. These numbers increased to 6.0 and 4.6 mm if the only PCL was reconstructed in a combined PCL–posterolateral corner injury. In addition, external rotation and varus angulation increased 14 and 7°, respectively. This study supports the reconstruction of both ligaments at the same setting in combined PCL–posterolateral corner injuries. If the ACL is also disrupted, it should be reconstructed either primarily or in a staged procedure, but the PCL and posterolateral corner should be considered to be a higher priority.[31]

Structural Properties of Ligaments and Commonly Used Grafts

The maximal stress that a ligament or graft can withstand prior to failure has been studied extensively. The ACL has been reported to have an average maximal tensile stress to failure of between 2160 and 2500 N. Many studies have found the PCL to have significantly more tensile strength than the ACL, but this is controversial.[31,46] The tensile strength of the MCL has been found to be twice as strong as the ACL in rabbit studies.[47]

Cooper et al. have shown that the tensile strength of grafts taken from the central third of the patellar tendon averages 4389 N for grafts 15 mm wide and 2977 N for grafts 10 mm wide. Twisting the graft 90° increased its strength approximately 30%. This study advocates using 10 mm central-third patellar tendon grafts for ACL reconstructions to avoid the risks of notch impingement and patellar fracture encountered with larger grafts.[48]

Over time, wear and degeneration cause ligaments and grafts to decrease in strength. This has been demonstrated in multiple studies by means of ACL and graft tensile tests. The biologic effects of aging, maturation, and immobilization may also affect the viscoelastic properties of a ligament or graft, leading to a decrease in biomechanical strength.[22]

Conclusions

Although rare, knee dislocations are severe injuries because they may result in disruption of multiple ligaments, surrounding musculature, and neurovascular structures.[49] Treatment of these injuries is controversial, and results following surgery are often poor. These injuries, owing to ligamentous disruption and surrounding soft tissue damage, may lead to a biomechanical disadvantage of the knee joint. To prevent abnormal translations and angulations in the reconstructed knee, surgeons performing reconstructions in patients with multiple ligament injuries must have a complete understanding of the normal anatomy and biomechanics of the knee. This knowledge should help optimize the timing of surgery, the order of ligamentous reconstruction, the anatomic placement of grafts, and the rehabilitation of the surrounding musculature.

References

1. Warren R, Arnoczky SP, Wickiewicz TL. Anatomy of the knee. In: Nicholas JA, Hershman EB, eds. The Lower Extremity and Spine in Sports Medicine. St. Louis, MO: CV Mosby; 1986:657–694.
2. Insall JN, Kelly MA. Anatomy. In: Insall JN, Windsor RE, Scott WN, Kelly MA, Aglietti P, eds. Surgery of the Knee. 2nd ed. New York: Churchill Livingstone; 1993:1–20.
3. Chapman MW, ed. Gray's Anatomy. 30th American ed. Philadelphia: Lea & Febiger; 1985.
4. Feagin JA. Isolated anterior cruciate injury. In: Feagin JA, ed. The Cruciate Ligaments. New York: Churchill Livingstone; 1988:15–23.
5. Smith BA, Livesay GA, Woo SL. Biology and biomechanics of the anterior cruciate ligament. Clin Sports Med 1993; 12:637–670.
6. Arnoczky SP. Anatomy of the anterior cruciate ligament. Clin Orthop 1983; 172:19–25.

7. Kennedy JC, Alexander IJ, Hayes KC. Nerve supply of the human knee and its functional importance. Am J Sports Med 1982; 10:329–335.
8. Shutte MJ, Dabezies EJ, Zimney ML, et al. Neural anatomy of the human anterior cruciate ligament. J Bone Joint Surg Am 1987; 69:243–247.
9. Harner CD, Xerogeanes JW, Livesay GA, Carlin GJ, Smith BA, Kusayama T, Kashiwaguchi S, Woo SLY. The human posterior cruciate ligament complex: an interdisciplinary study. Am J Sports Med 1995; 23:736–745.
10. Johnson CJ, Bach BR. Current concepts review. Posterior cruciate ligament. Am J Knee Surg 1990; 3:143–153.
11. Girgis FG, Marshall JL, Al Monajem ARS. The cruciate ligaments of the knee joint. Anatomic, functional, and experimental analysis. Clin Orthop 1975; 106:216–231.
12. Vladimirov B. Arterial sources of blood supply in the knee joint in man. Acta Med 1968; 47:1–10.
13. Warren LF, Marshal JL. The supporting structures and layers of the medial side of the knee. J Bone Joint Surg Am 1979; 61:56–62.
14. Chen FS, Rokito AS, Pitman MI. Acute and chronic posterolateral rotary instability of the knee. J Am Acad Orthop Surg 2000; 8:97–110.
15. Seebacher JR, Ingilis AE, Marshal JL, et al. The structure of the posterolateral aspect of the knee. J Bone Joint Surg Am 1982; 64:536–541.
16. Belzer JP, Cannon WD. Meniscal tears: treatment in the stable and unstable knee. J Am Acad Orthop Surg 1993; 1:41–47.
17. Miller MD, Warner JJP, Harner CD. Meniscal repair. In: Fu FH, Harner CD, Vince KG, eds. Knee Surgery. Baltimore, MD: Williams & Wilkins, 1994.
18. Last RJ. The popliteus muscle and the lateral meniscus. J Bone Joint Surg Br 1950; 32:93.
19. Miller MD, Gomez BA. Anatomy. In: Miller MD, ed. Review of Orthopaedics. 3rd ed. Philadelphia: WB Saunders; 2000:519–583.
20. Miller MD. Sports medicine. In: Miller MD, ed. Review of Orthopaedics. 3rd ed. Philadelphia: WB Saunders; 2000:195–240.
21. Burks RT, Schaffer JJ. A simplified approach to the tibial attachment of the posterior cruciate ligament. Clin Orthop 1990; 254:216–219.
22. Woo SLY, Debski RE, Withrow JD, Janaushek MA. Biomechanics of knee ligaments. Am J Sports Med 1999; 27:533–543.
23. Fu FH, Harner CD, Johnson DL, Miller MD, Woo SLY. Biomechanics of knee ligaments. J Bone Joint Surg Am 1993; 75:1716–1727.
24. Lafortune MA, Cavanaugh PR, Sommer HJ III, Kalenak A. Three-dimensional kinematics of the human knee during walking. J Biomech 1992; 25:347–357.
25. Andriacchi TP. Knee joint, anatomy and biomechanics. In: Pellicci PM, Tria AJ, Garvin KL, eds. Orthopaedic Knowledge. Update Hip and Knee Reconstruction 2. Rosemont, IL: American Academy of Orthopaedic Surgeons; 2000:239–249.
26. Mow VC, Ratcliffe A, Chern KY, Kelly MA. Structure and function relationships of the menisci of the knee. In: Mow VC, Arnoczky SP, Jackson DW, eds. Knee Meniscus: Basic and Clinical Foundations. New York: Raven Press; 1992:37–57.
27. Procter CS, Schmidt MB, Whipple RR, Kelly MA, Mow VC. Material properties of the normal medial bovine meniscus. J Orthop Res 1989; 7:771–782.
28. Fithian DC, Kelly MA, Mow VC. Material properties and structure–function relationships in the menisci. Clin Orthop 1990; 252:19–31.
29. Butler DL, Noyes FR, Grood ES. Ligamentous restraints to anterior–posterior drawer in the human knee. A biomechanical study. J Bone Joint Surg Am 1980; 62:259–270.
30. Butler DL, Guan Y, Kay MD, et al. Location-dependent variations in the material properties of anterior cruciate ligament subunits. Trans Orthop Res Soc 1991; 16:234.
31. Miller MD, Cooper DE, Warner JJP. Review of Sports Medicine and Arthroscopy. Philadelphia: WB Saunders; 1995:3–71.
32. Woo SLY, Adams DJ. The tensile properties of the human anterior cruciate ligament and ACL graft tissues. In: Daniel DM, Akeson WH, O'Conner JJ, eds. Knee Ligaments, Structure, Function, Injury, and Repair. New York: Raven Press; 1990:279–289.

33. Gollehon DL, Torzilli PA, Warren RF. The role of posterolateral and cruciate ligaments in the stability of the human knee. A biomechanical study. J Bone Joint Surg Am 1987; 69:233–242.
34. Covey DC, Sapega AA. Current concepts review. Injuries of the posterior cruciate ligament. J Bone Joint Surg 1993; 75:1376–1386.
35. Fox RJ, Harner CD, Sakane M, Carlin GJ, Woo SLY. Determination of the in situ forces in the human posterior cruciate ligament using robotic technology, a cadaveric study. Am J Sports Med 1998; 26:395–401.
36. Harner CD, Hoher J, Vogrin TM, Carlin GJ, Woo SLY. The effects of a popliteus muscle load on in situ forces of the posterior cruciate ligament and on knee kinematics. Am J Sports Med 1998; 26:669–673.
37. Burstein AH, Wright TM. Biomechanics. In: Insall JN, Windsor RE, Scott WN, Kelly MA, Aglietti P, eds. Surgery of the Knee, 2nd ed. New York: Churchill Livingstone; 1993:43–62.
38. Muller WD. Kinematics. In: Muller W, ed. The Knee, Form, Function, and Ligament Reconstruction. New York: Springer-Verlag; 1983:8–28.
39. Morrison JB. The mechanics of the knee joint in relation to normal walking. J Biomech 1970; 3:51.
40. Elftman H. The forces exerted by the ground in walking. Arb Physiol 1939; 10:485.
41. Satterwhite Y. The anatomy and biomechanics of the medial structures of the knee. In: Drez D, DeLee JC, eds. Operative Techniques in Sports Medicine. 1996; 4:134–140.
42. Coffer H. Mechanical function of the patella. J Bone Joint Surg Am 1971; 53:1551.
43. Goodfellow J, Hungerford D, Woods C. Patellofemoral joint mechanics and pathology of chondromalacia-patella. J Bone Joint Surg Br 1976; 59:291.
44. Last RJ. Anatomy: Regional and Applied. 6th ed. Edinburgh: Churchill Livingstone; 1978.
45. Desio SM, Burks RT, Bachus KN. Soft tissue restraints to the lateral patellar translation in the human knee. Am J Sports Med 1998; 26:59–65.
46. Prietto MP, Bain JR, Stonebrook SN, Settlage RA. Tensile strength of the human posterior cruciate ligament (PCL). Trans Orthop Res Soc 1988; 13:195.
47. Woo SLY, Newton PO, MacKenna DA, Lyon RA. A comparative evaluation of the mechanical properties of the rabbit medial collateral and anterior cruciate ligaments. J Biomech 1992; 25:377–386.
48. Cooper DE, Deng XH, Burstein AL, Warren RF. The strength of the central third patellar tendon graft, a biomechanical study. Am J Sports Med 1993; 21:818–823.
49. Meyers M, Harvey JJ. Traumatic dislocation of the knee joint: a study of eighteen cases. J Bone Joint Surg Am 1971; 53:16–29.

Chapter Two

Initial Assessment: Physical Examination and Imaging Studies

Jeff C. Brand, Jr, and Darren L. Johnson

Generally considered rare, from 0.001 to 0.013% per year at various institutions, the multiple ligament injured knee may be more common than we in the orthopaedic community appreciate.[1-8] A spectrum exists between the high velocity knee dislocation and the low velocity (bicruciate injuries) or sports-related multiple ligament injured knee. The multiple ligament injured knee can be missed, particularly by primary care physicians who increasingly provide care to this patient population.

Although a knee dislocation usually represents substantial damage to the anterior cruciate ligament (ACL), the posterior cruciate ligament (PCL), and one of the collateral ligaments, case reports have detailed injuries of only two ligaments. Four cases of complete knee dislocation without disruption of both cruciates have been described.[9] Toritsuka et al. noted a complete dislocation of the knee with a torn ACL, osteochondral fracture, bruise of the lateral femoral condyle, and torn lateral meniscus. Other ligamentous structures were intact.[10] A series of 53 patients had 5 patients with an intact PCL.[2] There have been reports of three complete anterolateral knee dislocations, requiring reduction, with an intact PCL.[11]

Classification

The tibia position and its relationship to the femur specify the type of knee dislocation as described by Kennedy.[12] An anterior dislocation (40%) is slightly more common than a posterior dislocation (33%). Lateral (18%), medial (4%), and rotational dislocations (5%) are much less predominant.[13] It is likely that a rotational component exists with displacement in either the coronal or sagittal plane.[14]

The position of the knee dislocation, although suspected, is not known with spontaneous reductions or dislocations reduced elsewhere. Wascher et al., noted the pattern of dislocation correlated poorly with the injured anatomic structures.[15] These concerns led Schenck to devise a classification scheme with five categories based on the ligamentous deficits and the neurovascular status (Table 2.1): "C" specifies an arterial injury and "N" a neural injury. For example, KDIIIL-CN is an ACL/PCL/PLC, where PLC stands for posterolateral corner with a vascular and a neural injury.[16] Wascher et al., based on their experience, described a similar classification scheme that accounts for periarticular fractures (Table 2.2).[15]

Open-knee dislocations deserve mention as a separate classification. Because of the high energy dissipated in the soft tissues, the amount of soft

Table 2.1. Schenck classification for the multiple ligament injured knee

Class	Injury
KDI	Lesion of ACL + MCL or LCL
KDII	Rupture of ACL + PCL with intact collateral ligament
KDIII	
IIIM	Rupture of ACL + PCL + MCL with intact LCL and posterolateral corner
IIIL	Rupture of ACL + PCL + LCL with intact MCL
KDIV	Rupture of ACL + PCL + MCL + LCL

Source: Data from Schenck.[16]
Note: See Table 3.1 for new class.

tissue injury exceeds that of the closed-knee dislocation, which in itself is a high energy injury. The incidence of neurovascular injury increases in the open-knee dislocation compared with the closed-knee dislocation. Additionally, wound healing difficulties approximated 42% in one report of open-knee dislocations.[17]

Although a timing classification scheme has yet to be established, most would agree that an injury seen within the first 3 weeks would be considered to be acute, an injury seen between 3 weeks and 3 months would be considered to be subacute, and one seen beyond 3 months may be considered to be chronic.[8,18]

History

Historically, knee dislocation occurs in young males participating in high velocity motorized activity, specifically, motor vehicle and motorcycle accidents.[19,20] Collisions between the more vulnerable pedestrians and motor vehicles are notable for producing knee dislocations. Seat belts remain the most effective restraint in the prevention of lower extremity trauma in the motor vehicle.[21]

Two groups of patients trend toward popliteal artery injuries. A noteworthy subset of anterior knee dislocations with a predilection toward popliteal artery thrombosis is represented by trampoline injuries. Traditionally, trampoline injuries have been considered unlikely to result in popliteal artery injuries.[22] Hagino et al. identified "spontaneous dislocations of the knee joint" in morbidly obese patients, those who were more than 100 lb over ideal body weight or a body mass index (BMI) greater than 35. This proved a pernicious injury. All 7 of these patients presented with popliteal artery disruption. No spontaneous dislocations occurred in nonobese patients.[14]

All manner of sporting activity can result in a low velocity bicruciate knee injury. Occasionally a trivial misstep results in a multiple ligament injury in older patients. Every series also includes patients who fell from a height.[23]

Table 2.2. Modification by Wascher et al.[15] of the Schenck classification

Injury pattern
ACL + PCL alone
ACL + PCL + MCL
ACL + PCL + posterolateral complex
ACL + PCL + posterolateral complex + MCL
ACL + PCL + major periarticular fracture

Source: Reprinted from Wascher,[15] with permission.

Anatomy

The cruciate ligaments consist of anatomically isolated bands combining to give a functional composite of the each ligament. This is particularly true in the posterior cruciate ligament. The anterolateral band provides stability of the knee in flexion to posterior tibial translation. It is six times stronger than the posteromedial band, which diminishes posterior translation of the tibia with respect to the femur when the knee is in the extended position.[24] The two PCL bands have separate femoral insertions, giving the composite PCL a broad femoral insertion: approximately 3 cm from cephalad to caudad and a full centimeter in depth. The anterior cruciate ligament consists of two bands: the anteromedial tightens in flexion and the posterolateral tightens in extension. They do not mimic the level of independent function seen in the PCL bands. The ACL is hourglass shaped, but the insertion sites are smaller than in the PCL, and the ACL is better suited for a single-band reconstruction.

The medial collateral ligament (MCL) is the primary restraint to valgus load. The mid-third of layer III, the deep layer of the medial knee, includes the deep portion of the MCL. The deep MCL proximal to the meniscus is the meniscofemoral ligament, and the portion distal is meniscotibial. Posterior to the mid-third of medial capsule and the deep MCL, layer III fuses with layer II to form the posterior oblique ligament. Further posterior the capsule is reinforced by the multiple insertions of the semimembranosus.[25] The deep ligament's origin lies directly distal and slightly posterior to the origin of the superficial MCL. The superficial MCL is vertical in extension, while the deep ligament runs obliquely from distal anterior to proximal posterior or nearly parallel to the ACL. In flexion, both the deep and superficial ligaments are vertical and perpendicular to the tibial plateau. The deep ligament parallels the superficial ligament in flexion because the femoral origin rotates from its posterior location in extension to an anterior position in flexion.[26] The deep portion of the ligament attaches with the capsule to the tibia at the joint line. The superficial portion of the ligament fans out distally to lie directly under the pes anserine tendons.

Functionally, the fibular collateral ligament (FCL), the popliteus complex, the mid-third lateral capsular ligament, and the popliteal fibular ligament (PFL) comprise the static stabilizers to varus stress and external tibial rotation. The FCL, the primary stabilizer to varus opening, extends from the midsection of the lateral fibular head to originate proximal and posterior to the lateral femoral epicondyle. The popliteus complex resists posterolateral rotation of the tibia. The popliteus tendon is one of two intra-articular tendons and also has the distinction of being upside down, with a proximal tendon insertion and a distal muscular origin. Its insertion resides in the anterior third of the popliteal sulcus, 2 cm anterior to the FCL origin. It has been noted to be avulsed off the femur in 33% of grade III posterolateral knee injuries. The popliteal fibular ligament, a static stabilizer of external tibial rotation, connects the musculotendinous portion of the popliteus to the medial aspect of the posterior fibular styloid (posterior division) and the anterior medial downslope of the styloid (anterior division). The mid-third lateral capsular ligament, the secondary stabilizer to the varus opening, consists of a thickening of the lateral midline capsule, equivalent to the deep MCL. The meniscofemoral portion attaches between the FCL and the popliteus and is infrequently injured. The meniscotibial portion, the more frequently injured portion of the mid-third lateral capsular ligament, is the site of the Segond and soft tissue Segond injuries. The dynamic stabilizer of the posterolateral corner is the biceps femoris complex. Multiple components comprise the short head biceps femoris with attachments to the fibular styloid, posterolateral capsule and through the anterior tibial arm to the anterior tibia. Also, the long head biceps femoris consist of five components whose main attachments are to the fibular styloid.[27]

Failure to recognize and address damage to secondary restraints is a common cause of failure in ACL reconstruction and is presently receiving recognition as the leading cause of PCL postreconstruction laxity. In decreasing order of importance, the secondary restraints of the ACL are the medial collateral ligament (MCL), the illiotibial band (ITB), the midmedial capsule, the midlateral capsule, and the lateral collateral ligament (LCL).[28] Similarly, the secondary restraints to the PCL in decreasing order of importance are the posterior lateral capsule and the popliteus, the MCL, the posterior medial capsule, the LCL, and the midmedial capsule.[28] Unrecognized posterolateral corner damage presently is implicated in PCL graft laxity after reconstruction. Therefore, meticulous evaluation of this structure at the time of reconstruction is mandatory.

Associated Injuries

Many knee dislocation patients are multiple injury patients. Injuries throughout the body and injuries about the same extremity should be avidly pursued. Treiman et al., who cataloged the associated fractures concomitant with the knee dislocation, found that 53% of knee dislocations were accompanied by a fracture. These associated fractures were, in order of prevalence, tibial plateau, distal femur, tibia/fibula, isolated fibula, and isolated tibia.[29] Tibial plateau rim fractures, although common in their association with knee dislocation, do not often alter management. On the other hand, intra-articular fracture displacement requires aggressive fixation and may necessitate staged reconstruction. Preoperative planning and discussion with the patient should include recognition of osteochondral fractures.

Extensor mechanism injuries, quadriceps tendon disruptions, patellar fractures, and patellar tendon ruptures should not be overlooked. Fortunately, extensor mechanism injuries are revealed with magnetic resonance imaging (MRI).

Proximal tibiofibular joint dislocation can accompany a knee dislocation. This injury should be sought, since it is often unrecognized.[30,31]

Nerve Injuries

Nerve injuries comprise 16 to 40% of knee dislocations. Owing to the peroneal anchorage at the fibula head, peroneal nerve injuries occur more commonly than tibial nerve injuries. Injuries that apply tensile load to the lateral knee architecture create more peroneal nerve injuries.

Neural injuries are managed expectantly, serial electromyograms give information regarding extent of damage and prognosis. However, with or without surgical repair, the chance of functional return may not be much better than 50%. Many peroneal nerve injuries occur under tension, such as posterolateral knee dislocations. Peroneal nerve injuries commonly accompany popliteal artery damage. Complete disruption of the nerve is rare. Even with an intact nerve sheath, profound interstitial nerve damage precludes end-to-end repair. Consequently the functional nerve defect requires nerve grafting, usually with a sural nerve graft. Inconsistent results with nerve grafting encourage proponents of tendon transfers to recommend transfers for their patients.

Arterial Injuries

According to Wascher et al., vascular injury occurred just as frequently in bicruciate ligament injuries as in knee dislocations.[15] Therefore, arterial examination cannot be ignored in the low velocity injuries. The incidence of arterial injury concomitant with knee dislocation is noted in Table 2.3. The same authors stated that the direction of the knee dislocation predicted neither ligament injury pattern nor the presence of arterial injuries, wrote Wascher et al.[15] Yet not all writers on the topic of knee dislocation would agree with this assertion. Treiman et al. noted that "no patient with an isolated lateral, medial, or rotational dislocation had an arterial injury."[29] Popliteal arterial injury pattern corresponds to the direction of dislocation, and an anterior dislocation with a hyperextension mechanism classically stretches the artery with intimal injury or arterial contusion.[13] In contrast, the posterior dislocation occurring with a posteriorly displaced tibial injury likely transects the artery in a sharp manner.[32]

"Arteriography is recommended in all cases of complete dislocation of the knee," wrote Welling et al. in 1981 in the *Journal of Trauma*.[33] As recently as 1994, McNeil and McGee stated: "Arteriography should be done for all trauma patients with a grossly unstable knee joint or knee dislocation and palpable pedal pulses."[34] Case reports have detailed intimal arterial damage with a pseudoaneurysm, even though each patient had "normal" pulses and a well-perfused foot.[35,36] However there is considerable evidence to support the use of selective arteriography (Table 2.3). Signs of ischemia include hypothermia, a tense calf with hypoesthesia, and diminished motor function.[23] The absence of pedal pulses and a frankly ischemic foot after knee reduction demands immediate operative repair by a trained vascular surgeon. The arteriogram is a delay in this treatment plan. Indeed, at the University of Southern California Medical Center, arteriography typically required 3h, which reflected the time delay necessary to call in the arteriography team for emergency studies.[29] Delay beyond 6 to 8h in arterial reconstruction has been associated with an increase in the likelihood of lower limb amputation.[37] Amputation rate with an arterial repair before 6 to 8h was 11%, but in one reported series it was 86% if the repair occurred

Table 2.3. Incidence of arterial injury concomitant with knee dislocation

Authors	Year	Patients[1]	Vascular injuries[2]	False positive[3]	False negative[4]	Recommendation
Kendall et al.[20]	1993	35/37	6 (37%)	0	0	Selective arteriography
Treiman et al.[29]	1992	115	27 (23%)	6	4[5]	Selective arteriography
Kaufman et al.[23]	1992	19	6 (32%)	0	2[5]	Radiologist's discretion[6]
McCoy et al.[71]	1987	4	4 (100%)	0	3	Routine arteriography

[1] Number of patients in each report, followed by the number of knee dislocations experienced by the patient population in the study.
[2] Number of vascular injuries in the study population, followed by the percentage of total number of knee dislocations.
[3] Abnormal clinical examination for arterial injury but no arterial injury with arteriogram or exploration.
[4] Normal clinical examination for arterial injury but an arterial injury reported after arteriogram or exploration.
[5] Patients with normal pulses and an intimal flap of the artery treated nonoperatively without vascular complications.
[6] Investigation performed in the Department of Radiology.

more than 8 h after the injury.[13] For a prolonged ischemic event, fasciotomies must accompany the vascular repair or grafting.[22,32]

At the other end of the clinical spectrum is the patient with normal pulses, a healthy appearing foot, and Doppler signals of normal amplitude. Kendall et al. noted, "In absence of these findings (ischemia or absent or diminished pulses), no patient was found to have an arterial injury"[20] (Table 2.3). A review by Applebaum et al. of 22 patients with knee dislocation and complex long-bone fractures who underwent routine arteriography identified three arterial injuries, none of which required operative intervention. For all patients in their study, two variables, pulse deficit and delayed capillary refill, strongly correlated ($p < 0.05$) with arteriographic demonstration of an arterial injury.[38]

Between these two extremes in the clinical spectrum, the arteriogram improves the diagnosis of an arterial injury. Postreduction, a patient may have present, but diminished, pulses with a warm, perfused foot. In this instance an arteriogram, along with a vascular consultation, may be indicated. A closed head injury or other injuries requiring lengthy operative attention may also prompt an arteriogram.

Physical Examination

Technological advances such as MRI do not relieve the clinician of the responsibility of performing a thorough physical examination.[21] Progression in an orderly fashion through the many steps of the physical examination avoids omitting pertinent patient factors. Initial emphasis must be placed on the neurovascular aspects discussed earlier, for the knee dislocation and indeed the bicruciate injured knee are limb-threatening conditions.[13,39,40]

Acute

Careful observation aids early detection of knee dislocation or bicruciate injured knee. How uncomfortable is the patient? Although a knee dislocation represents a significant injury, patients can be surprisingly comfortable and possess a sense of resignation. A writhing, grimacing, anxious patient suggests a vascular injury and possible compartment syndrome. Is the skin about the knee mottled or pale? Transient skin discoloration promptly resolves with knee reduction. Does the foot appear flaccid? The flail and toneless foot is symptomatic of a significant nerve injury and possible arterial injury. How much swelling presents in the limb, and where is it located? Rupture of the capsule decreases the swelling around the knee, so swelling underestimates the soft tissue trauma.

A dimple sign at the medial joint line heralds an irreducible posterolateral knee dislocation. A buttonhole is created as the medial femoral condyle folds the medial capsule into the joint, pulling the skin into the telltale dimple. Although an irreducible posterolateral dislocation occurs about as often as Halley's comet, the dimple sign is regarded as pathognomonic.[41] Recognition and expedient open reduction may be limb saving.

Knee positioning cues the experienced examiner to the direction of the dislocation and the expected ligamentous deficits. Excessive varus suggests posterolateral complex damage (Figure 2.1). A positive Godfrey sign (Figure 2.2) is indicative of a grade III posterior cruciate ligament injury. Patella location points to an extensor mechanism injury. A quadriceps tendon rupture manifests as baja. Patellar tendon rupture presents with alta.

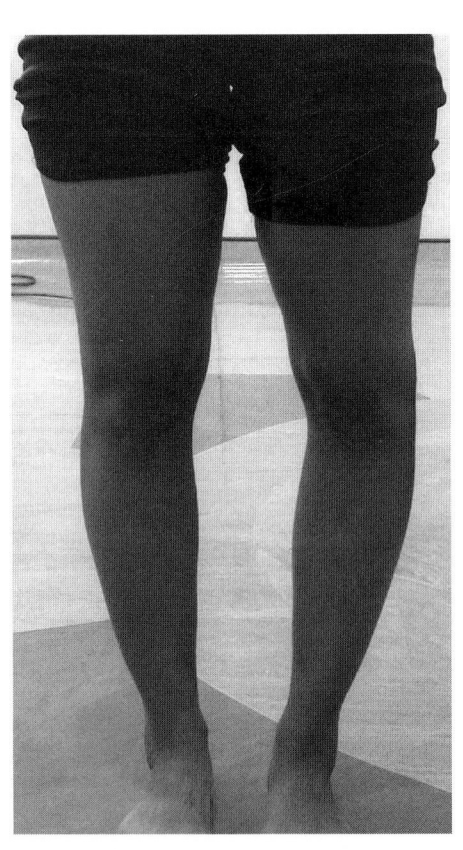

Fig. 2.1. Woman in the standing position demonstrating a varus thrust from her PLC injury.

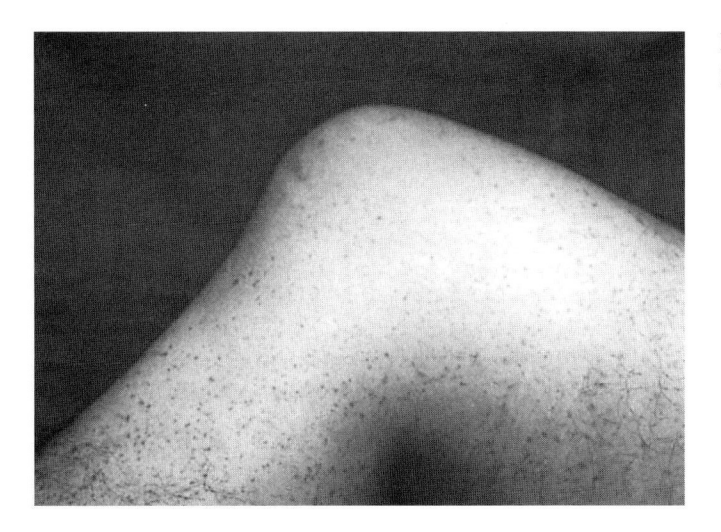

2. Initial Assessment: Physical Exam and Imaging

Fig. 2.2. Patient with a sag of the tibia posterior to the femur, or the Godfrey sign.

Ligamentous examination, performed immediately after reduction with some degree of anesthesia, accurately portrays the ligamentous deficits. Reduction and anesthesia minimize muscular guarding. With these markedly unstable knees, establishing a neutral point for the stability examination, in both the coronal and sagittal plane represents a real challenge. Determination of collateral ligament and capsular damage may be more important than definition of the cruciate ligament damage. The vast majority of these knees are bicruciate injured. Medial-sided injuries often can be treated with cruciate ligament reconstruction alone, while lateral injuries usually require a separate operative approach.[42,43]

The stability examination, like good detective work, is thorough and necessary for further decisions. When given a choice between relying on clinical information and radiographic findings, the advantage lies with clinical findings. Radiographic findings should supplement and refine clinical findings.

Anteior Cruciate Ligament

The Lachman's, an anteriorly directed vector applied to the tibia with the knee in 20 to 30° of flexion, is the most sensitive test for ACL deficiency, given that the correct knee neutral point is established. Both the end point (mushy or absent) and the length of excursion f > 5 mm) determine a positive result of the Lachman's. Displaced bucket handle meniscal tears and hamstring spasm will diminish tibial excursion. A third-degree MCL tear will increase the excursion. The MCL is a secondary stabilizer to anterior tibial motion, and its absence may cause a false positive Lachman's in the hands of an inexperienced examiner.

For the drawer sign, the examiner's hands are placed on the patient's hamstring muscles to assess the degree of muscular guarding preceding the anterior drawer testing. Restoring the tibial step-off with respect to the femoral condyles serves as reference point to the neutral knee position in the sagittal plane (Figure 2.3). Grade I laxity is defined as from 0 to 5 mm, grade II ranges from 6 to 10 mm, and grade III is more than 10 mm of motion for the anterior drawer. The posterior drawer and the varus and valgus stress test share the same measurement scale for knee laxity. The drawer tests can be evaluated with the knee in rotation. Increased laxity with the tibia

Fig. 2.3. The examiner's thumbs palpate the soft spot between the anterior tibial plateau and the femoral condyles.

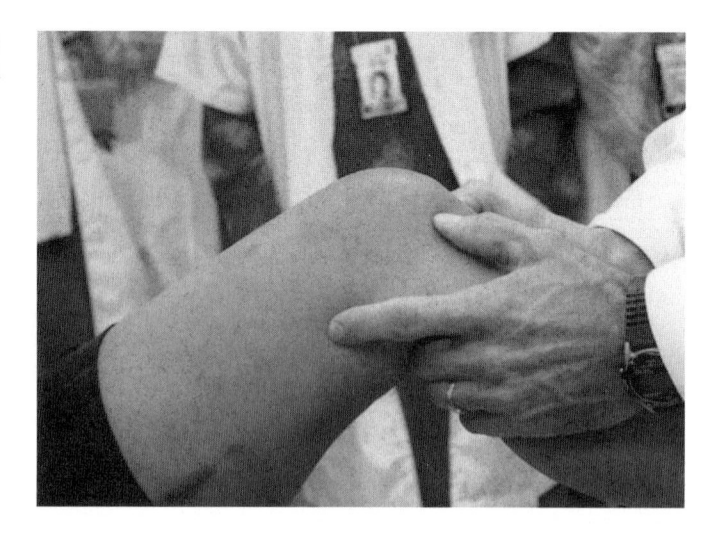

internally rotated suggests a posterolateral corner injury. Increased laxity with the tibial externally rotated indicates a posteromedial capsule injury.[44]

The sine qua non of anterolateral rotatory instability associated with ACL deficiency is the pivot shift. Ivar Palmer in 1938 created a movie of the subluxation maneuver.[45] The pivot shift more accurately represents anterolateral rotatory instability in the chronic condition or under some degree of anesthesia. Apprehension effectively extinguishes the pivot shift, since it is similar to the apprehension test in the unstable shoulder. The positive pivot shift is impossible with a complete MCL tear.

Although variation exists between the different described techniques, some principles emerge. The knee is reduced in the flexed position and subluxed in the extended position. In extension the iliotibial band snaps over the lateral femoral condyle as it moves anterior to the center of joint rotation, producing an anteriorly directed force to the tibia, and the subluxation clunk appears. In flexion, the iliotibial band moves posterior to the center of joint rotation, applying a posterior-directed force to the tibia that reduces the knee. The knee reduces again with full extension or hyperextension as a result of the screw home mechanism. The clunk appears at 20 to 40° of knee flexion depending on the test performed. Tibial internal rotation exaggerates the finding, and neutral or external tibial rotation diminishes the clunk. A valgus force is applied to the knee as the test is performed. Grading consists of 0 (absent), 1+ (rolling or slip), 2+ (moderate slip), and 3+ (momentary locking).[44–46]

The pivot shift maneuver is tested with the patient supine and initiated with the knee in slight flexion. The jerk test of Hughston occurs in reverse order of the pivot shift. The supine patient's knee initially is held in 90° of flexion and gradually extended, subluxation of the knee joint occurs at 30 to 40° of flexion.[47] Losee modified the tibial translation test. The test is initiated with external tibial rotation at 45° of knee flexion. In this position the knee is reduced. With knee extension and a valgus force at the knee, subluxation occurs at 20° of flexion with a clunk.[48] The Slocum variation of the pivot shift is performed with the patient in the lateral decubitus position with the affected side up. The patient's pelvis is rotated 30° posteriorly, and the medial side of the foot rests on the examination table. This position rotates the tibia internally and places the knee in valgus. The knee flexes with the examiner's index fingers anteriorly placed on the joint line and the thumbs placed posteriorly. The knee reduces at 25 to 45° of flexion. Acutely, the Slocum maneuver may be more accurate, owing to patient relaxation and reduced pain associated with the lateral position.[44,49]

Posterior Cruciate Ligament

A quadriceps active test allows a patient to demonstrate posterior laxity. Lying supine with the hip flexed 70° and the knee at 60°, the patient performs an active contraction of the quadriceps muscle that slides the tibia anterior to the femur in absence of a PCL. The patient's foot should be fixed flat to the table.[50] This sign is more easily expressed in the chronic situation.

The posterior drawer, the most sensitive test for PCL laxity, is best performed in the same position as the quadriceps active test. The examiner's thumbs palpate the tibial step-off with respect to the femoral condyles (Figure 2.3). The absence of a symmetric tibial step-off to that of the uninvolved knee implies that the tibia lies posterior to the femur. The tibia should be restored to its normal position under the femur before the extent of posterior laxity to evaluated. The laxity is graded I to III in the same manner as the anterior drawer.

Medial Collateral Ligament

A valgus stress test applied with the knee in extension and 30° of flexion estimates the amount of MCL laxity. Pain degrades accuracy in the acute setting owing to tension exerted to the injured medial collateral ligament. The same grading scheme applies to the valgus stress test. Significant valgus laxity in knee extension implies a complete tear of the ACL, since this is a secondary restraint to the MCL. As with all laxity tests, the other knee serves as an internal control.

Posterolateral Complex

Varus testing describes fibular collateral ligament and mid-third lateral capsular ligament laxity. Grade III laxity in full knee extension suggests concomitant cruciate ligament injury. The fibular collateral ligament can be palpated and compared to the contralateral FCL with the leg in the figure-of-four position.

Knee recurvatum (Figure 2.4) is a frequent, subtle presentation of a PLC injury. With more extensive PLC injuries, the examiner may note varus and external rotation at the knee with lifting the patient's leg by grasping the great toe.

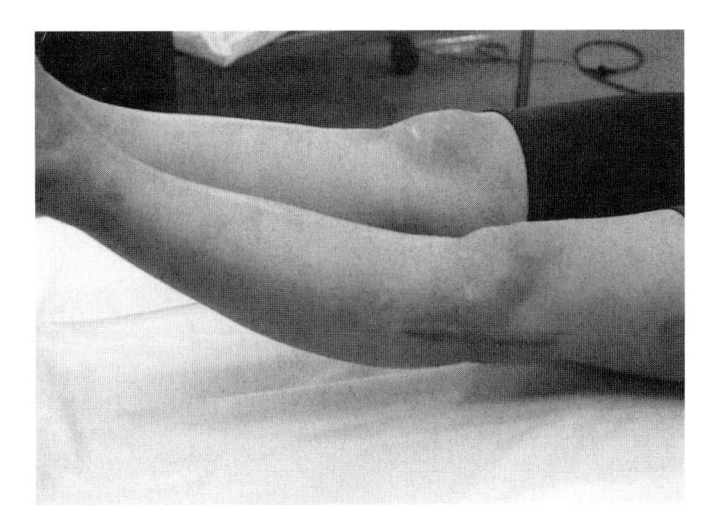

Fig. 2.4. Young female patient who has had a failed PLC reconstruction of the left knee with residual recurvatum of the knee.

Presence of a reverse pivot shift indicates a PLC injury. With this maneuver, the knee reduces in extension but subluxes in the flexed position. However, the positive clunk is less noticeable than the clunk associated with a pivot shift. Initially the patient is positioned supine with the knee flexed at least 45° and the foot placed in external rotation. As the knee extends, the examiner applies a valgus load. The knee reduces with an audible clunk at approximately 20° of the flexion.

Arguably the most easily elicited evidence of grade II or III PLC may be the spin-out or dial sign. It can be tested in the prone or supine position. External tibial rotation at both the knee and the ankle with the knee at 30° and 90° determines the extent of PLC injury. A side-to-side difference of more than 10° indicates pathologic laxity.[46]

The drawer sign gives evidence of a significant PLC injury. Evaluating the posterior drawer sign with the foot in external rotation, internal rotation, and neutral rotation demonstrates capsular injury. The anterior drawer fails to tighten with the foot in the internally rotated position with a grade III PLC injury.

Chronic

Anterior Cruciate Ligament

In the chronic multiple ligament injured knee, the result of Lachman's test is seldom altered by muscular guarding. Recognizing a posteriorly placed tibia in the PCL-injured knee allows an accurate estimation of anterior laxity. An associated chronic MCL injury will exaggerate the extent of anterior laxity owing to its role as a secondary restraint to anterior tibial excursion in absence of the ACL.

Accuracy and reliability improve in the chronic situation with the anterior drawer. Consequently, the anterior drawer yields better information in the chronically injured knee.

The chronically injured MCL lax knee displays a false negative pivot shift. The pivot shift is frequently elicited in the knee with chronic anterolateral rotatory instability, once. After one subluxation event, muscular guarding usually extinguishes the pivot shift sign.

Posterior Cruciate Ligament

Both the posterior drawer and the quadriceps active test are accurate in the examination of the chronically PCL lax knee. Centering the knee in the sagittal plane for the posterior drawer test is the key to successful evaluation of the degree of PCL laxity.

Medial Collateral Ligament

Determining the neutral position of the knee in the coronal plane is the primary challenge when one is evaluating the degree of MCL injury. Significant laxity of both medial and lateral ligamentous structures, although rare, markedly complicates the evaluation of these structures.

Posterolateral Corner

Muscle relaxation eases the examination of the fibular collateral ligament and the PLC in the chronic situation. Consequently, knee recurvatum (Figure 2.4), varus external rotation recurvatum, reverse pivot shift, spin-out sign, and posterior drawer test occur readily in the chronically injured multiple ligament deficient knee.

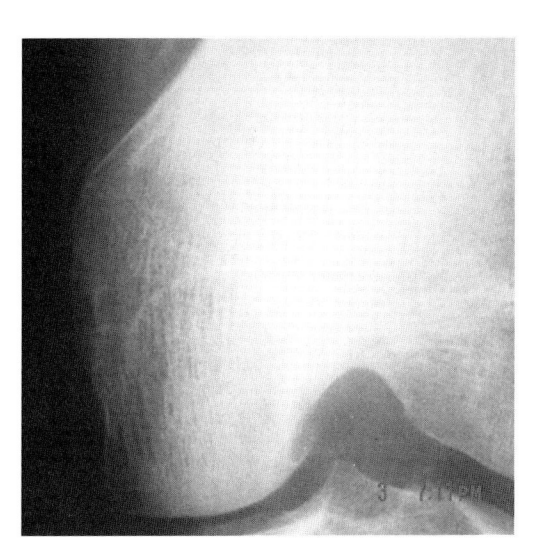

Fig. 2.5. AP radiograph depicting an MCL avulsion from the medial femoral epicondyle known as the Pellegrini–Stieda sign.

Imaging Studies

Radiographs

Acutely, anteroposterior (AP) and lateral views suffice to make the diagnosis and direct the knee reduction. In addition to the AP and lateral, postreduction views should include a sunrise view of the patella and a notch view. Accessory views, as indicated by concomitant injuries, consist of oblique views and an AP view angled 10° caudad. The routine AP and lateral plain radiographs confirm a concentric reduction. An incomplete or nonconcentric reduction suggests interposed structures such as the meniscus. Avulsion injuries off the medial femoral epicondyle (Figure 2.5) or the tip of the fibula imply collateral ligament injury. A patellar sunrise view may reveal a patellar avulsion fracture that suggests retinacular damage or osteochondral injuries. Osteochondral injuries of the distal femoral articular surface may be demonstrated with the notch view. Segond injuries (Figure 2.6), lateral capsular avulsion fractures, proximal tibial–fibular dislocations, and tibial plateau fractures may all be shown to advantage with the various oblique plain radiographs. Tibial plateau fracture displacement may be elucidated with an AP view angled 10° caudad.

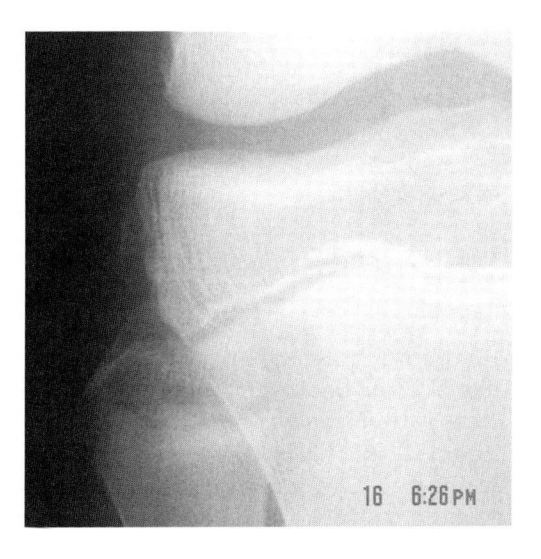

Fig. 2.6. The lateral capsular avulsion sign or the Segond injury.

Fig. 2.7. Lateral stress radiograph showing recurvatum associated with a PLC injury.

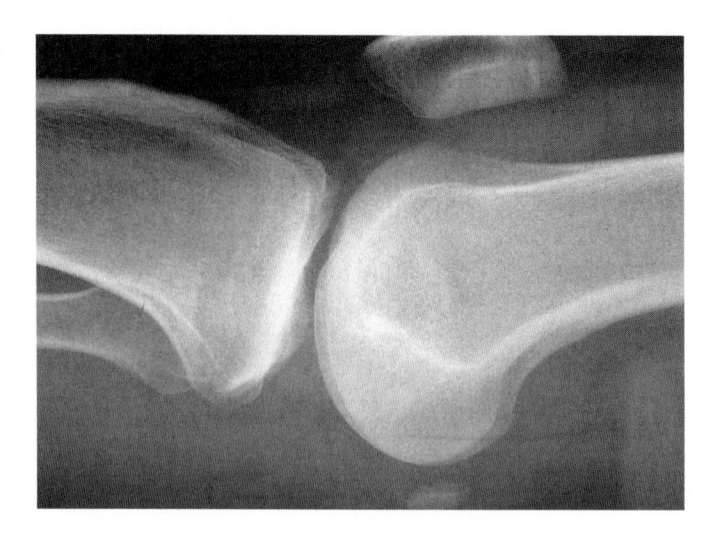

The role of stress radiographs in most centers has diminished as MRI image clarity, resolution, and software have improved. When the clinical examination and MRI findings do not agree, or when the extent of a ligament injury is ill defined, however, stress radiographs with defined parameters can be diagnostic (Figure 2.7).

Magnetic Resonance Imaging

Delineation of extensor mechanism injuries or disruption improves with MRI. Reconstruction of the multiple ligament injured knee demands a number of grafts. Damage to the extensor mechanism precludes using this as a donor site. Extensive patellar tendon rupture with marked interstitial damage may require separate allograft reconstruction.

An experienced examiner can determine the ACL status in the isolated ACL-deficient knee. Therefore, MRI offers little advantage in the diagnosis of an isolated ACL rupture.[51] The accuracy of clinical examination for the cruciate ligaments is yet to be decided in the multiple ligament injured knee, but it may not be as accurate as the diagnosis of isolated cruciate ligament tears.[52] Sensitivity and specificity of MRI for the cruciate ligaments in reported series have been excellent. Primary findings (abnormal signal intensity, abnormal course, discontinuity) and secondary findings (bone bruise in lateral compartment, anterior tibial displacement, uncovering of the posterior horn of the lateral meniscus, the configuration of the PCL[53]) have proven reliable in the diagnosis of ACL injury.[54,55] Anterior tibial displacement is measured by drawing a tangent to the posterior margin of the cortex of the lateral femoral condyle and parallel to the long axis of the tibia in the midsagittal plane of the lateral femoral condyle. A second vertical tangential line to the proximal tibial condyle is created. Anterior tibial translation of more than 5mm between the two lines defines an anteriorly positioned tibia.[56] As the tibia subluxes anteriorly, the inferior margin of the lateral meniscus is exposed. A line drawn tangential to the proximal tibial condyle discussed earlier passes through the lateral meniscus in the midsagittal plane of the lateral femoral condyle.[57,58]

Extensive PCL damage indicated by indistinct margins, abnormally thick diameter, and ligament discontinuity visualizes well with MR imaging (Figure 2.8).[59] Difficulty may arise in the gray area of partial ligament injury, albeit an uncommon situation in the multiple ligament injured knee. Phys-

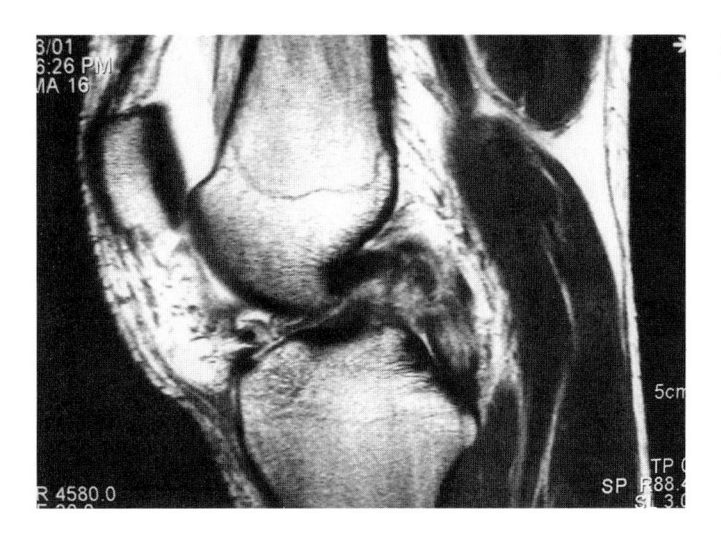

Fig. 2.8. MRI of a knee with a complete rupture of the PCL.

ical examination and examination under anesthesia must be the tiebreaker when the MRI and its interpretation prove inconclusive. MRI may be most helpful in discerning avulsion injuries of the cruciate ligaments from midsubstance cruciate injuries. Evidence suggests that repair of cruciate large bony avulsions, particularly of the PCL, facilitates superior results to ligament reconstruction (Figure 2.9).[60,61]

The MRI appearance of a chronic cruciate ligament tear can be misleading. Shelbourne et al. noted that "all partial PCL tears and most (86%) complete tears will regain continuity without surgery." The follow-up MRI occurred at a mean of 3.2 years after the index injury. Unfortunately, the authors did not evaluate knee stability at follow-up.[62]

Posterolateral corner injuries can be defined with MRI by using correct sequences including thin-slice coronal oblique T1-weighted images through the fibular head. Although many of the PLC structures lie oblique to standard planes, sensitivity, specificity, and accuracy were acceptable in a clinical study. Surgically validated grade III injuries of the popliteal–fibular ligament, popliteus, mid-third lateral capsular ligament, fibular collateral ligament (Figure 2.10), and biceps femoris tendon could all be discerned with MRI (Table 2.4).[63] Three of 6 patients with complete popliteal tendon tears in one investigation also suffered from peroneal nerve injuries.[64]

Such MRI signs as ligament discontinuity, focal disruption, fluid, and loss of demarcation between the MCL and adjacent fat are "questionably accurate" for grade I and II injuries and "inaccurate" for grade III lesions. Bone bruises accompanied one quarter of isolated MCL injuries.[65] The extent of the medial collateral ligament injury reveals itself more completely with clinical examination in the relaxed state.

Diagnostic accuracy of the report of an experienced examiner for an isolated meniscal injury approaches 69% for both the medial and lateral meniscus. Not surprisingly, the MRI was more accurate for the diagnosis of an injured medial meniscus (84%) and lateral meniscus (82%) in the same study.[51] The accuracy for the MRI diagnosis of meniscal injury approaches 90% for each meniscus.[66–68] Diagnostic accuracy of meniscal injury based on clinical examination likely diminishes when there is suspicion of other concordant knee injuries, such as ACL injuries.[69] Meniscal damage may not be as common in the multiple ligament injured knee as it is in the knee with an isolated cruciate ligament tear. The energy dissipated in the soft tissues typically results in capsular damage rather than meniscal damage in the knee

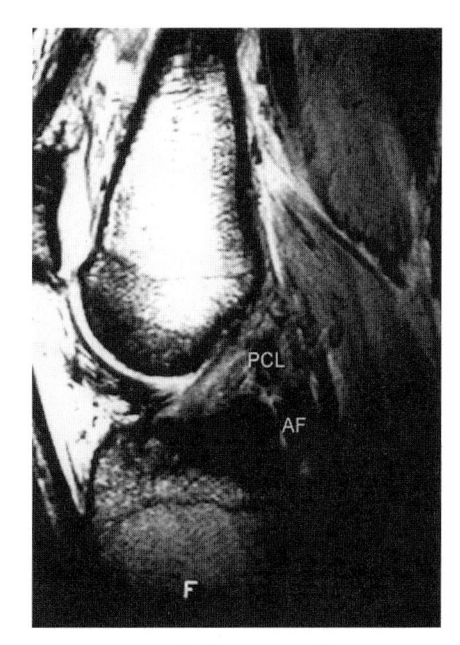

Fig. 2.9. Sagittal plane MRI demonstrating a large chronic PCL avulsion: AF, avulsed PCL tibial fracture fragment; F, fibular collateral ligament.

Fig. 2.10. Coronal plane MRI of a patient demonstrating a complete femoral rupture of the fibular collateral ligament: LFC, lateral femoral condyle; F, fibular collateral ligament.

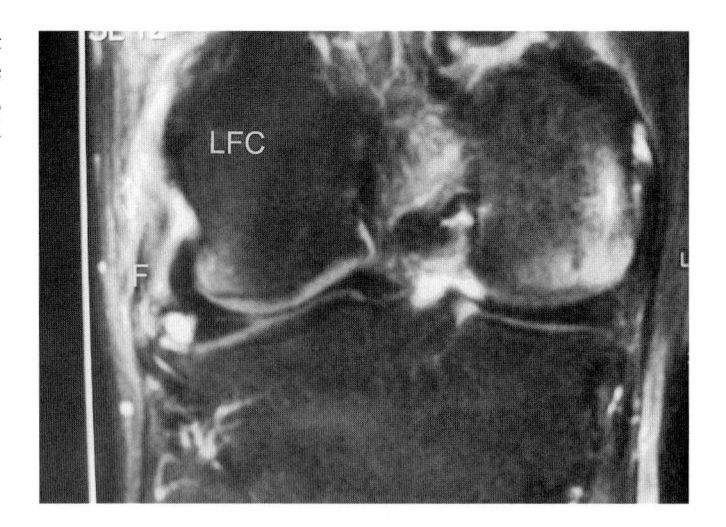

dislocation. Therefore, MRI may be more accurate than clinical examination in the diagnosis of meniscal injury in the multiple ligament injured knee.

The MR examination of the medial meniscus is more accurate than imaging of the lateral meniscus.[67] The anatomy of the posterior horn of the lateral meniscus includes the meniscofemoral ligaments and the popliteus tendon. These structures lead to confusion in interpreting MR images. MRI visualizations of meniscocapsular separations, which may be more common in the multiple ligament injured knee images, correspond poorly with arthroscopy findings.[67]

Bone bruises serve to map a history of the forces applied to the knee. The lateral femoral condyle (LFC) sulcus terminalis bone bruise in the knee with the isolated ACL-deficient knee is pathognomonic. This marker of ACL injury may be associated with a kissing lesion on the posterior aspect of the lateral tibial plateau. Bone bruises are a common occurrence in the isolated PCL-injured knee, since approximately 83% have an associated bone bruise. The bone bruises are typically located on the compression side of the knee from applied force. A knee in which a valgus load has been experienced would possess kissing LFC and lateral tibial plateau lesions. A varus load to the knee would produce a medial-sided bone bruise.[70] In patellar dislocations, a bone bruise is often found where the patella contacts the LFC at the time of dislocation. Cartilage lesions often overlie bone bruises. Diligence in reviewing the articular surfaces on MR images reveals these occasionally subtle lesions.

Knee dislocations are frequently associated with ipsilateral fractures about the knee (see earlier section on associated injuries). Occult fractures, particularly metaphyseal fractures, will be demonstrated on MRI. A com-

Table 2.4. Sensitivity, specificity, and accuracy of MRI for surgically documented grade III injuries of the posterolateral corner components

Structure	Sensitivity (%)	Specificity (%)	Accuracy (%)
Fibular collateral ligament	94.4	100	95
Popliteofibular ligament	78.6	66.7	75
Popliteofemoral origin	93.3	80	90
Mid-third lateral capsular ligament	93.8	100	95
Short head biceps	80	100	85
Anterior arm			
Direct arm	81.3	100	85

Source: Data from LaPrade.[63]

puted tomography (CT) series with narrow widths between slices may better define the amount of fracture displacement.

Conclusions

A spectrum exists between the high velocity knee dislocation and the low velocity (bicruciate injuries) or sports-related multiple ligament injured knee. Failure to recognize and correctly address damage to secondary restraints is a frequent cause of failure in ACL reconstruction and is receiving recognition as the leading cause of PCL postreconstruction laxity. Many knee dislocation patients have multiple injuries: that is, other injuries are present elsewhere and on the same limb as the knee dislocation, and these should be avidly pursued.

Neural injuries may be managed expectantly; serial electromyograms give information regarding extent of damage and prognosis. However, with or without surgical repair, the chance of functional return may not be much better than 50%. The arterial status of the majority of patients with the multiple ligament injured knee falls into two groups. Postreduction, the first and largest group of patients demonstrates normal pedal pulses with no evidence of overt ischemia. According to the studies quoted in this chapter, patients in this group will not have an arterial injury. The second group has an arterial injury expressed with overt ischemia and absent or diminished pulses. For patients between these two extremes in the clinical spectrum, the arteriogram may improve the diagnosis of arterial injury.

MR imaging and other technological advances do not relieve the clinician of the responsibility of performing a thorough physical examination.[21] A dimple sign at the medial joint line heralds an irreducible posterolateral knee dislocation. Recognition and expedient open reduction may be limb saving.

Ligamentous examination immediately performed postreduction with some degree of anesthesia more accurately reveals the ligamentous deficits. With these markedly unstable knees, establishing a neutral point for the stability examination, in both the coronal and sagittal planes, represents a real challenge. Determination of collateral ligament and capsular damage is critical, given that most knees experience bicruciate injuries.

Plain radiographs reveal the direction of the dislocation and predict ligamentous deficits that guide orthopaedic management. Postreduction views should be carefully scrutinized for avulsion injuries and fractures. Clinical examination trumps MRI of the cruciate ligaments. Conversely, MRI scanning of the menisci is more accurate than clinical examination, particularly in the multiple injured knee. Identification of avulsion injuries, occult fractures, bone bruises, and other soft tissue injuries about the knee proves MRI indispensable for evaluation of the bicruciate ligament injured knee. However, MCL, PLC, and capsular injury discrimination on MRI may be imprecise because some of these structures are oblique to standard planes.

The multiple ligament injured knee offers a challenging examination. Attention to detail, patience, and extensive knowledge of the ligament examination comprise the clinician's armamentarium to meet this challenge. The suspected ligament deficits should be defined with clinical examination. Plain radiographs and MRI refine the diagnosis. Only then may further treatment of the patient start.

References

1. Hoover N. Injuries of the popliteal artery associated with fractures and dislocations. Surg Clin North Am 1962; 41:1099–1112.

2. Meyers M, Harvey J. Traumatic dislocation of the knee joint. J Bone Joint Surg Am 1971; 53:16–29.
3. Meyers M, Moore T, Harvey J. Follow-up notes on articles previously published in the journal: traumatic dislocation of the knee joint. J Bone Joint Surg Am 1975; 57:430–433.
4. Quinlan A, Sharrad W. Posterolateral dislocation of the knee with capsular interposition. J Bone Joint Surg Br 1958; 40:660–663.
5. Shelbourne K, Porter D, Clingman J, et al. Low-velocity knee dislocation. Orthop Rev 1991; 20:995–1004.
6. Shields L, Mital M, Cave E. Complete dislocation of the knee: experience at the Massachusetts General Hospital. J Trauma 1969; 9:192–215.
7. Klimkiewiez J, Petrie R, Harner C. Surgical treatment of combined injury to anterior cruciate ligament, posterior cruciate ligament, and medial structures. Clin Sports Med 2000; 19:479–492.
8. Borden P, Johnson D. Initial assesment of the acute and chronic multiple ligament-injured knee. Sports Med Arthrosc Rev 2001; 9:178–184.
9. Bratt H, Newman A. Complete dislocation of the knee without disruption of both cruciate ligaments. J Trauma 1993; 34:383–389.
10. Toritsuka Y, Horibe S, Hiro-oka A. Knee dislocation following anterior cruciate ligament disruption without any other ligament tears. Arthroscopy 1999; 15:522–526.
11. Shelbourne K, Pritchard J, Rettig A, et al. Knee dislocations with intact PCL. Orthop Rev 1992; 21:607–611.
12. Kennedy J. Complete dislocation of the knee joint. J Bone Joint Surg Am 1963; 45:889–904.
13. Green N, Allen B. Vascular injuries associated with dislocation of the knee. J Bone Joint Surg Am 1977; 59:236–239.
14. Hagino R, DeCaprio J, Valentine R. Spontaneous popliteal vascular injury in the morbidly obese. J Vasc Surg 1998; 28:458–462.
15. Wascher D, Dvirnak P, DeCoster T. Knee dislocation: initial assessment and implications for treatment. J Orthop Trauma 1997; 11:525–529.
16. Schenck R. The dislocated knee. Instr Course Lect 1994; 43:127–136.
17. Wright D, Covey D, Born C, et al. Open dislocation of the knee. J Orthop Trauma 1995; 9:135–140.
18. Marin E, Bifluco S, Fast A. Obesity: a risk factor for knee dislocation. Am J Phys Med Rehabil 1990; 69:132–134.
19. Alberty R, Goodfried G, Boyden A. Popliteal artery injury with fractural dislocation of the knee. Am J Surg 1981; 142:36–38.
20. Kendall R, Taylor D, Slavian A, et al. The role of arteriography in assessing vascular injuries associated with dislocations of the knee. J Trauma 1993; 35:875–878.
21. Brautigan B, Johnson D. The epidemiology of knee dislocations. Clin Sports Med 2000; 19:387–397.
22. Kwolek C, Sundaram S, Schwarcz T, et al. Popliteal artery thrombosis associated with trampoline injuries from anterior knee dislocations in children. Am Surg 1998; 64:1183–1187.
23. Kaufman S, Martin L. Arterial injuries associated with complete dislocation of the knee. Radiology 1992; 184:153–155.
24. Race A, Amis A. The mechanical properties of the two bundles of the human posterior cruciate ligament. J Biomech 1994; 27:13–24.
25. Warren L, Marshall J. The supporting structures and layers on the medial side of the knee. J Bone Joint Surg Am 1979; 61:56–62.
26. Jobe C, Wright M. Anatomy of the knee. In: Fu F, Harner C, Vince K, eds. Knee Surgery. Vol 1. Baltimore, MD: Williams & Wilkins; 1994:1–54.
27. LaPrade R, Wentorf F, Engebretsen L, et al. Current concepts on posterolateral knee injuries: anatomy, diagnosis, biomechanics and acute and chronic reconstructions. ISAKOS, Montreux, Switzerland, April 18–22, 2001.
28. Fu F, Harner C, Johnson D, et al. Biomechanics of knee ligaments. Basic concepts and clinical application. J Bone Joint Surg 1993; 75-A:1716–1727.
29. Treiman G, Yellin A, Weaver F, et al. Examination of the patient with a knee dislocation. The case for selective arteriography. Arch Surg 1992; 127:1056–1062.

30. Fallon P, Virani N, Bell D, et al. Delayed presentation: dislocation of the proximal tibiofibular joint after knee dislocation. J Orthop Trauma 1994; 8: 350–353.
31. Hegyes M, Richardson M, Miller M. Knee dislocation: complications of nonoperative and operative management. Clin Sports Med 2000; 19:519–543.
32. Peck J, Eastman A, Bergan J, et al. Popliteal vascular trauma: a community experience. Arch Surg 1990; 125:1339–1344.
33. Welling R, Kakkasseril J, Cranley J. Complete dislocations of the knee with popliteal vascular injury. J Trauma 1981; 21:450–453.
34. McNeil J, McGee G. Popliteal artery injury in a lumberjack. South Med J 1994; 87:958–960.
35. Gable D, Allen J, Richardson J. Blunt popliteal artery injury: is physical examination alone enough for evaluation? J Trauma 1997; 43:541–544.
36. Siani A, Intrieri F, Jabbour J, et al. Lesioni traumatiche dell'arteria poplitea da lussazione posteriore del ginocchio. Minerva Cardioangiol 2001; 49:221–226.
37. Downs A, MacDonald P. Popliteal artery injuries: civilian experience with sixty-three patients during a twenty-four year period (1960 through 1984). J Vasc Surg 1986; 4:55–62.
38. Applebaum R, Yellin A, Weaver F, et al. Role of routine arteriography in blunt lower-extremity trauma. Am J Surg 1990; 160:221–224.
39. Reynolds R, McDowell H, Diethelm A. The surgical treatment of blunt and penetrating injuries of the popliteal artery. Am Surg 1983; 49:405–410.
40. O'Donnell T, Brewster D, Darling C, et al. Arterial injuries associated with fractures and/or dislocations of the knee. J Trauma 1977; 17:775–782.
41. Huang F, Simonian P, Chansky H. Irreducible posterolateral dislocation of the knee. Arthroscopy 2000; 16:323–327.
42. Fanelli G, Giannotti B, Edson C. Arthroscopically assisted combined anterior and posterior cruciate ligament reconstruction. Arthroscopy 1996; 12:5–14.
43. Fanelli G, Giannotti B, Edson C. Arthroscopically assisted combined PCL/posterolateral complex reconstruction. Arthroscopy 1996; 12:521–530.
44. Ritchie J, Miller M, Harner C. History and Physical Examination. In: Fu F, Harner C, Vince K, eds. Knee Surgery. Vol 1. Baltimore, MD: Williams & Wilkins; 1994:253–273.
45. Eriksson E. Legends in Sports Medicine: Ivar Palmer—master of knee ligaments. ISAKOS, Montreux, Switzerland, April 18–22, 2001.
46. Fanelli G, Maish D. Knee ligament injuries: epidemiology, mechanism, diagnosis, and natural history. In: Fitzgerald R, Kaufer H, Malkani A, eds. Orthopaedics. Mosby, St. Louisule, MO, 2002:619–636.
47. Hughston J, Andrews J, Cross M, et al. Classification of knee ligament instabilities. II: The lateral compartment. J Bone Joint Surg Am 1976; 58:173–179.
48. Losee R, Johnson T, Southwick W. Anterior subluxation of the lateral tibial plateau: a diagnostic test and operative repair. J Bone Joint Surg Am 1978; 60:1015–1030.
49. Slocum D, James S, Larson R, et al. Clincal test for anterolateral rotary instability of the knee. Clin Orthop 1976; 118:63–69.
50. Daniel D, Stone M, Barnett P, Sachs R. Use of the quadriceps active test to diagnose posterior cruciate-ligament disruption and measure posterior laxity of the knee. J Bone Joint Surg Am 1988; 70:386-391.
51. Alioto R, Browne J, Barnhouse C, et al. The influence of MRI on treatment decisions regarding knee injuries. Am J Knee Surg 1999; 12:91–97.
52. Twaddle B, Hunter J, Chapman J, et al. MRI in acute knee dislocation. J Bone Joint Surg Br 1996; 78:573–579.
53. Liu S, Osti L, Dorey F, et al. Anterior cruciate ligament tear: a new diagnostic index on magnetic resonance imaging. Clin Orthop 1994; 302:147–150.
54. Lee K, Siegel M, Lau D, et al. Anterior cruciate ligament tears: MR imaging–based diagnosis in a pediatric population. Radiology 1999; 213: 697–704.
55. Brandser E, Riley M, Berbaum K, et al. MR imaging of anterior cruciate ligament injury: independent value of primary and secondary signs. Am J Radiol 1996; 167:121–126.
56. Vahey T, Hunt J, Shelbourne K. Anterior translocation of the tibia at MR imaging: a secondary sign of anterior cruciate ligament tear. Radiology 1993; 187:817–819.

57. McCauley T, Moses M, Kier R, et al. MR diagnosis of tears of anterior cruciate ligament of the knee: importance of ancillary findings. AJR Am J Roentgenol 1994; 162:115–119.
58. Tung G, Davis L, Wiggens M, et al. Tears of the anterior cruciate ligament: primary and secondary signs at MR imaging. Radiology 1993; 188:661–667.
59. Patten R, Richardson M, Zink-Brody G, et al. Complete vs partial-thickness tears of the posterior cruciate ligament: MR findings. J Comput Assist Tomogr 1994; 18:793–799.
60. Sisto D, Warren R. Complete knee dislocation: a follow-up study of operative treatment. Clin Orthop 1985; 198:94–101.
61. Wascher D, Becker J, Dexter J, et al. Reconstruction of the anterior and posterior cruciate ligaments after knee dislocation: results using fresh-frozen nonirradiated allografts. Am J Sports Med 1999; 27:189–196.
62. Shelbourne K, Jennings R, Vahey T. Magnetic resonance imaging of posterior cruciate ligament injuries. Am J Knee Surg 1999; 12:209–213.
63. LaPrade R, Bollom T, Gilbert T, et al. The MRI appearance of individual structures of the posterolateral knee: a prospective study. Paper presented at: 25th Annual Meeting of the American Orthopaedic Society for Sports Medicine; June 19–22, 1999; Traverse City, MI.
64. Yu J, Goodwin D, Salonen D, et al. Complete dislocation of the knee: spectrum of associated soft-tissue injuries depicted by MR imaging. Am J Radiol 1995; 164:135–139.
65. Schweitzer M, Tran D, Deely D, et al. Medial collateral ligament injuries: evaluation of multiple signs, prevalence and location of associated bone bruises, and assessment with MR imaging. Radiology 1995; 194:825–829.
66. Rangger C, Klestil T, Kathrein A, et al. Influence of magnetic resonance imaging on indications for arthroscopy of the knee. Clin Orthop 1996; 330:133–142.
67. Rubin D. MR imaging of the knee menisci. Radiol Clin North Am 1997; 35:21–44.
68. Otani T, Matsumoto H, Suda Y, et al. Proper use of MR imaging in internal derangement of the knee (orthopaedic surgeon's view). Semin Musculoskelet Radiol 2001; 5:143–145.
69. Shelbourne K, Martini D, McCarroll J. Correlation of joint line tenderness and meniscal lesions in patients with acute anterior cruciate ligament tears. Am J Sports Med 1995; 23:166.
70. Mair S, Schlegel T, Gill T, et al. Incidence and location of bone bruises after acute posterior cruciate ligament injury. Paper presented at: 25th Annual Meeting of the MI American Orthopaedic Society for Sports Medicine; June 19–22, 1999; Traverse City, MI.
71. McCoy GF, Hannon DG, Barr RJ, et al. Vascular injury associated with low-velocity dislocations of the knee. J Bone Joint Surg Br 1987; 69:285–287.

Chapter Three

Classification of Knee Dislocations

Robert C. Schenck, Jr.

The concept of a dislocated knee has changed over the past 20 years to include a wide variety of injury patterns. Although a dislocation is still defined as the complete displacement (even momentary) of the tibia and femur from their articulation, the presence and acceptance of spontaneously reduced dislocations and cruciate-intact (PCL or ACL) knee dislocations make the concept of a "dislocation" somewhat limited (Figure 3.1). Combining this change in the definition of a dislocation with the current understanding of functional anatomy of the knee gives the clinician wishing to find the proper treatment of a "knee dislocation" a much more accurate understanding of what is injured. The need for an accurate and reproducible classification system for knee dislocations is extremely important in the management of knee dislocations. The description of a knee dislocation based on the position of the tibia on the femur has limited clinical application. Position description says nothing about what is torn (i.e., cruciate intact vs complete bicruciate injuries) and cannot be applied at all to most traumatic dislocations that are spontaneously reduced. Thus classifying a knee dislocation by indicating what is torn is important and will be described in detail in this chapter.

The incidence of knee dislocations is probably underreported. In separate reports, investigators noted the presence of spontaneously reduced knee dislocation that is suspected to occur in over 20% of patients eventually diagnosed with a dislocated knee.[1-3] Furthermore, a clinician's exposure to a spontaneously reduced dislocation will depend upon the practice environment as well as the individual level of suspicion during patient evaluation. The relative rarity of knee dislocations in the sporting population makes the understanding of this injury an important clinical area for the practicing sports medicine physician. Unlike anterior cruciate ligament (ACL) dislocations, the rarity of knee dislocations (<1.2% of orthopaedic trauma in one series) adds to the difficulty of treating an already complex knee injury in which multiple ligaments are torn. The varying injury patterns, including complete corner injuries, musculotendinous injuries, ligament avulsions, nerve and vascular injuries, association with multitrauma, and the possibility of soft tissue and open injuries, as well as the different management opting for bicruciate injuries, including the decision and timing of surgery, and postoperative rehabilitation, underscore the many difficulties encountered in the treatment of a knee dislocation (KD).[1-15] For these reasons, a classification system is important for the clinician. Classification systems should be fairly universal and reproducible, and they should give information to the clinician that will be helpful in making treatment decisions as

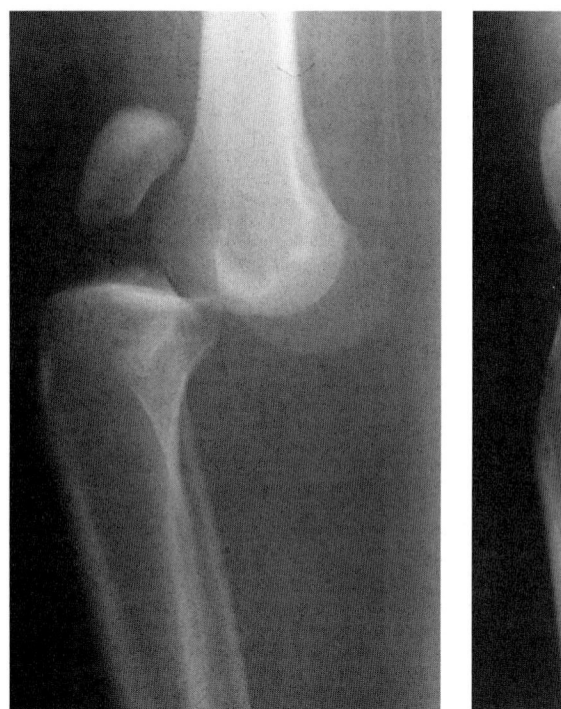

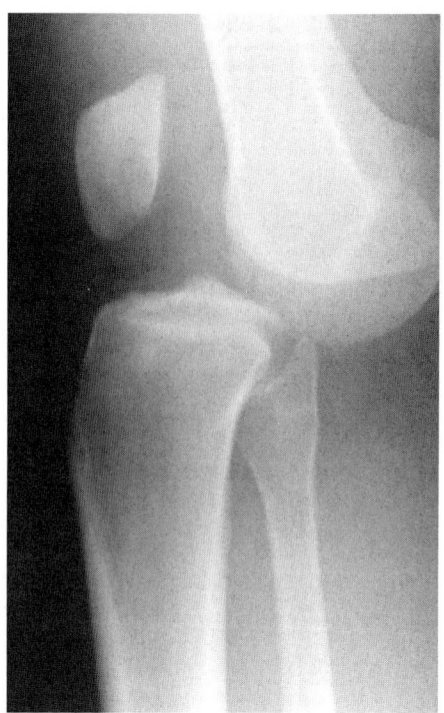

Fig. 3.1. Lateral radiographs of different presentations of knee dislocations in two different patients: (A) a PCL-intact knee dislocation and (B) a complete bicruciate ligament knee dislocation. Note the parallel alignment of the patellofemoral joint with the femur in (B) and the relatively more close proximity of the femur and tibia in (A), the PCL-intact knee dislocation. (From Schenck RC, Injuries of the knee. In: Heckman JD, ed. Rockwood and Green. 5th ed. Philadelphia: Lippincott, Williams & Wilkins. By permission of the publisher.)

well as in developing prognoses for injuries. Several classification systems exist including those based on position, level of energy, and anatomy. This chapter reviews current classification systems that allow for better communication concerning the injury, as well as guidelines for direct treatment and aid in predicting outcomes.

Anatomy

In knee dislocation, multiple structures can be injured in combination in definite patterns of injury commonly seen.[1,7,8] As discussed in Chapter 1, the anatomy and biomechanics of the knee are clearly defined, and the successful classification and treatment of a dislocated knee requires a thorough understanding of knee functional anatomy. The classification of knee dislocations is most accurately determined by the ligaments torn (the anatomic system) rather than by joint position; hence, knowledge of the functional anatomy of ligaments is very important in classifying and defining an injury pattern. Adding to the variability of structures torn during a knee dislocation are the association of disruption of musculotendinous structures (extensor mechanism, iliotibial band, biceps femoris, gastrocnemius, and popliteus tendons) and the importance of associated injuries. Last, the bony architecture is important since joint surface fractures can occur with a knee dislocation. Depending on the size of fracture fragments, the knee injury can be classified as a fracture-dislocation when associated with a large condyle fracture rather than a pure ligamentous injury as implied by the term *knee dislocation*.[2,16]

Conceptually, defining the anatomy of the knee into four simply definable structures (two cruciates and two collaterals, including the corners) is very useful. The ACL and PCL can be either torn together (bicruciate injury), separately (ACL- or PCL-intact knee dislocations) or, rarely, not torn at all (cruciate intact knee dislocations) (Figure 3.2). The injuries to the collaterals are frequently complete, with involvement of the structures related to the ligamentous corners. In my experience, the sidedness and determination of a complete or partial collateral and corner injury in a dislocation strongly determines the acuity of surgery (within 7 days vs delayed with initial range of motion). Hence, the ability to perform an accurate functional examination of ligaments is crucial in classifying and treating a dislocated knee.

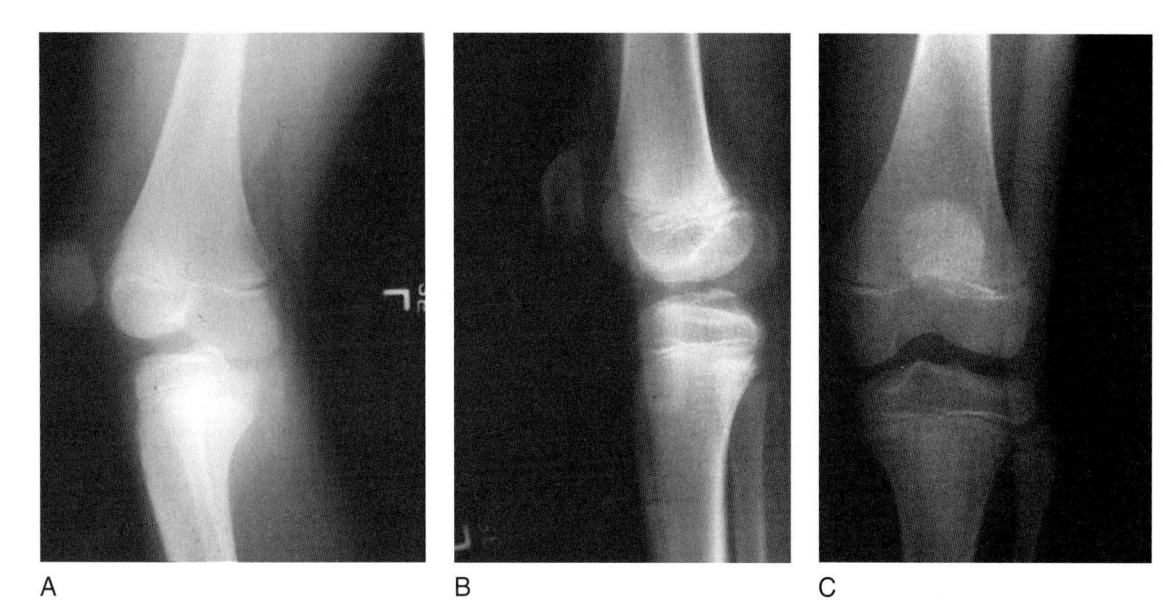

A thorough working knowledge of knee anatomy is crucial because virtually any structure about the knee can be injured, be it ligamentous, meniscal, neurovascular, and/or musculotendinous. As has been discussed elsewhere, surgical dissection for an open reconstruction is frequently simplified in the dislocated knee as soft tissue and anatomic planes are created by the injury.[12,17] The ligamentous variations of the posterolateral and medial corners, as well as the varying associated injuries, make surgical treatment of each dislocated knee challenging and unique. With the great advances in arthroscopic ACL surgery, an open approach to the knee is rarely required. PCL surgery and dislocations are also relatively rare in the routine sports orthopaedic practice, so open collateral/corner surgery can be challenging to the uninitiated orthopaedic surgeon.[18] Clearly the need to approach and reconstruct the posterolateral corner in a complete combined injury in a dislocated knee makes familiarity with this complex structure important for a successful reconstruction. The surgeon should be very familiar with the ligamentous structures about the knee outside the commonly seen intra-articular landmarks of the cruciates with which sports orthopaedic surgeons are familiar.

Fig. 3.2. Knee dislocations present with varying ligamentous injury patterns. (A) Radiograph of a knee in an adolescent with a cruciate intact rotatory dislocation of the tibiofemoral joint (note the anteroposterior view of the femur and lateral view of the tibia. (B) Reduction lateral and (C) anteroposterior radiographs of the knee. Postreduction MRI revealed integrity of both cruciate and collateral ligaments. (From Schenck RC, Injuries of the knee. In: Heckman JD, ed. Rockwood and Green. 5th ed. Philadelphia: Lippincott, Williams & Wilkins. By permission of the publisher.)

Mechanism of Injury

The mechanism of injury in knee dislocations is an important area of discussion and can be broken down into energy of injury and direction of forces. Knee dislocations occur in either low or high velocity settings: a sporting injury would be low velocity, and a motor vehicular injury would be high. Certainly, crossover of energy types occurs in both vehicular and sporting injuries. What is frequently worrisome is the knee dislocation occurring in football: a low energy injury is suspected, and a vascular tear due to a high energy injury is missed. Thus even though there are gray areas in distinguishing energy of injury in vehicular and sporting injuries, the concept of energy is an important one in classifying knee dislocations, especially in describing associated injuries, such as neurovascular injuries.[18–21]

With respect to force application, exaggerated hyperextension of the knee is a commonly seen mechanism of injury in knee dislocations. A varus or valgus directed force in combination with hyperextension produces the variability of collateral ligaments torn. Last, the knee positioned in flexion (most commonly 90° while seated in a motor vehicle) with a posteriorly directed force (also in combination with either a varus or valgus force) is another common injury mechanism in high velocity motor vehicle knee dislocation traumas. In my experience, the PCL avulsion with a large bony fragment most often occurs with this mechanism of injury to the knee positioned in 90° of flexion. In contrast, peel-off lesions of the PCL (stripping of the PCL with little to no bony fragments from the femoral origin), are more often seen in hyperextension.

In the classic study by Kennedy on complete knee dislocations, the anterior knee dislocation was produced by hyperextension. Specifically, Kennedy and his colleagues used 10 cadaveric knee specimens to create exaggerated hyperextension. In hyperextension, the ACL was torn first, followed by rupture of the PCL and posterior capsule at 30° hyperextension, and, last, by tearing of the popliteal artery at 50° hyperextension. Hyperextension of the knee, with or without abduction or adduction forces, produces an initial tear of the ACL. As will be seen, the clinical findings of hyperextension imply an injury involving the ACL that must occur before tearing of the PCL (see Figure 3.3). Last, with rupture of both cruciate ligaments, tibiofemoral displacement occurs unchecked and the popliteal artery is at risk for injury.

Knee dislocations have a high incidence of avulsion injury patterns for both ligamentous and tendinous structures. Two reports have documented a high incidence of cruciate ligament avulsions in knee dislocations. Sisto and Warren, and Frassica et al. in a separate series, noted similar percentages of PCL (88 and 77%, respectively) and ACL (63 and 46%, respectively) avulsions.[13,22,23] Upon combining both series, PCL avulsions were noted in approximately 80% of knee dislocations, and ACL avulsions were noted in approximately 50% of dislocated knees. Although the relative incidence of ligamentous avulsions is due in part to the energy of the injury, and clinically, depending on one's practice, one may see midsubstance tears of the PCL (i.e., patient population is sporting rather than victims of high energy trauma) rather than the preponderance of avulsions noted in the two series quoted,[13,22,23] the suspicion for an avulsion is important in both appropriate classification and treatment of any knee dislocation. Avulsions in knee dislocations should be contrasted with the high frequency of midsubstance tears seen in the isolated injuries to the ACL. As noted in the knee dislocation literature, the possibility of cruciate ligament avulsion directs and simplifies the treatment plan of the knee dislocation.[7,8,24]

The effect of strain rate on the failure properties of the ACL and ligaments in general was investigated by Noyes and colleagues studying bone–ligament–bone preparations. The primary mode of failure in this study was tibial avulsion at slow rates (0.67%/s strain) and midsubstance failure at faster rates (67%/s strain). In a similar strain rate study, Kennedy and colleagues noted that the primary mode of failure of all ACL tears was midsubstance under both slow (40%/s) and faster (140%/s) strain rates. Although these laboratory strain rates are termed slow and fast, in reality,

3. Classification of Knee Disorders

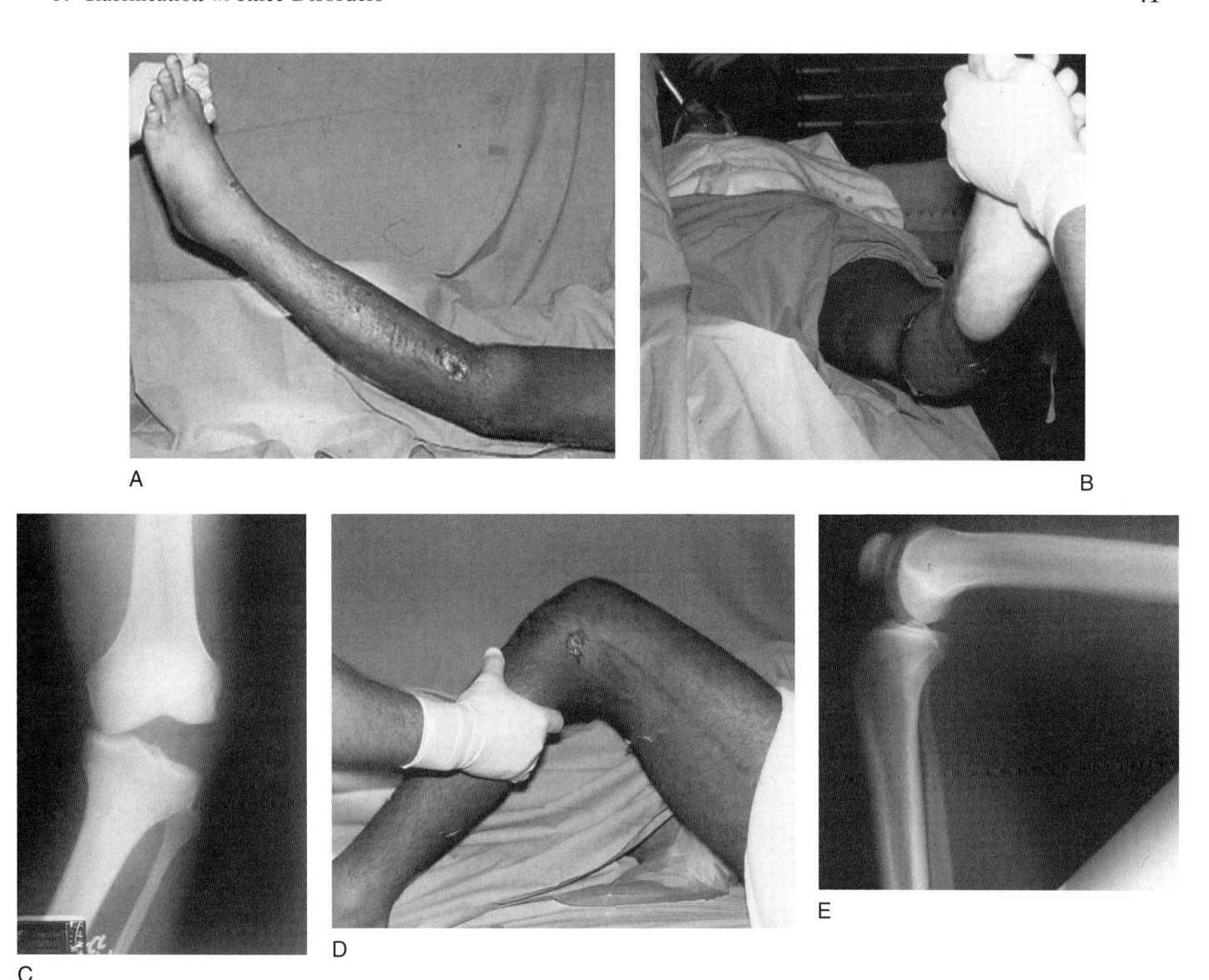

Fig. 3.3. Hyperextension recurvatum test as described by Jack Hughston. (A–C) The leg is held by the great toe, producing varus and hyperextension of the knee. (D) Posterior drawer testing reveals a normal positioned tibia relative to the femur. (E) Posterior drawer stress radiograph verifies a functioning PCL. (From Schenck RC, Injuries of the knee. In: Heckman JD, ed. Rockwood and Green. 5th ed. Philadelphia: Lippincott, Williams & Wilkins. By permission of the publisher.)

when viewed from a clinical perspective, they are both slow. In an attempt to create clinically applicable strain rates in a cadaveric cruciate ligament injury model in knee hyperextension, Schenck and colleagues noted a variation in injury pattern of the PCL when evaluated with change of strain rate or velocity that is more clinically realistic. Ten cadaveric knees were tested in hyperextension with MTS loading creating a strain rate of 100%/s in straight knee hyperextension. These were compared to a higher strain rate in knee hyperextension created by dropping 22.67 kg from a height of 4 ft (Figure 3.4). The higher strain rate calculated for the PCL at approximately 5400%/s produced a stripping lesion of the femoral attachment of the PCL that correlated well with the peel-off lesion of the PCL seen clinically in hyperextension knee dislocation following motor vehicular trauma. In that cadaveric study, the "stripping" or "peel-off" lesions occurred in an avulsion pattern with minimal bony fragments present tearing through Sharpey's fibers. With the low velocity model (100%/s strain), the PCL tore in a more consistent midsubstance pattern. The ACL was variable in its pattern of injury but tore in midsubstance in both high and low velocity injury rates, appearing to be less affected by strain rate.

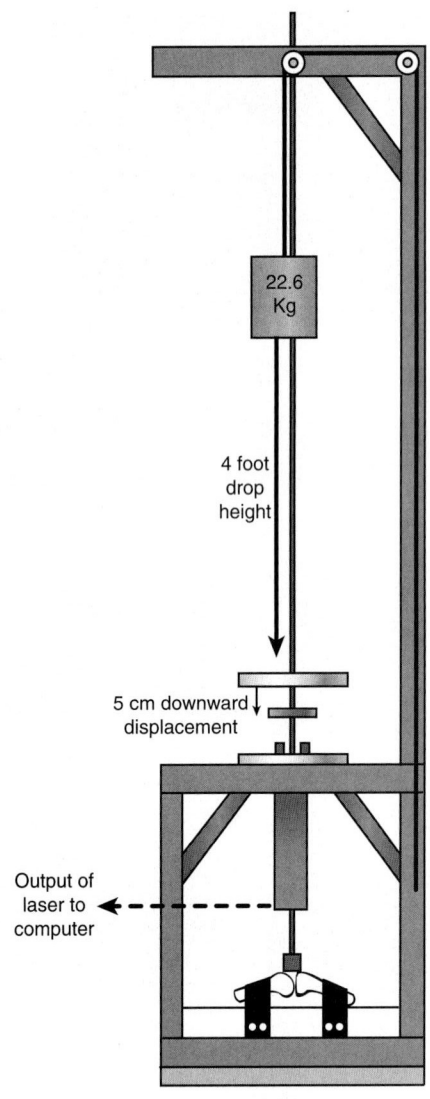

Fig. 3.4. Drop tower mechanism designed to produce high energy/fast strain rate knee hyperextension injury.

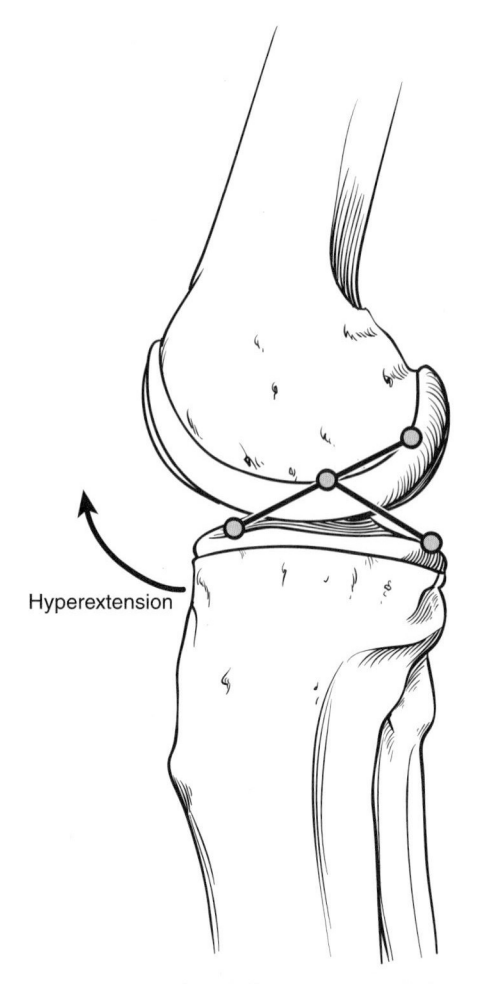

Fig. 3.5. Four-bar linkage system of the cruciate ligaments. Hyperextension produces distraction forces in parallel, with the PCL fibers making the PCL more strain rate sensitive than the ACL in this mechanism.

The authors theorized that the cruciate injury patterns are created by the action of the femoral notch. The ACL classically is torn by impaction of the notch transverse to the ligamentous fibers, whereas in the cadaveric study the PCL was torn with forces in parallel to the ligament, theoretically making the PCL more strain rate sensitive than the ACL in the injury model of hyperextension (Figure 3.5).[25] In summary, the mechanism through which multiple ligaments are injured in a knee dislocation is varied but commonly involves hyperextension.

Classification

Several authors have questioned the long-held opinion that both cruciate ligaments must be torn for a knee dislocation to occur. As early as 1971, Meyers et al. referred to the knee dislocation with an intact posterior cruciate ligament (PCL). Shelbourne et al. and Cooper et al. have recently reported on patients with a radiographically defined knee dislocation that, upon reduction

3. Classification of Knee Disorders

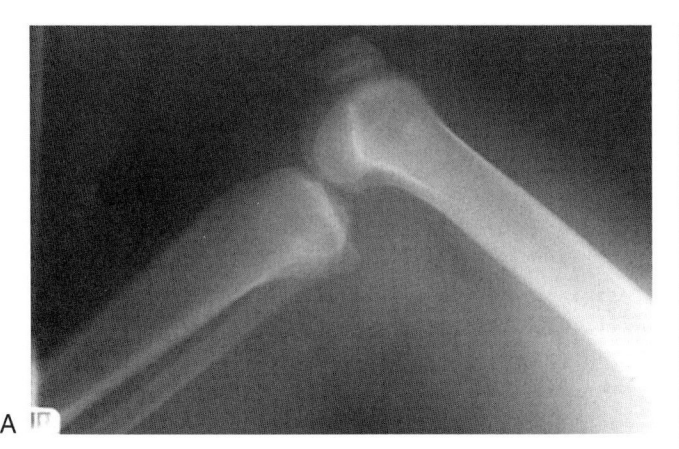

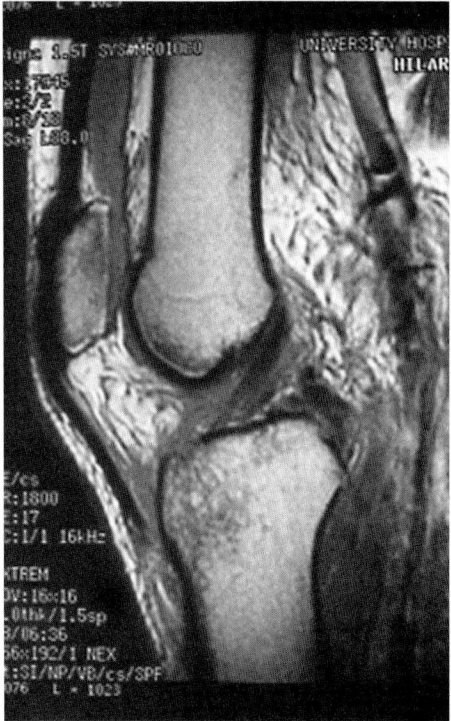

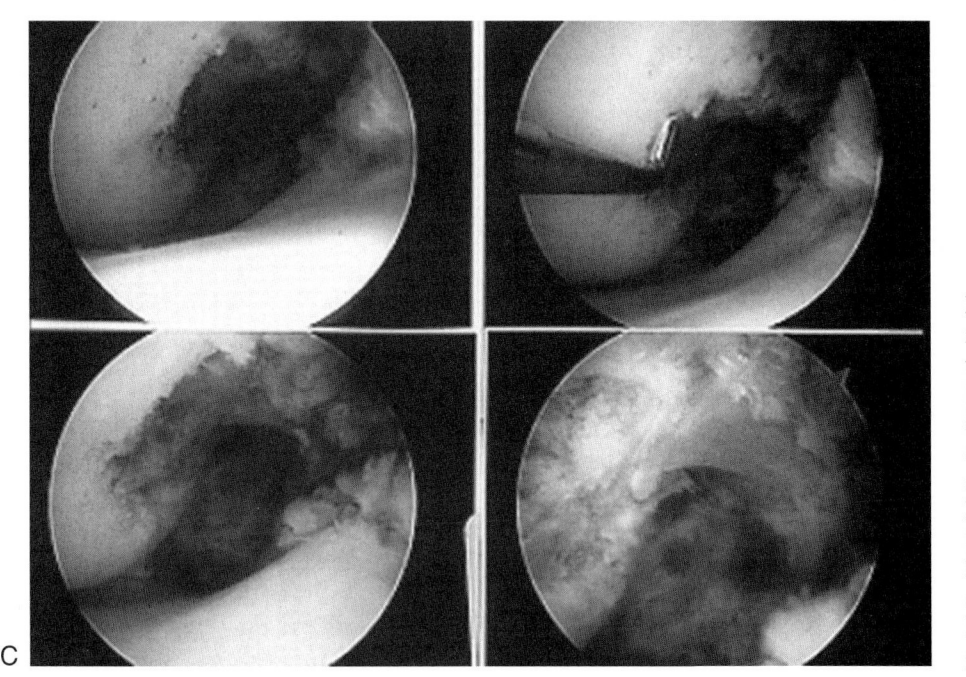

Fig. 3.6. (A) Anterior cruciate ligament (ACL) intact knee dislocation with a posterior tibiofemoral position. (B) Magnetic resonance image revealing an intact ACL and the tibial stump of the PCL. (C) Arthroscopic preparation of the femoral side of the PCL reconstruction. (See color insert.) (From Schenck RC, Injuries of the knee. In: Heckman JD, ed. Rockwood and Green. 5th ed. Philadelphia: Lippincott, Williams & Wilkins. By permission of the publisher.)

or operative exploration, demonstrated a functioning PCL.[4–8,26] Although some of these patients were noted to have suffered partial PCL tears, the presence of a functioning PCL changes the ligamentous makeup of the dislocated knee and its eventual treatment. A PCL-intact knee dislocation is usually an anterior knee dislocation with common involvement of the medial or lateral collateral ligament (MCL or LCL). In a similar type of cruciate intact knee dislocation, ACL intact knee dislocations occur with the tibia posteriorly positioned on the femur with complete tearing of the PCL. Although relatively rare, it is a well-accepted clinical phenomenon that the knee can dislocate with an intact ACL or PCL (Figure 3.6; see color plate for part C).

Although there is complete displacement of the tibia on the femur, a PCL-intact knee dislocation differs greatly from a classic knee dislocation in which both cruciates are torn. The presence of a functioning PCL changes surgical management to the more simple treatment of a single cruciate ligament injury. Although the surgeon must decide between immediate and delayed cruciate ligament reconstruction, the entire treatment plan for a PCL-intact knee dislocation is different from and much simpler than that for a complete bicruciate injury. Furthermore, a functioning PCL, in theory, would appear to protect the popliteal artery, since tibiofemoral distraction is limited. The PCL-intact knee dislocation should be considered to be a distinct entity from one that has experienced complete tears of both cruciate ligaments. Thus, description of a knee injury as a dislocation does not clearly define the injury or the treatment. Classification of such an injury must include specifically what is torn.

Fracture-Dislocation

Fracture-dislocation of the knee as described by Moore in 1981 involves a ligamentous injury to the knee in association with a fracture of the tibial or femoral condyles. This entity is distinguished from the purely ligamentous definition of a knee dislocation as discussed in this chapter. Schenck and colleagues described an additional fracture-dislocation of the knee involving the femoral condyle (Hoffa fragment) and an associated knee ligament injury.[27] This subset of injuries was termed "femoral-sided" fracture-dislocation and should be considered in the description of a knee fracture-dislocation. Avulsion injuries are frequently seen in purely ligamentous knee dislocations (Segond's fractures, fibular head avulsion fractures, cruciate avulsions) but should be considered to be ligamentous injuries and not condylar injuries such as joint destabilization fractures seen in a fracture-dislocation of the knee. Although understanding of this concept of fracture-dislocation is useful in treating the spectrum of injuries involving the knee, it should be distinguished from what is being discussed in this book. Fracture-dislocations can occur with fractures of either the tibial or femoral condyles; treatment usually involves fixation of the fracture and repair of the ligamentous injury (Figure 3.7; see color plate for part C).

Position Classification

In 1963 Kennedy classified knee dislocations in terms of tibial position with respect to the femur; that is, an anterior knee dislocation implies that the tibia is dislocated straight anterior to the femur. He noted five main types of dislocation: anterior, posterior, lateral, medial, and rotatory. Rotatory dislocations are classified into four groups: anteromedial, anterolateral, posteromedial, and posterolateral, with posterolateral being the most frequently described type of rotatory knee dislocation. This classification system has been widely utilized in the literature.[19]

Although the least common of knee dislocation types, the posterolateral dislocation is well described and still has applicability today. The hallmark of this condition is its irreducibility: it is a true complex joint dislocation in which the medial femoral condyle buttonholes through the medial capsule and the medial collateral ligament invaginates into the knee joint, preventing closed reduction. A transverse furrow seen on the medial aspect of the knee is the distinguishing feature of this knee dislocation type and the reason

3. Classification of Knee Disorders

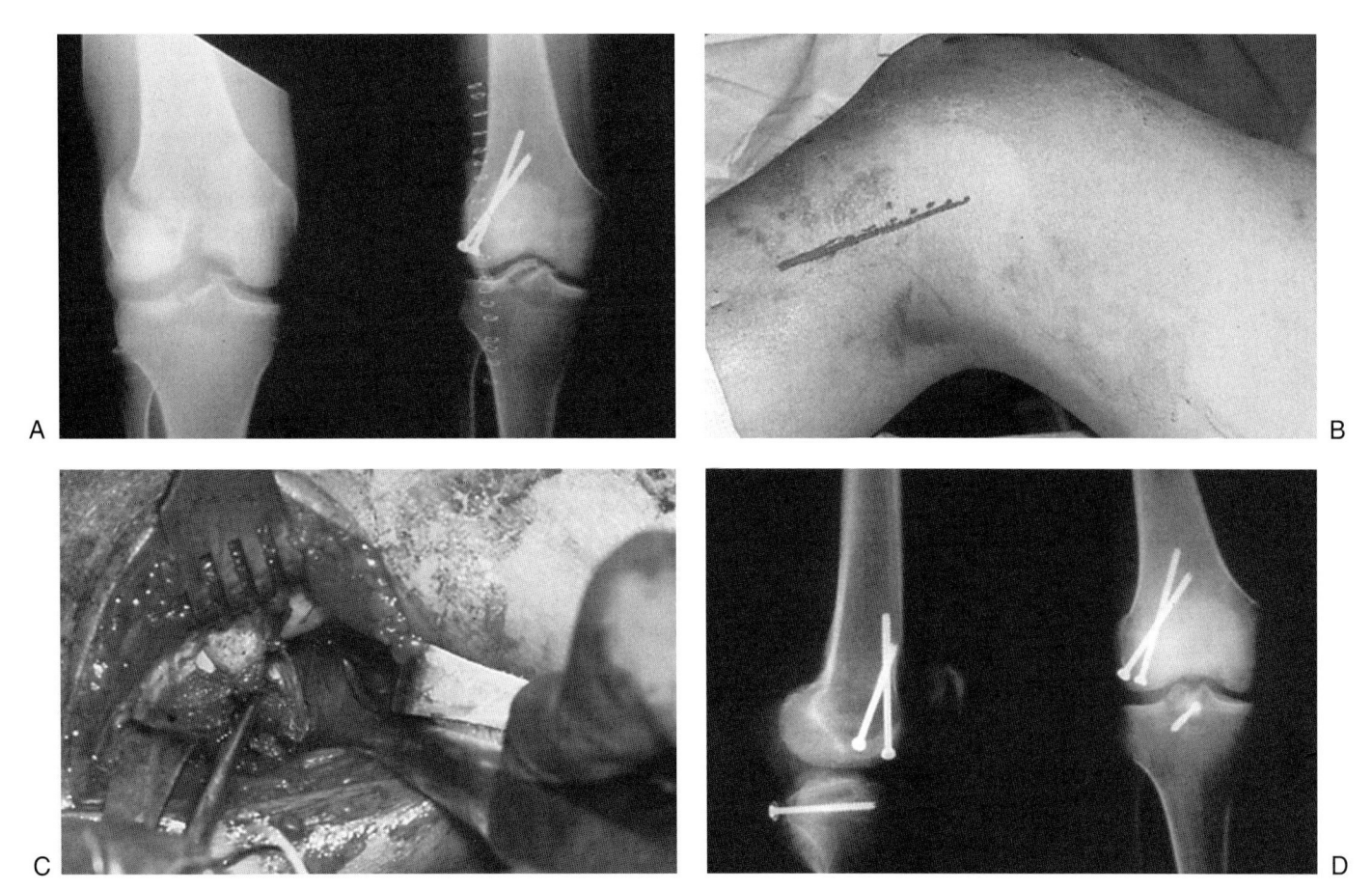

for its irreducibility. The mechanism of injury as described by Quinlan and Sharrard is that of an abduction force to the flexed knee coupled with internal rotation of the tibia.[28] Peroneal nerve palsy, resulting from a traction injury to the nerve over the lateral femoral condyle, is frequently associated with this type of dislocation. Skin necrosis secondary to pressure from the medially displaced femur has been reported.

The position classification system of knee dislocations is well established and very useful in alerting the physician to the reduction maneuver needed and to potential associated injuries such as are found in the scenario of the posterolateral dislocation. Nonetheless, the position classification system has limitations. In various series of knee dislocations, 20 to 50% of the knee injuries were reduced at the time of medical evaluation and thus are considered to be spontaneously reduced, hence unclassifiable by the position system. Second, position classification only suggests possible ligamentous involvement. With the possibility of a PCL-intact knee dislocation, tearing of both cruciate ligaments is not guaranteed in a knee dislocation. As seen earlier in Figure 3.1, the anterior knee dislocation creates two different ligamentous injuries requiring completely different treatment plans. In addition to lack of knowledge of cruciate involvement, the exact status of the collateral ligaments is not defined with a position classification system. The knee ligamentous anatomy is complex, with many combinations of cruciate and collateral disruptions possible when knee dislocation occurs. Thus, it is useful to classify knee dislocations in terms of ligaments involved, and this is best performed at the time of injury (if tolerated) with a careful examination as well as during examination under anesthesia.[29,30]

Fig. 3.7. Sequential images of a femoral-sided fracture dislocation of the knee with a lateral femoral condyle fracture and a tibial avulsion of the PCL. (A) Anteroposterior radiographic images of the knee with initial open reduction and internal fixation of the lateral femoral condyle. (B,C) Open approach to the PCL: avulsion with open reduction and internal fixation using a 4.0 mm cannulated anterior oblique screw through a posteromedial approach. (D) Final lateral and anteroposterior knee radiographs postfixation. (See color plate.) (From Schenck RC, Injuries of the knee. In: Heckman JD, ed. Rockwood and Green. 5th ed. Philadelphia: Lippincott, Williams & Wilkins. By permission of the publisher.)

Anatomic System

This classification system is termed the anatomic system and is based upon ligament function (that is, what is torn) and is very useful in deciding upon treatment and operative incision. One should be able to identify one of at least five possible injury patterns based upon an anatomic classification (Table 3.1). The higher the number, the greater the injury to the knee, and in most scenarios, the greater the velocity of injury. Additional labels of "C" and "N" are utilized for associated injuries: "C" indicates an arterial injury such as used with classification of open tibial fractures, and "N" indicates a neural injury, be it the tibial or, more commonly, the peroneal nerve. Thus a KDIIILCN implies a complete bicruciate injury: the LCL and the posterolateral corner are torn, with an injury of the popliteal artery and most commonly the peroneal nerve. Further subsets will identify injuries to the menisci, injuries to tendons (i.e., patellar tendon rupture or ITB avulsion). In a series of 13 dislocations by Walker and colleagues and further follow-up of 28 dislocations by Eastlack and colleagues, investigators used the anatomic system to classify injuries and direct treatment.[2,3] In those series, KDIIIL injuries fared worse than KDIIIM dislocations, with greater incidence of postoperative arthrofibrosis, longer disability, greater laxity on KT-1000 testing, poorer scores on outcome measures using the sickness impact profile, and poorer scores on objective measures with the modified Lysholm and International Knee Documentation Committee (IKDC) scales. In these series, the KDIII was the most common injury type and KDIIIM (ACL, PCL, MCL torn, posterolateral corner grossly intact) the most common injury pattern in dislocated knees (Figure 3.8; see color plate for part B). KDIV (all four ligaments torn) was rarer and usually involved high energy motor vehicular trauma. The anatomic system is useful because it requires the clinician to focus on what is torn, thereby directing treatment of what is torn, especially directing repair of the corner and collateral ligament involved. It also allows accurate discussion of injuries between clinicians and allows for comparisons of like injuries in the wide spectrum of knee dislocations.

One recent study looked at the use of MRI in the evaluation of the dislocated knee.[30] Indeed, several authors have commented on the utility of the MRI in evaluation of ligaments involved in knee dislocations. In contrast, Lonner and colleagues noted inaccuracies when MRI was used to correlate with functional examination of the knee.[29] The anatomic classification is applied during examination under anesthesia (EUA), since this determines what is torn and, simplistically speaking, implies what needs to be fixed. However, I find MRI extremely useful in preoperative planning prior to performing the EUA as well as distinguishing avulsion versus substance tears. The needs for allograft availability and for ligament or muscular re-attachments are well delineated by a preoperative MRI exam.[27,30,31] It is

Table 3.1. Anatomic classification of knee dislocations

Class[a]	Injury
KDI	Cruciate intact knee dislocation
KDII	Both cruciates torn, collaterals intact
KDIII	Both cruciates torn, one collateral torn; subset KDIIIM or KDIIIL
KDIV	All four ligaments torn
KDV	Periarticular fracture-dislocation

[a] Additional abbreviations as follows: C, arterial injury; N, nerve injury.

3. Classification of Knee Disorders

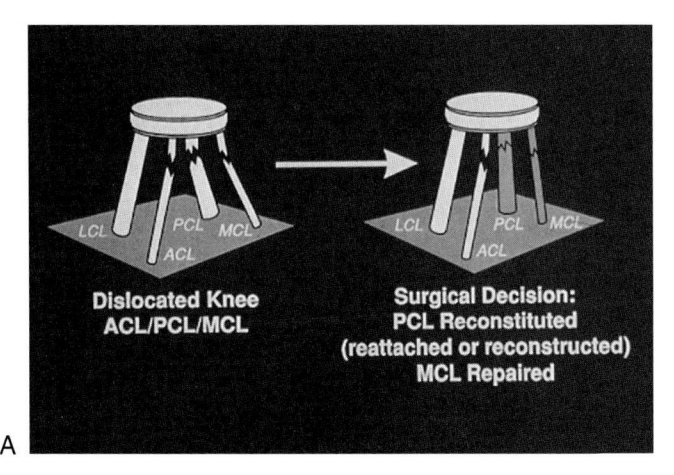

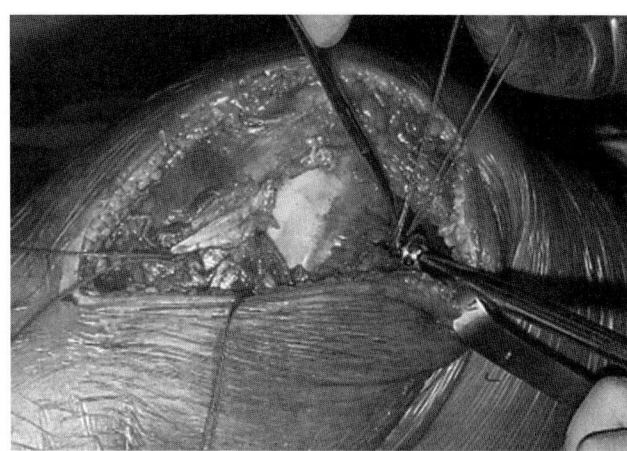

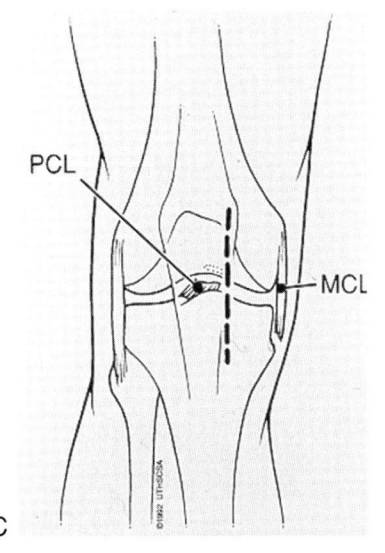

Fig. 3.8. (A) The injured ligaments in a KCDIIIM pattern of knee dislocation with avulsion of the PCL on MRI. (B,C) Medial exposure of the knee for reattachment of the posterior, anterior, and medial collateral ligaments. (See color plate.) (From Schenck RC, Injuries of the knee. In: Heckman JD, ed. Rockwood and Green. 5th ed. Philadelphia: Lippincott, Williams & Wilkins. By permission of the publisher.)

important to emphasize that a physical examination determines the anatomic classification. The entity of a KDIIIM will have a functionally intact posterolateral corner but frequently will have some MR evidence of mild injury of the posterolateral corner. EUA determines the anatomic classification and, in turn, what needs to be repaired at surgery. Nevertheless, preoperative MRI is extremely useful in the management of the dislocated knee and is recommended by this author.

Conclusions

Successful treatment of the dislocated knee requires an understanding of the knee injury on multiple levels. The multiple presentations and injury patterns that can occur with dislocation of the tibiofemoral joint dictate individualizing the injury. Classifying knee dislocation is best performed based on what structures are torn, and use of the anatomic system enhances communication and surgical planning. MRI is useful preoperatively to determine ligament injury type and position and presence of avulsions.

Acknowledgment

The author would like to thank Ms. Sandra Mosher for her assistance in the preparation of this chapter.

References

1. Wascher DC, Dvirnak PC, DeCoster TA. Knee dislocation: initial assessment and implications for treatment. J Orthop Trauma 1997; 11(7):525–529.
2. Walker DN, Hardison R, Schenck RC. A baker's dozen of knee dislocations. Am J Knee Surg 1994; 7(3):117–124.
3. Eastlack RK, Schenck RC, Jr., Guarducci C. The dislocated knee: classification, treatment, and outcome. US Army Med Department J 1997; 11(12):2–9.
4. Meyers M, Harvey JP. Traumatic dislocation of the knee joint. J Bone Joint Surg Am 1971; 53:16–29.
5. Meyers M, Moore T, Harvey JP. Follow-up notes on articles previously published in the journal. Traumatic dislocation of the knee joint. J Bone Joint Surg Am 1975; 57:430–433.
6. Cooper DE, Speer KP, Wickiewicz TL, Warren RF. Complete knee dislocation without posterior cruciate ligament disruption. A report of four cases and review of the literature. Clin Orthop 1992; 284:228–233.
7. Schenck RC. Knee dislocations. Instr Course Lect American Academy of Orthopaedic Surgeons. 1994; 43:127–136.
8. Schenck RC, Hunter R, Ostrum R, et al. Knee dislocations. Instr Course Lect 1999; 48:515–522.
9. Green NE, Allen BL. Vascular injuries associated with dislocation of the knee. J Bone Joint Surg Am 1977; 59:236–239.
10. Taylor AR, Arden GP, Rainey HA. Traumatic dislocation of the knee: a report of forty-three cases with special references to conservative treatment. J Bone Joint Surg Br 1972; 54:96–109.
11. Fanelli GC, Giannotti BF, Edson CJ. Arthroscopy assisted combined anterior and posterior cruciate ligament reconstruction. Arthroscopy 1996; 12:5–14.
12. Schenck RC. Management of PCL injuries in knee dislocations. Techniques Sports Med 1993; 1(2):143–147.
13. Sisto DJ, Warren RF. Complete knee dislocation. A follow-up study of operative treatment. Clin Orthop 1985; 198:94–101.
14. Jones RE, Smith EC, Bone GE. Vascular and orthopaedic complications of knee dislocation. Surg Gynecol Obstet 1979; 149:554–558.
15. McCutchan JDS, Gillhan NR. Injury to the popliteal artery associated with dislocation of the knee. Palpable distal pulses do not negate the requirement for arteriography. Injury 1989; 5:307–310.
16. Moore TM. Fracture-dislocation of the knee. Clin Orthop 1981; 156:128–140.
17. Schenck RC. Injuries of the knee. In: Heckman JD, ed. Rockwood and Green. 5th ed. Philadelphia: Lippincott, Williams & Wilkins; 2001:1843–1937.
18. Shelbourne KD, Porter DA, Clingman JA, et al. Low velocity knee dislocations. Orthop Rev 1991:995–1004.
19. Kennedy JC. Complete dislocation of the knee joint. J Bone Joint Surg Am 1963; 45:889–904.
20. Wascher DC, Becker JR, Dexter JG, et al. Reconstruction of the anterior and posterior cruciate ligaments after knee dislocation. Results using fresh-frozen nonirradiated allografts. Am J Sports Med 1999; 27(2):189–196.
21. Muscat JO, Rogers W, Cruz AB, et al. Arterial injuries in orthopaedics: the posteromedial approach for vascular control about the knee. J Orthop Trauma 1996; 10(7):476–480.
22. Frassica FS, Franklin HS, Staeheli JW, et al. Dislocation of the knee. Clin Orthop 1992; 263:200–205.
23. Krackow KA, Thomas SC, Jones LC. A new stitch for ligament–tendon fixation: brief note. J Bone Joint Surg Am 1986; 68:764–768.
24. Walker D, Rogers W, Schenck RC. Immediate vascular and ligamentous repair in a closed knee dislocation: a case report. J Trauma 1994; 35(6):898–900.
25. Berg EE. Positive cruciate ligament tibial inlay reconstruction. Arthroscopy 1995; 11:69–76.

26. Shelbourne KD, Pritchard J, Rettig AC, et al. Knee dislocations with intact PCL. Orthop Rev 1992; 5:607–611.
27. Schenck RC, McGanity PLJ, Heckman JD. Femoral-sided fracture-dislocations of the knee. J Orthop Trauma 1997; 11(6):416–421.
28. Quinlan A, Sharrad W. Posterolateral dislocation of the knee with capsular interposition. J Bone Joint Surg Br 1958; 40:660–663.
29. Lonner JH, Dupuy DE, Siliski JM. Comparison of magnetic resonance imaging with operative findings in acute traumatic dislocations of the adult knee. J Orthop Trauma 2000; 14(3):183–186.
30. Schenck RC, DeCoster T, Wascher D. MRI and knee dislocations. Sports Med Rep 2000; 2(12):89–96.
31. Wascher DC, DeCoster TA, Schenck RC. 10 commandments of knee dislocation. Orthop Special Ed 2001; 7(2):28–31.

Chapter Four

Nonoperative Treatment of the Acutely Dislocated Knee

Bradley F. Giannotti

A dislocation is defined as disruption of a joint so complete that the articular surfaces are no longer in contact.[1] Brautigan and Johnson assert that the term *knee dislocation* is a misnomer in the orthopaedic literature because a knee with multiply injured ligaments or the multidirectionally unstable knee has been imprecisely labeled as a knee dislocation.[1] For the purposes of this chapter, *knee dislocation* will be used to denote a radiographically confirmed knee disarticulation as well as the multiple ligament injured knee. This dual use is somewhat important, since the physical examination will confirm multiple ligament insufficiency in a knee that spontaneously reduced at the time of injury. Defining terms such as dislocation may seem purely academic, but because of this inconsistency, it has been difficult to draw conclusions from the knee dislocation literature on the success or failure of treatment options. Despite these difficulties, there has now been enough written on the topic to obtain a modern consensus on the nonoperative treatment of the acutely dislocated knee.

Historically, reports of a dislocated knee have been very rare. Shields and others evaluated the Massachusetts General Hospital experience with dislocated knees and found an incidence of 26 cases over a 27-year period.[2] The true incidence is probably higher, since many knee dislocations spontaneously reduce. Moreover, knees with multiply injured ligaments are often not immediately recognized in the polytraumatized patient.[3] Because of the relatively small incidence of acute knee dislocations, historical reports of treatment outcomes are somewhat varied, with brief case reports providing much of the early data.

Associated Injuries

A complete knee dislocation is a devastating injury with various combinations of ligamentous disruption reported. Yu et al. reported on 17 knee dislocations evaluated preoperatively by magnetic resonance imaging (MRI) and confirmed at the time of surgical intervention. All 17 patients had complete tears of the anterior cruciate ligament (ACL), 15 had complete tears of the posterior cruciate ligament (PCL), 9 patients had tears of the medial collateral ligament (MCL), 9 patients had concomitant tears of the biceps femoris tendon and fibular collateral ligament.[4] Sisto and Warren, in a follow-up study of 20 knee dislocations, reported similar findings.[5]

Nerve injuries are also common in acute knee dislocations. The majority of cases in which there is neurologic injury involve the common peroneal nerve, largely because of its superficial and relatively well fixed location.[6] Approximately 25% of all knee dislocations involve injury to the common peroneal nerve.[1,6,7] Detailed clinical examination is crucial, and documentation of neurovascular injury is of utmost importance. With or without direct surgical intervention such as repair or neurolysis, however, the prognosis for recovery of the peroneal nerve is poor.[8]

Vascular injury at the time of knee dislocation is obviously the most limb-threatening condition, requiring preferential and speedy evaluation and management. Because of its limited mobility, the popliteal artery is especially vulnerable to injury at the time of knee dislocation. The popliteal artery is tethered proximally by the adductor hiatus and distally by the soleus arch before bifurcating into the anterior and posterior tibial arteries.[7] Several injury mechanisms can occur. The artery can be stretched, directly contused by the tibial plateau, or completely disrupted. Intimal tears can occur as well. A reasonable approximation of popliteal injury with a dislocated knee is 30 to 35%.[7,9,10] A safe assumption is that a poor result can be expected when popliteal artery injury is treated nonoperatively; once such an injury is recognized, emergent operative intervention, ideally by a vascular surgeon, is needed. Therefore, this chapter discusses treatment modalities of the acutely dislocated knee only as these pertain to ligamentous disruption.

As recognition of the specific ligament injury has evolved, so too have treatment modalities. Now, more than ever, largely because of decades of trial and error, conclusions can be drawn on the effectiveness (or lack thereof) of nonoperative treatment, especially in the active population. What follows is an up-to-date historical review of acute knee dislocations treated without surgery.

Kennedy described his experience with 22 complete knee dislocations.[11] Twelve were treated without ligamentous reconstruction, 5 received "selective" ligament reconstruction, and 5 necessitated acute amputation. Despite lacking functional knee score data or rating scales, the author suggests that functional results were good in both reconstructed and nonreconstructed patients.

Nine years later, Taylor and colleagues took a firmer position toward nonoperative treatment. In that study, 26 patients were treated with cast immobilization for a period of 3 to 12 weeks followed by physical therapy. The authors asserted that 18 had good results and subsequently concluded that conservative management was the treatment of choice for uncomplicated traumatic knee dislocation.[12] Careful analysis of that study reveals that only 3 patients in the operative group actually underwent ligamentous reconstruction with operative treatment that included wound management as well.

In a small study of 10 patients, Thomsen and colleagues, reported on operative ligament repair versus conservative treatment in traumatic knee dislocations.[13] They used the same grading scale as Taylor et al., in which a good result is defined as a stable, painless knee with 90° of flexion or more; a fair result is slight stress instability, no pain, and flexion of 60 to 90°; a poor result the remainder.[12] The authors reported similar outcomes in both the operative and nonoperative groups at average 6-year follow-up.[13]

The controversy between operative and nonoperative intervention for the dislocated knee that is neurovascularly intact has waxed and waned through the mid-1980s. Many have since questioned earlier reports of success with nonoperative treatment because of the lack of objective or combined subjective/objective clinical outcomes data and performance ratings.

Using the knee diagnostic score, which gives both a subjective and objective rating, Sisto and Warren sought to refine and quantify the comparison between operative and nonoperative treatment of the dislocated knee.[5] In their study, 13 knees treated by ligamentous repair and evaluated at an average follow-up of 24 months were found to have an average knee diagnostic score of 43 out of a possible 50. Though no results were reported on 4 knees that underwent nonoperative management, and though recognizing the limitations of a relatively small study population, the authors concluded that early operative ligamentous repair is the treatment of choice in the young, active population.

Roman and colleagues evaluated 20 knee dislocations at average 2-year follow-up.[14] The authors treated the majority of patients with ligamentous repair, suggesting that nonoperative intervention was, for the most part, unsuccessful. Of the 5 treated by nonoperative means, all had 2+ or greater instability with a range of motion of 0 to 90°. Though stiffness was sometimes associated with operative intervention, the authors recommended operative repair in young, active patients.[14]

In another series by Almekinders and colleagues, 16 patients with dislocated knees were evaluated.[15] Though the authors did not not outline the specific operative intervention used, the operative group fared better than the nonoperative group with regard to range of motion, varus/valgus instability, and anteroposterior instability as measured by means of the KT 1000 arthrometer (MEDmetric, San Diego, CA). The authors went on to discuss long-term results; they found no difference radiographically between the two groups, with both groups showing similar degenerative changes. Also, the ability to return to full activities was essentially the same for both groups.[15] As discussed throughout this book, there is evidence to suggest that as specific arthroscopic reconstructive techniques become more refined and widespread, not only will objective data improve, but patients' ability to resume their preinjury lifestyle will improve as well.

More recently, Montgomery and colleagues retrospectively reviewed knee dislocations treated from 1973 to 1990.[16] Of this group, 25 were available for average 5-year follow-up. Not surprisingly, earlier study subjects were treated nonoperatively; essentially, vascular injuries were treated operatively and ligamentous disruption nonoperatively. The subjects in the study treated more recently more often than not received operative intervention, utilizing, for the most part, open techniques of ligament reconstruction. The average Lysholm knee score for the nonreconstructed group was 66 (95–100, excellent, 84–94, good; 65–83, fair; below 65, poor). Closed treatment consisted of cast immobilization or external fixation with the knee held in 10 to 20° of flexion for 6 weeks followed by vigorous physical therapy. When various modes of open ligamentous direct repair and graft reconstructive techniques were used, the operative group average Lysholm score was 80. Furthermore, range of motion, stability, and subjective ease of daily activity were better in the operative group.[16]

Knee reconstruction, specifically arthroscopic anterior and posterior cruciate ligament reconstructive techniques, has been dramatically refined, as has postreconstruction rehabilitation. One may infer from Montgomery's review that open treatment for the dislocated knee offers a potentially improved outcome over closed management. Perhaps the more specific arthroscopic techniques, though technically demanding, may offer even more improvement both objectively and subjectively.[17,18]

Most studies presented thus far have been based on small patient populations, with the results of various modes of operative and nonoperative treatment analyzed retrospectively. This combination does, perhaps, make it difficult to establish firm conclusions. In an effort to end the controversy between nonoperative and operative treatment, Dedmond and Almekinders performed a meta-analysis literature review.[19] The authors extracted raw data from several other studies so that a total of 206 knee dislocations were evaluated: 74 of these knee dislocations were treated nonoperatively and 132 were treated operatively. The average Lysholm knee score for the operative group was 85.2 and for the nonoperative group 66.5.[19] Interestingly, results were similar to those from Montgomery's earlier, smaller review.[16] The limitation of a meta-analysis, however, is that conclusions cannot be drawn regarding the type of surgical treatment; rather, there is a gross measurement of operative success. Chapters 6, 7, and 8 will provide a benchmark of specific operative techniques.

Conclusions

Perhaps the most confusing issue in the preceding literature review entails the use of the terms "good" or "excellent" to describe results. In the 1960s and 1970s, before the wide application of functional knee scores, an outcome was considered to be "good" if the patient was able to achieve 90° of flexion and had only "moderate" instability. Now that outcomes studies are more complete in compiling objective and subjective data, evolving techniques can be appropriately assessed. This author believes that the indications for nonoperative intervention in the dislocated knee are quite narrow. Perhaps nonoperative treatment is satisfactory for the elderly and/or sedentary population without vascular involvement. Ligament reconstruction should be strongly considered for the remainder of the population, with or without vascular injury.

References

1. Brautigan B, Johnson DL. The epidemiology of knee dislocations. Clin Sports Med 2000; 19:387–397.
2. Shields L, Mital M, Cave EF. Complete dislocations of the knee: experience at the Massachusetts General Hospital. J Trauma 1969; 9:192–212.
3. Kremchek TE, Welling RE, Kremchek EJ. Traumatic dislocation of the knee. Ortho Rev 1989; 18:1051–1057.
4. Yu JS, Goodwin D, Salonen D, et al. Complete dislocation of the knee: spectrum of associated soft-tissue injuries depicted by MR imaging. AJR Am J Roentgenol 1995; 164:135–139.
5. Sisto DJ, Warren RF. Complete knee dislocation: a follow-up study of operative treatment. Clin Orthop 1985; 198:94–101.
6. Good L, Johnson RJ. The dislocated knee. J Am Acad Orthop Surg 1995; 3:284–292.
7. Hegyes MS, Richardson MW, Miller MD. Knee dislocation: complications of nonoperative and operative management. Clin Sports Med 2000; 19:519–543.
8. Taft TN, Almekinders LC. The dislocated knee. In: Fu F, ed. Knee Surgery. Baltimore, MD: Williams & Wilkins; 1994:837–857.
9. Frassica FJ, Sim FH, Staeheli JW, et al. Dislocation of the knee. Orthop Clin North Am 1991; 263:200–205.
10. O'Donnell TF, Brewster DC, Darling RC, et al. Arterial injuries associated with fractures and/or dislocations of the knee. J Trauma 1977; 17:775–783.
11. Kennedy JC. Complete dissociation of the knee joint. J Bone Joint Surg Am 1963; 45:889–904.
12. Taylor AR, Arden GP, Rainey HA. Traumatic dislocation of the knee. J Bone Joint Surg Br 1972; 54:96–102.
13. Thomsen PB, Rud B, Jensen UH. Stability and motion after traumatic dissociation of the knee. Acta Orthop Scand 1984; 55:278–283.

14. Roman PD, Hopson CN, Zenni EJ. Traumatic dislocation of the knee: a report of 30 cases and literature review. Orthop Rev 16; 1987:917–924.
15. Almekinders LC, Logan TC. Results following treatment of traumatic dislocations of the knee joint. Clin Orthop 1991; 284:203–207.
16. Montgomery TJ, Savoie FH, White JL, et al. Orthopedic mangagement of knee dislocations: comparison of surgical reconstruction and immobilization. Am J Knee Surg 1995; 8:97–103.
17. Fanelli GC, Giannotti BF, Edson CJ. Arthroscopically assisted combined anterior and posterior cruciate ligament reconstruction. Arthroscopy 1996; 12:5–14.
18. Fanelli GC, Giannotti BF, Edson CJ. Arthroscopically assisted combined posterior cruciate ligament/posterior lateral complex reconstruction. Arthroscopy 1996; 12:521–530.
19. Dedmond BT, Almekinders LC. Operative versus nonoperative treatment of knee dislocations. Am J Knee Surg 2001; 14:33–38.

Chapter Five

Graft Selection

Kevin R. Willits and Walter R. Shelton

The treatment of knee injuries involving multiple ligaments must be carefully planned. Injury history, physical examination, and imaging are all important tools used to evaluate the injured knee. Careful assessment of each ligament for the location and extent of injury is crucial in planning the appropriate type of repair or reconstruction.

The number of ligaments injured and the extent of each injury will have a direct impact on treatment options including the number and type of grafts required. Avulsion or partial tears can be treated either with direct repair or with repair plus graft augmentation.[1] Midsubstance tears usually require reconstruction, with a graft capable of restoring the mechanical properties of the injured ligament.[2,3] Careful evaluation of preoperative imaging helps construct a preoperative plan that ensures the availability of appropriate graft materials at the time of surgery. All surgical plans for knees with multiple ligament injuries should include contingencies for finding more severe damage than preoperative assessment had indicated. Planning for harvesting a graft from the opposite extremity or having additional allograft materials available may often prove essential.

Theoretical Considerations

Knees with multiple ligament tears often require the surgeon to decide between additional surgery on an injured knee to obtain ligament grafts or the use of other options such as contralateral graft harvest or allografts. The main concern for ipsilateral graft harvest is the additional morbidity inflicted on the injured knee and its potential for compromising the final outcome.

Ipsilateral Autografts

When multiple grafts are required, one choice is to harvest two from the injured extremity.[2] This approach has the disadvantage of adding further insult to the knee, but it allows for graft harvest through the same or minimally increased incisions without violating the contralateral extremity or incurring the risks of using allografts.[4] When two grafts are required, ipsilateral graft combinations include quadriceps tendon and patellar tendon, quadriceps tendon and hamstring tendons, and patellar tendon and hamstring tendons. Harvest of all three of these grafts from the ipsilateral extremity would increase donor site morbidity significantly enough to make the use of other options advisable.

Contralateral Autografts

In recent years, graft harvest from the contralateral extremity has been advocated.[5] An excellent autograft can be obtained without further insulting the injured knee. The practice does result in morbidity to the normal knee, however, and in the immediate postoperative period may decrease the patient's mobility. Combining ipsilateral and contralateral graft harvests may be necessary when the use of an allograft has been excluded.

An important role of the contralateral graft is that of creating a universal backup plan. If this graft is included in preoperative plans, any unexpected intraoperative findings can be treated. This option requires obtaining preoperative consent for possible contralateral graft harvest, and the opposite extremity must be included in the surgical field. In this fashion, the contralateral limb can play an important role in the treatment of multiple ligament knee injuries.

Allografts

A popular way to treat multiple ligament tears is with the use of allografts.[6–13] The advantage of eliminating graft site morbidity is appealing.[14] Allografts provide a readily available source of tissue that can be prepared simultaneously before or during the surgical procedure. Efficient time management is important in multiple ligament tears, where fluid extravasation and tourniquet time are concerns. Allografts also offer versatility in treating a variety of ligament tears. The wide variety of allograft choices allows a more anatomic reproduction of the injured ligament.

Disadvantages of allografts include the slight but definite risk of disease transmission. This risk has been reported to be 1 in 1.67 million,[11,15] but it is dependent on the preparation and sterilization processes used. The risk should be thoroughly explained to the patient during preoperative planning. The incorporation of allografts proceeds more slowly than that of autografts,[7] and rehabilitation protocols may need to be modified.

Surgeons using allografts should have a thorough and complete understanding of the processing procedures used by the tissue bank supplying the grafts. Standards may vary, and one must be comfortable that the grafts to be used have been properly tested and screened.

Autografts

Patellar Tendon

The bone–patellar tendon–bone (BPTB) graft is the most commonly used graft in anterior cruciate ligament reconstructions (Figures 5.1 and 5.2; see color plates).[2] It offers the surgeon familiarity and reliability in addressing multiple ligament injuries. The BPTB graft can also be utilized to reconstruct the posterior cruciate ligament as well as the lateral collateral ligament (LCL) if necessary. Combinations of the BPTB graft with quadriceps tendon (QT) or hamstring tendon (HT) grafts are appropriate when multiple grafts are necessary.

Quadriceps Tendon

The QT graft has been used to reconstruct the ACL and the PCL.[13,16,17] It has the advantages of providing superior length, bulk, and strength in com-

5. Graft Selection

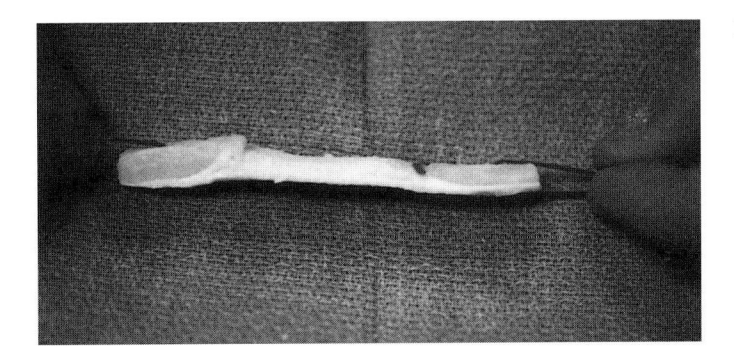

Fig. 5.1. BPTB graft. (See color plate.)

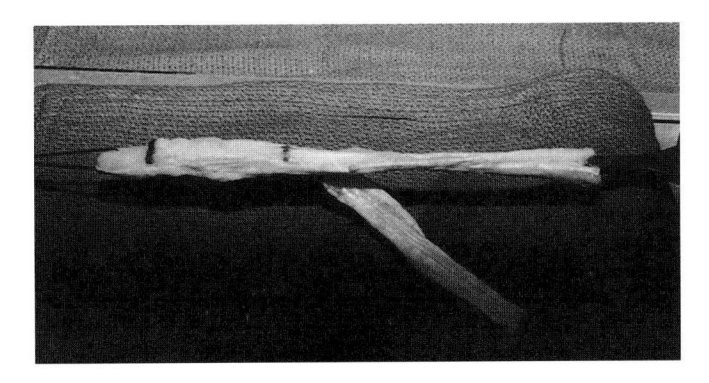

Fig. 5.2. Quadriceps tendon graft. (See color plate.)

parison to BPTB grafts.[13] The QT graft can be divided into vastus intermedius and rectus femoris bundles allowing for a two-bundle reconstruction (Figures 5.1 and 5.2). In addition to reconstructing the ACL and PCL, the QT can be used to reconstruct or augment the LCL of the posterolateral corner. This versatility makes the QT a good option to combine with hamstring tendon autografts or allografts when one is reconstructing multiple ligaments.

Hamstring Tendons

The hamstring tendons (semitendinosus and gracilis) are also commonly used for ACL and PCL reconstructions.[18-21] They offer the surgeon a familiar graft source and significant flexibility in treating partial ligament injuries and avulsion or "peel-off" injuries to the ACL or PCL (Figure 5.3; see color plate). Augmentation of the repair with a single- or double-strand hamstring graft provides stability early in healing and limits stretching out of the repaired ligament.[1] In ACL reconstruction, a three- or four-strand graft is required to achieve necessary strength and bulk.

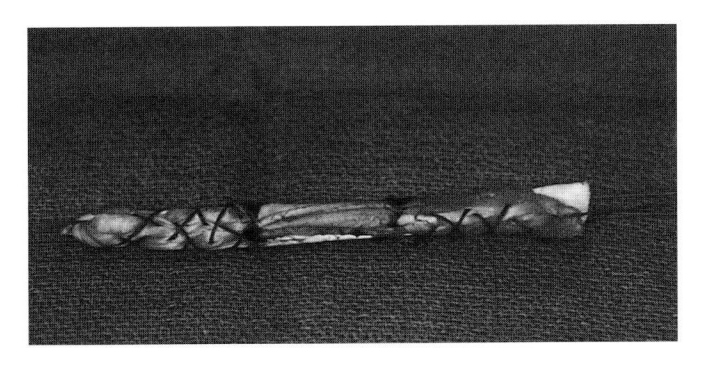

Fig. 5.3. Hamstring graft. (See color plate.)

The hamstring tendons also provide an excellent source of graft material for injuries to the LCL or PLC. Ligament repairs on the lateral side of the knee can be augmented with a single hamstring graft to enhance stability. PCL reconstructions require four-strand grafts for adequate bulk and strength.

The hamstring graft can be used in combination with either QT or BPTB grafts without incurring undue donor site morbidity.

Fascia Lata

The fascia lata (FL) graft has been used for the reconstruction of a variety of ligament injuries.[9,21] Although not commonly used at present for ACL or PCL reconstructions, it is recognized as a viable option for injuries to the LCL or PLC. It has the advantage of minimal graft site morbidity as well as utility in combination with many other graft options. The FL graft can be combined with ipsilateral QT, HT, or BPTB grafts.

Allografts

Achilles Tendon

Achilles tendon allografts (ATA) have been used extensively in the reconstruction of knee ligament injuries.[2,6,7,12] They are commonly used for reconstructing the PCL but have increasingly been used in multiple ligament knee injuries (Figure 5.4; see color plate). This graft source has the advantage of supplying abundant graft material capable of allowing two-bundle reconstructions. The ATA can be chosen for ACL, PCL, LCL, and PLC injuries. A single AT graft may provide enough graft tissue for reconstruction of the ACL or PCL in addition to the PLC or LCL, if necessary.

The ATA graft can be used in combination with all the autograft options, as well as other allograft options. Although graft incorporation is a consideration in all allograft applications, this factor can be offset by the substantial graft volume and mechanical strength afforded by the AT graft.

Quadriceps Tendon

The quadriceps tendon allograft (QTA) has gained popularity for both isolated and combined ligament injuries.[13] Its bulk, strength, and length have encouraged its use in reconstructing the ACL, PCL, and PLC. Often a quadriceps tendon allograft can provide enough tissue to fashion two complete grafts. It can be used with all other autograft and allograft options to reconstruct multiple ligaments.

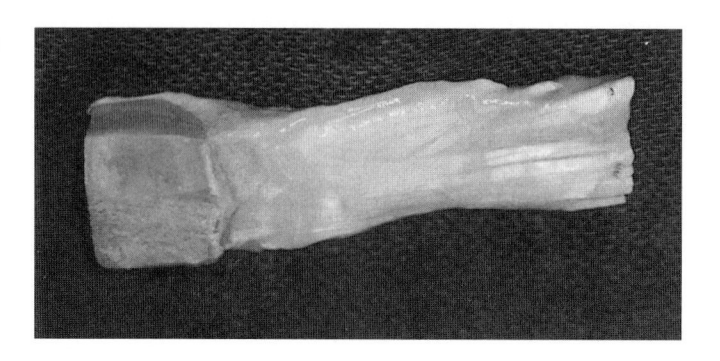

Fig. 5.4. Allograft (Achilles tendon, QT, etc.). (See color plate.)

Hamstring Tendon

Hamstring tendon allografts (HTA) are gaining popularity, particularly in the multiple ligament injured knee. The HTA has the advantage of familiarity for surgeons who use this graft for ACL or PCL reconstructions. Its use as an allograft avoids the donor site morbidity associated with hamstring harvest. HTA can be used to reconstruct the ACL, PCL, LCL, PLC, and MCL. It can be used in combination with all other allograft and autograft choices.

Fascia Lata

The fascia lata allograft (FLA) has been used for a variety of reconstructive procedures.[9] Once again, it has the advantage of good mechanical properties and versatility in application. Although the FLA could potentially serve in the reconstruction of most knee ligaments, it most commonly has been used to reconstruct the LCL or PLC and to augment these structures following repair.

Conclusions

Effective and successful treatment of multiple knee ligament tears requires careful preoperative planning, meticulous attention to the surgical detail, and proper rehabilitation. Identifying the extent and specific characteristics of each torn ligament allows the acquisition of grafts that will adequately address these injuries.

Each graft choice has specific advantages and disadvantages. Applying this knowledge when choosing which graft to use in reconstructing multiple ligament tears is the first important step toward a successful outcome.

References

1. Sgaglione NA, Warren RF, Wickiewicz TL, Gold DA, Panariello RA. Primary repair with semitendinosus tendon augmentation of acute anterior cruciate ligament injuries. Am J Sports Med 1990; 18:64–73.
2. Fu FH, Bennett CH, Lattermann C, Ma CB. Current trends in anterior cruciate ligament reconstruction. 1: Biology and biomechanics of reconstruction. Am J Sports Med 1999; 27:821–830.
3. Noyes FR, Butler DL, Grood ES, Zernicke RF, Hefzy MS. Biomechanical analysis of human ligament grafts used in knee ligament repairs and reconstructions. J Bone Joint Surg Am 1984; 66(3):344–352.
4. Kartus J, Stener S, Lindahl S, Eriksson BL, Karlsson J. Ipsi- or contralateral patellar tendon graft in anterior cruciate ligament revision surgery. A comparison of two methods. Am J Sports Med 1998; 26(4):499–504.
5. Shelbourne KD, Klootwyk TE, Wilckens JH, et al. Ligament stability two to six years after anterior cruciate ligament reconstruction with autogenous patellar tendon graft and participation in accelerated rehabilitation program. Am J Sports Med 1995; 23:575–579.
6. Harner CD, Olson E, Irrgang JJ, Silverstein S, Fu FH, Silbey M. Allograft versus autograft anterior cruciate ligament reconstruction: 3 to 5 year outcome. Clin Orthop 1996; 324:134–144.
7. Jackson DW, Grood ES, Goldstein JD, et al. A comparison of patellar tendon autograft and allograft used for anterior cruciate ligament reconstruction in the goat model. Am J Sports Med 1993; 21:176–185.
8. Nin JR, Leyes M, Schweitzer D. Anterior cruciate ligament reconstruction with fresh-frozen patellar tendon allografts: sixty cases with 2 years' minimum follow-up. Knee Surg Sports Traumatol Arthrosc 1996; 4(3):137–142.

9. Noyes FR, Barber SD, Mangine RE. Bone–patellar-ligament–bone and fascia lata allografts for reconstruction of the anterior cruciate ligament. J Bone Joint Surg Am 1990; 72:1125–1136.
10. Noyes FR, Barber-Westin SD. Reconstruction of the anterior cruciate ligament with human allograft. Comparison of early and later results. J Bone Joint Surg Am 1996; 78(4):524–537.
11. Roberts TS, Drez D, McCarthy W, Paine R. Anterior cruciate ligament reconstruction using freeze-dried, ethylene oxide sterilized, bone–patellar-tendon–bone allografts. Two year results in thirty-six patients. Am J Sports Med 1991; 19:35–41.
12. Shapiro MS, Freedman MJ. Allograft reconstruction of the anterior and posterior cruciate ligaments after traumatic knee dislocation. Am J Sports Med 1995; 23(5):580–587.
13. Shelton WR, Papendick L, Dukes AD. Autograft versus allograft anterior cruciate ligament reconstruction. Arthroscopy 1997; 13(4):446–449.
14. Kartus J, Magnusson L, Stener S, Brandsson S, Eriksson BI, Karlsson J. Complications following arthroscopic anterior cruciate ligament reconstruction. A 2–5 year follow-up of 604 patients with special emphasis on anterior knee pain. Knee Surg Sports Traumatol Arthrosc 1999; 7(1):2–8.
15. Buck BE, Malinin TI, Brown MD. Bone transplantation and human immunodeficiency virus: an estimated risk of acquired immunodeficiency syndrome (AIDS). Clin Orthop 1989; 240:129–136.
16. Chen CH, Chen WJ, Shih CH. Arthroscopic anterior cruciate ligament reconstruction with quadriceps tendon–patellar bone autograft. J Trauma 1999; 46(4):678–682.
17. Howe JG, Johnson RJ, Kaplan MJ, et al. Anterior cruciate ligament reconstruction using quadriceps patellar tendon graft. I: Long-term follow-up. Am J Sports Med 1991; 19:447–457.
18. Aglietti P, Buzzi R, Zaccherotti G, et al. Patellar tendon versus doubled semitendinosus and gracilis tendons for anterior cruciate ligament reconstruction. Am J Sports Med 1994; 22:211–218.
19. Lipscomb AB, Johnston RK, Snyder RB, Warburton MJ, Gilbert PP. Evaluation of hamstring strength following use of semitendinosus and gracilis tendons to reconstuct the anterior cruciate ligament. Am J Sports Med 1982; 10:340–342.
20. Maeda A, Shino K, Horibe S, et al. Anterior cruciate ligament reconstruction with multistranded autogenous semitendinosus tendon. Am J Sports Med 1996; 24:504–509.
21. Zarins B, Rowe CR. Combined anterior cruciate ligament reconstruction using semitendinosus tendon and iliotibial tract. J Bone Joint Surg Am 1986; 68:160–177.

Chapter Six

Surgical Treatment of Acute and Chronic ACL/PCL/Medial Side Injuries of the Knee

Craig H. Bennett, Kevin E. Coates, Corey Wallach, and Ronald A. Hall

This chapter discusses management of the acute and chronic knee injury that can occur with any type of knee dislocation. The focus is on anterior cruciate ligament (ACL), posterior cruciate ligament (PCL), and medial side knee injuries following dislocation.

Classification

Current classification schemes for the dislocated knee include an assessment of (1) the direction of the displaced tibia relative to the femur, (2) the severity of the initial injury, as either high or low energy trauma, (3) whether the dislocation spontaneously reduces or requires reduction, (4) whether it is a closed or open injury, and (5) whether there is an associated neurovascular injury. Although knee dislocations may occur via a low energy mechanism, they usually follow high velocity trauma, such as motor vehicle accidents, contact sport injuries, and significant falls. In regard to displacement of the tibia, knee dislocations are classified as anterior, posterior, medial, lateral, or rotational (Figure 6.1). The rotational category is further subdivided into anteromedial, posteromedial, anterolateral, and posterolateral. Generally, a knee dislocation involves the disruption of at least two major ligaments. Regardless of whether the knee requires reduction at the initial evaluation, tearing of both cruciate ligaments is considered to constitute a knee dislocation.

Regarding direction, a straight anterior dislocation is the most common type, occurring in approximately 40% of knee dislocations. This is followed by posterior dislocations in 35%, lateral dislocations in 15%, and medial and rotational dislocations in approximately 5% each.[1] The mechanism of injury in an anterior dislocation is thought to be hyperextension, and the PCL is frequently disrupted as well. The anterior cruciate ligament is always disrupted and frequently, but not always, associated with a PCL injury. There is usually partial injury to one or both collateral ligaments, and this damage is often clinically significant.

With posterior knee dislocations, the most common mechanism is a direct blow to the proximal anterior tibia with the knee in a flexed position. This is classically associated with a dashboard injury during a motor vehicle accident. The dislocation results in disruption of the PCL, and there is frequent disruption of the ACL. As with the anterior dislocations, there is usually some degree of collateral ligament damage.

Fig. 6.1. Radiographic example of (A) medial and (B) posterior knee dislocation.

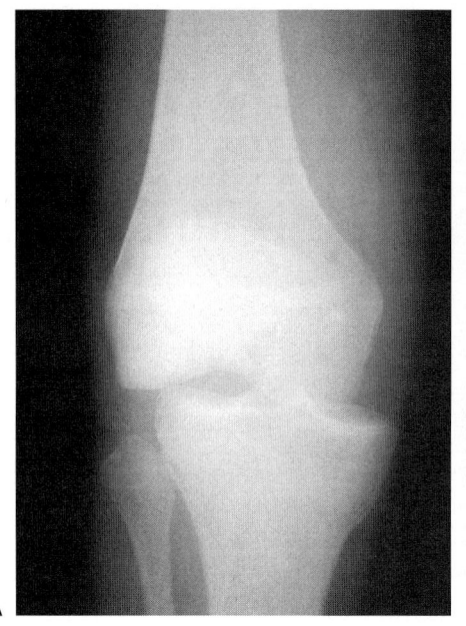

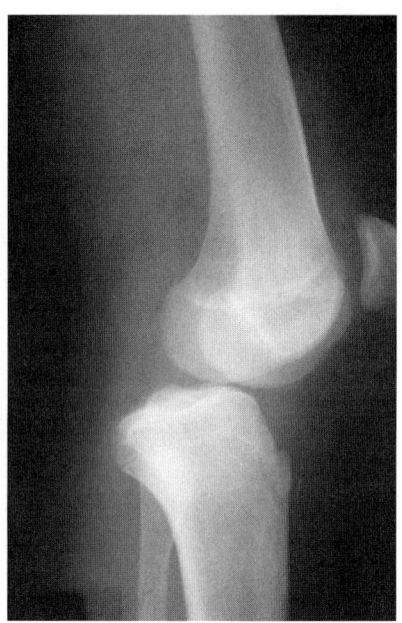

Lateral and medial dislocations of the tibia are significantly less common. Most of these injuries involve violent valgus or varus force. Many patients with these injuries also sustain distal femoral or proximal tibial fractures. In true medial and lateral dislocations, there is complete disruption of both collaterals and at least one of the cruciates.[1]

Rotatory dislocations are much less common, accounting for approximately 5% of knee dislocations.[1] These dislocations are produced by a twisting force on the knee. The most common rotatory dislocation, posterolateral, can produce significant anterior, posterior, and medial side knee damage. Quinlan and Sharrard proposed a mechanism of extreme valgus stress combined with internal tibial rotation in the flexed, non-weight-bearing limb.[2] The posterolateral dislocation is often irreducible by closed means, secondary to incarceration of the medial capsule and deep medial collateral ligament (MCL) into the joint. There may also be button-holing of the medial femoral condyle through the medial capsule, appreciated as skin dimpling along the medial joint line.

Associated Injuries

In addition to disruption of the cruciate and collateral ligaments, a knee dislocation can damage other structures within or about the knee, including the menisci, articular cartilage, muscles, tendons, bone, and proximal neurovascular structures. Fractures, including but not limited to the supracondylar femur and the tibial plateau, may also occur. Additionally, there may be disruption of the extensor mechanism, including the quadriceps and patellar tendons. Injury to the popliteal artery is the most serious potential complication associated with knee dislocations.

Vascular Injuries

It is estimated that one third of all patients with a knee dislocation have an associated vascular injury.[1] The popliteal artery courses directly posterior to the knee joint, anchored superiorly at the adductor hiatus and inferiorly by the fibrous arch of the soleus. Because of this anatomic relationship, the artery is particularly susceptible to injury when the knee is dislocated. For this reason, attention to vascular injury must take precedence when one is evaluating the dislocated knee. The direction of the dislocation and the resultant deformity are important factors in determining the likelihood and magnitude of neurovascular injury. Vascular damage is more often associated with anterior (39%) and posterior (44%) dislocations than with the lateral, medial, or rotatory type. Anterior dislocations are usually hyperextension injuries in which the vessels are stretched, which may result in extensive damage and possible thrombosis. With posterior dislocations, the tibia disrupts the popliteal artery, usually just beyond the point at which it penetrates the medial intramuscular septum at Hunter's canal.[1]

Even in cases of spontaneous reduction, occult vascular injuries may still exist, and a high index of suspicion is required. A range of injury patterns exists, and the artery may either be stretched, transected, or crushed. In the case of arterial transection, the loss of circulation may be immediate. In stretch or crush injuries, the outer layers (the adventitia and muscularis layers) of the vessel may remain intact, with only the intimal being injured (Figure 6.2). The loss of circulation may be gradual in these cases, since the progression of thrombosis slowly occludes the artery. Loss of circulation may occur hours or days following the injury. As a result, frequent vascular exams are mandatory when the knee is dislocated, especially when no arteriogram has been performed. If it is unclear whether a pulse difference exists, ankle–brachial pressure measurements can be obtained. If the ankle–brachial index (ABI) is less than 0.1, then an arteriogram is mandatory.[3] It is our preference to obtain an arteriogram in the majority of cases, particularly when operative intervention is planned or when frequent pulse checks are not possible. The arteriogram can identify an intimal tear that may not necessarily demonstrate a deficit in distal pulse during the initial evaluation.

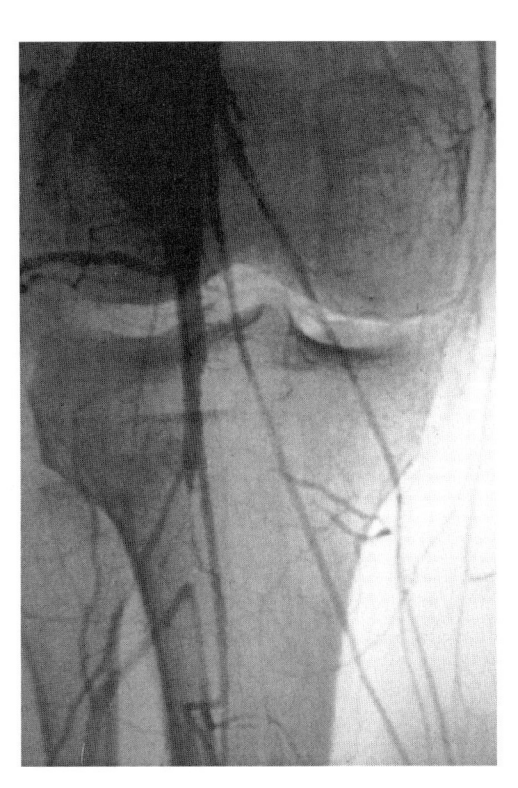

Fig. 6.2. Representative arteriogram.

When vascular flow is compromised, expedient vascular repair within 6 to 8 h of the time of injury is critical. Further delay increases the likelihood that amputation will be required. Green and Allen demonstrated that when arterial repair was completed within the 6 to 8 h window, there was an amputation rate of 11%; with repair after 8 h, the amputation rate was 86%. With ischemia time surpassing 6 h, two thirds of patients developed muscle fibrosis, contracture, and chronic vascular insufficiency.[1]

Nerve Injuries

Nerve injuries are considerably less common, occurring in 15 to 40% of knee dislocations. A reasonable mean incidence is approximately 25%.[4,5] Nerve damage is most often associated with posterolateral dislocations. The peroneal nerve, which is tightly anchored around the fibula, is much more likely to be injured than the tibial nerve, which runs freely through the popliteal space. Severity of injury can range from transient palsy to complete transection.

Fractures

Fractures can be associated with the knee dislocation as well. These include tibial plateau fractures, small avulsion fractures of the proximal tibia or distal femur, and fractures of the fibular head. The incidence of these fractures is not known; however, there is a high association of such injuries with medial and lateral dislocations.[6]

Initial Patient Workup

The initial patient workup begins with the vascular examination. This is followed by a reduction of any obvious knee dislocation (Table 6.1). The distal pulses are reassessed following any reduction, and a neurologic evaluation is performed as well. Paticular attention is paid to assessment of common peroneal nerve function. Knee radiographs are then obtained to rule out fracture and to verify the adequacy of knee reduction. Once the radiographs have been reviewed, a more detailed lower extremity exam is performed. This begins with an evaluation of straight leg raise and palpation of quadriceps and patellar tendons, followed by gentle Lachman test. Ligamentous

Table 6.1. Initial Evaluation and Treatment of the Acutely Dislocated Knee

1. Vascular examination.
2. Reduction: if obvious dislocation, reduce with axial traction.
3. Repeat vascular with addition of neurologic exam postreduction.
4. X-ray (to determine adequate reduction and rule out fracture):
   AP
   Lateral
5. Secondary physical examination:
   Extensor mechanism.
   Assess varus and valgus laxity at full extension:—if 3+ opening with varus/valgus stress, probable cruciate and collateral ligament damage.
   If moderate to mild swelling, posterior drawer (90°) and Lachman exam (at 30°).
6. Assess extremity for compartment syndrome.
7. Immobilization:
   Splinting
   Brace
   External fixation
8. Arteriogram (rule out intimal tear).
9. Completion of imaging:
   MRI
   Additional x-rays: ensure reduction; rule out fracture and patella alta.

6. Surgery for ACL/PCL/Medial Side Knee Injuries

laxity, in the varus/valgus plane, is evaluated at full extension and 30° of knee flexion. If there is 3+ opening with varus/valgus stress at full extension, there is significant cruciate and collateral ligament damage (Figure 6.3; see color plate). The magnitude of effusion is quantified, followed by determination of the active and passive knee range of motion. Additional stability evaluation is then performed, including anterior and posterior drawer testing, if the knee is comfortably ranged to 90°. Aggressive examination maneuvers, including the pivot and reverse pivot shift examinations, should be avoided in the setting of the acutely dislocated knee.

When the secondary survey, including evaluation for an open knee dislocation, is performed, the leg should be evaluated for evidence of compartment syndrome, which should be expeditiously addressed if found. The extremity should be immobilized by using a splint, brace or external fixator. After immobilization, repeat radiographs should be performed to check the adequacy and maintenance of reduction. Further studies, arteriograms, and MR images are obtained on the basis of clinical suspicion.

Magnetic Resonance Imaging

While surgeons debate the usefulness of MRI in the setting of an obvious knee dislocation, our preference is to obtain such images when there is obvious knee dislocation, as well as when the ligamentous exam suggests a spontaneously reduced dislocation. The MRI examination allows for visualization of the cruciate and collateral ligaments. Damage to the menisci can be assessed, as can damage to the bony/chondral surfaces (Figure 6.4). The MR images can help localize damage to the posterior cruciate ligament. While the magnitude of posterior laxity must be assessed by examination under anesthesia, surgical decision making can also be affected by localization of the PCL. In the sagittal plane, MRI is useful in detection of femoral side PCL avulsion injuries (Figure 6.5). The coronal view is helpful in localization of medial side damage. For example, medial capsule damage may be extensive, at times even resulting in the extrusion of the medial meniscus (Figure 6.6; see color plate for part B). Since the aforementioned findings affect surgical decision making, the authors recommend an MRI exam in addition to plain radiographs in the setting of the acute knee dislocation.

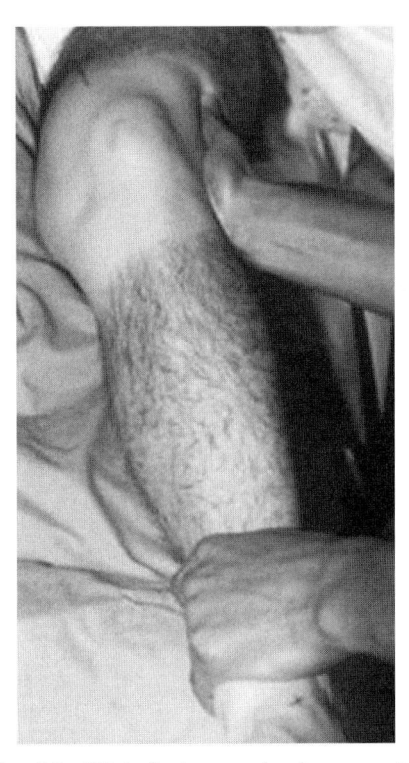

Fig. 6.3. Clinical picture of valgus opening in extension. (See color plate.)

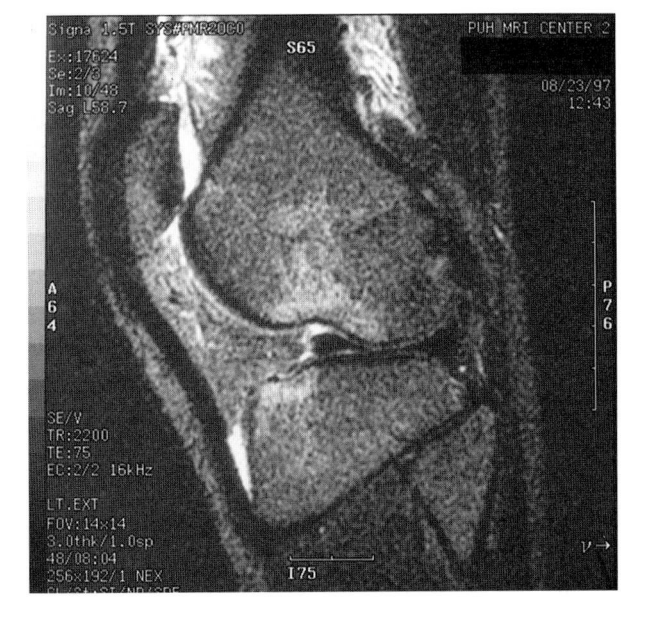

Fig. 6.4. Sagittal T2-weighted MR image demonstrating femoral and tibial bone bruising after knee dislocation.

Fig. 6.5. MR image demonstrating femoral side PCL avulsion.

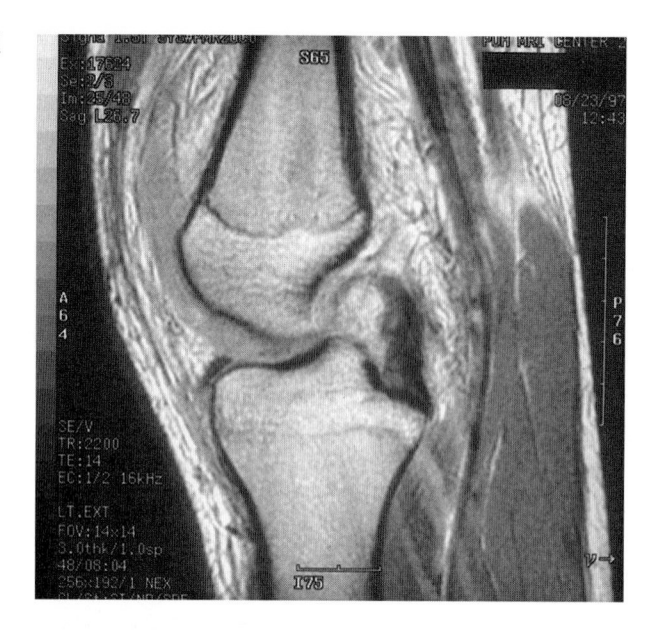

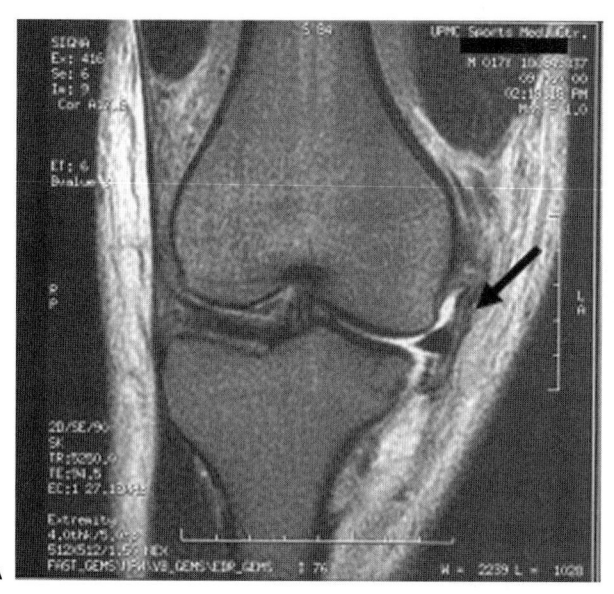

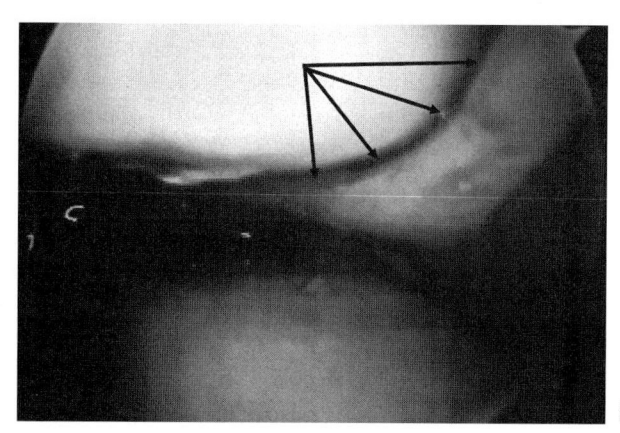

Fig. 6.6. (A) MR image of knee dislocation with associated medial meniscal extrusion (arrow) and (B) arthroscopic image of floating medial meniscus (arrows). (See color plate.)

This is helpful in surgical planning, especially in choosing between an arthroscopic or open approach.

Surgical Indications for Acute Injuries

Emergency Surgery

There are three absolute indications for emergent surgical intervention for the dislocated knee. These are injury to the popliteal artery, an open dislocation, and an irreducible dislocation.

Popliteal Artery Injury

If pulses are absent upon presentation, manual reduction should be performed immediately, and the vascular status reassessed. If after reduction the pulses continue to be absent or abnormal, immediate vascular repair, without an arteriogram, should be considered. When the pulse continues to be diminished but the limb appears to be vascularized, an emergent arteriogram is warranted. The orthopaedic surgeon usually does not have sufficient expertise to manage complex vascular injuries, and vascular surgical consultation should be sought.

The vascular surgeon usually performs the repair with an interpositional vein graft, since it is rare for such an injury to be amenable to direct suture repair. It has also been suggested that concomitant popliteal vein injuries be repaired to reduce the risk of venous thrombosis and pulmonary embolism.[1] Although the vascular surgeon performs the arterial repair, the orthopaedic surgeon should remain involved in the decision making, particularly in regard to selection of appropriate positioning of surgical incisions.

Following revascularization, the compartment pressures should be assessed, and if elevated or if clinical suspicion is high, four-compartment fasciotomies of the leg should be performed, using a two-incision technique. Cruciate ligament and extensive collateral ligament reconstruction should not be performed at the time of revascularization. If significant medial side knee injury exists, consideration can be given to distally extending the medial incision, used for vascular repair, to repair a torn or avulsed medial collateral ligament or medial capsule, and to address an extensive posteromedial capsular injury. Additional incisions to address other injured ligamentous structures should not be made at the time of revascularization. Orthopaedic repair and/or reconstruction should be delayed approximately 7 to 10 days until it is clear that the leg is well perfused and swelling of the knee and calf has decreased. The decision about whether the knee can tolerate the positioning and mobilization required to perform a cruciate reconstruction is based upon the vascular surgeon's confidence in the repair.

Open Dislocations

Open dislocations warrant immediate surgical attention. Approximately 20 to 30% of knee dislocations are open[7,8] and should be treated in accordance with the same general principles as other open injuries. Within 4 to 6h of injury, the knee should be irrigated with pulse lavage containing antibiotics, and all necrotic tissue should be debrided. Appropriate parenteral systemic antibiotics should be administered. If the soft tissue wounds are large and the knee is widely exposed, then collateral ligaments can be repaired with sutures. Reconstruction should be delayed for at least 2 months until the wounds and soft tissues have had an opportunity to heal and the potential for sepsis has diminished. Finally, any massive open wound with significant soft tissue damage should be left open for delayed primary closure or possible later flap coverage.

Irreducible Dislocations

With irreducible knee dislocations, the risks of neurovascular compromise and soft tissue necrosis mandate immediate open reduction. The most common irreducible dislocation is the posterolateral dislocation, in which the medial capsule and the medial collateral ligament are incarcerated in the joint. The medial femoral condyle may buttonhole through the medial capsule, and on physical exam there is a dimpling of the skin along the medial joint line. The medial femoral condyle may be palpable just under the skin in the subcutaneous soft tissue. Attempts at closed reduction often extenuate the defect as the medial structures are drawn deeper into the knee joint. While popliteal artery disruptions are uncommon in this setting, there is a relatively high risk of peroneal nerve injury and a significant risk of skin sloughing of the anteromedial soft tissues.

The patient should be taken to the operating room for open reduction with a medial utility incision. If the patient is otherwise a candidate for ligamentous reconstruction, acute reconstruction of the cruciate ligaments, medial meniscus, medial capsule, and medial collateral ligament should also be performed.

Surgical Indications for Combined ACL, PCL, and Medial Side Knee Injuries

Trends in managing the acute knee dislocation have changed over the past several decades from cast immobilization to operative ligament repair to ligamentous reconstruction for the cruciate ligaments, combined with repair for the collateral ligament damage. The most recent study advocating cast immobilization for treatment of the dislocated knee was published in 1972 by Taylor et al. Although these authors advocated nonoperative treatment, nearly one third of their patients had flexion of less than 90° at follow-up.[9] Other authors have noticed decreased motion or severe instability following nonoperative management.[4,10]

The largest series of patients who underwent primary operative repair of all ligaments was recorded by Meyers and Harvey.[8,11] In their series, 16 patients were available for 1-year follow-up. Those who underwent primary repair had better results than those treated nonoperatively. In another series by Sisto and Warren in 1985,[5] 13 patients underwent complete ligamentous repair followed by 6 weeks of cast immobilization. Pain and loss of motion were significant in 6 of the patients, who eventually required operative manipulation to improve flexion.

More recently, ligament reconstruction has replaced direct ligament repair as the standard treatment of isolated cruciate ligament injuries. The trend has likewise shifted toward ligament reconstruction for the management of injuries associated with knee dislocation.[12–17] Shelbourne and colleagues reported experience in the management of low velocity dislocations, recommended autograft patellar tendon reconstruction of the PCL with primary repair of the MCL and lateral structures.[12] Tears of the ACL either were not treated or were addressed later if symptomatic instability developed. In addition, the authors recommended delaying ligamentous reconstruction when the medial structures are involved (with a normal lateral side) until the patient achieves greater than 90° of flexion, near full extension, and good strength. Satisfactory results were reported in 9 patients treated in this manner, and the belief that the potential arthrofibrosis associated with concurrent ACL reconstruction or acute MCL repair may be avoided was expressed. A study by Yeh et al. also reports isolated reconstruction of the PCL after knee dislocation.[17] Twenty-two patients with knee dislocations were treated with autologous patellar tendon reconstruction of the PCL and acute debridement of the ACL. One patient received an allograft patellar tendon PCL reconstruction. Collateral ligament, capsule, and meniscal repairs were performed "as necessary." All reconstructions were performed within 25 days of the injury. The authors reported good subjective functional results with a mean Lysholm score of 84 and average flexion of 129.6°. In this series, however, 3 of the 22 patients required arthroscopic lysis of adhesions. Manipulations were not performed because of the potential for "various complications." Shapiro and Freedman reported satisfactory functional results in 6 of 7 patients evaluated an average of 4 years following a knee dislocation treated with allograft reconstruction of anterior and posterior cruciate ligaments.[13] The surgeries occurred on an average of 9.6 days after injury. The mean flexion was 118°, and 3 patients had flexion contractures of 5° or less. The average Lysholm score was 74.7. The Meyer ratings were as follows: 3 excellent, 3 good, and 1 fair. Four of the 7 patients required operative manipulation for arthrofibrosis.

Fanelli et al.[14] reported successful cruciate ligament reconstruction of 20 patients; they used either patellar tendon autografts or fresh-frozen allografts after knee dislocation. Ten patients received operations acutely, and 10 patients underwent delayed reconstruction. The authors did not note differences between the acutely and chronically treated groups. Therefore, they recommended delayed reconstruction of the ACL, PCL, and posterolateral corner injuries for at least 2 to 3 weeks and delayed reconstruction of ACL, PCL, and medial collateral ligament (MCL) injuries for 6 weeks to allow healing in a brace. Postoperative Lysholm scores in their series averaged 91.3. Wascher et al.[16] reported on 13 patients who underwent anterior and posterior cruciate ligament allograft reconstruction. Nine patients had acute ligament reconstruction and 4 had surgical repair of chronic injuries. Improved results were noted in patients with early, rather than late reconstructions. Mild residual laxity of the PCL was common. Meyer scores were excellent or good for 85% of the patients. Lysholm scores averaged 88. International Knee Documentation Center (IKDC) overall ratings were nearly normal for 6 knees, abnormal for 5 knees, and severely abnormal for 1 knee. Two patients required postoperative manipulation and lysis of adhesions for arthrofibrosis.

Authors' Recommendation

The authors' present recommendation is for early combined reconstruction of complete cruciate ligament injuries with fresh-frozen allograft tissues. Reconstruction of both cruciate ligaments allows patients to have a single operation and allays concerns for late anterior instability associated with reconstruction of the PCL alone. In addition, the ACL and PCL have vastly different functions. Combined reconstruction provides the best reproduction of normal knee kinematics without causing significantly decreased range of motion. We also advocate early primary repair of complete medial collateral ligament injuries. In our experience, this has not significantly changed the development of arthrofibrosis compared with delayed MCL repair. Appropriate physical therapy and rehabilitation seem to be more important factors for postoperative mobilization after reconstruction of the ACL and repair of the MCL than the timing of the surgery.

While the following description of the surgical technique for the combined ACL, PCL, medial side knee injury will address the use of both allograft and autograft tissue, in the authors' preferred method allograft tissues are used for the dislocated knee to avoid the additional surgical morbidity and increased surgical time associated with graft harvesting. Histologically, allografts undergo a similar process of revascularization and remodeling.[18] However, with allograft, this process has been noted to be slower than observed with most autografts.[19] Despite concerns over early graft failure, fresh frozen-allografts have been shown to have good clinical results for ACL reconstruction.[20-24] Authors favoring autograft commonly use patellar tendon for reconstruction. When using a transtibial PCL technique, we favor Achilles allograft over the patellar tendon autograft because the former provides more collagen to fill the bone tunnels.[25]

Surgical Indications and Protocol

The Anterior Cruciate Ligament

For the anterior cruciate ligament, tears are reconstructed with graft tissue. The authors' preference is allograft bone–patellar tendon–bone. However, autograft bone–patellar tendon–bone option is also reasonable. The decision depends, in part, on whether the extensor mechanism is damaged, as well as on the surgeon's overall approach to the knee, including PCL reconstruction preferences.

While autograft quadruple-stranded semitendinosus and gracilis hamstring tendons have been well described for use in the ACL-deficient knee, we do not recommend the use of autograft hamstrings in the ACL, PCL, medial side knee injury. Harvesting of the medial hamstrings sacrifices a secondary medial stabilizer for the knee. When there is extensive MCL damage or chronic medial laxity, the medial hamstring can be used to reconstruct the medial side of the knee.

While reconstruction of the anterior cruciate ligament provides a better result than direct repair, the ACL is amenable to primary repair in cases of tibial side avulsion injury. Tibial eminence fractures with displacement can be repaired by various methods. The bony fragment can be reattached with either a metal or a bioabsorbable screw. In addition, sutures can be passed through transtibial drill holes and tied over a bony bridge. The authors recommend recessing the tibial eminence fracture by a few millimeters because there is usually a component of intrasubstance stretching of the anterior cruciate ligament in cases of bony avulsion injuries. Recessing the bone may allow enhanced anterior stability upon fracture healing. With this type of injury, it is common for the anterior horn of the lateral meniscus to be trapped within the fracture site. Repair is occasionally necessary. With proper treatment, these injuries typically have a favorable outcome. The results of ACL avulsion injuries without an attached bone fragment are not as favorable. Owing to the uncertainty of bone-to-tendon healing with the ACL, a bone–tendon–bone graft reconstruction is preferred with the nonbony avulsion injuries.

The Posterior Cruciate Ligament

For treatment of the posterior cruciate ligament injury, examination under anesthesia is critical. While MRI can help determine the extent and location of the PCL tear, MRI does not help determine the magnitude of posterior laxity; hence, the examination under anesthesia is of increased utility. The most accurate clinical test is the posterior drawer with the knee flexed at 90°.[26] With a posteriorly directed force applied to the anterior tibia, the distance (usually 1 cm) between the anterior portion of the medial tibial plateau and the anterior portion of the medial femoral condyle is determined (Figure 6.7; see color plate). A grade I posterior drawer indicates a palpable, but decreased, anterior step-off of 0 to 5 mm. With a grade II posterior drawer, there is a loss of the anterior tibial step-off and the medial tibial plateau can be pushed flush with the medial femoral condyle (5–10 mm of diminished step-off). A grade III posterior drawer indicates that the anterior medial tibia can be pushed beyond the medial femoral condyle (>10 mm of increased laxity). In this latter case there will be a positive sag or Godfrey sign (Figure 6.8).

This grading system is useful in determining whether the significance of the PCL injury warrants operative reconstruction. With injuries that have a grade III posterior drawer, the recommendation is PCL reconstruction, particularly in the face of a midsubstance PCL tear. With a grade I posterior

6. Surgery for ACL/PCL/Medial Side Knee Injuries

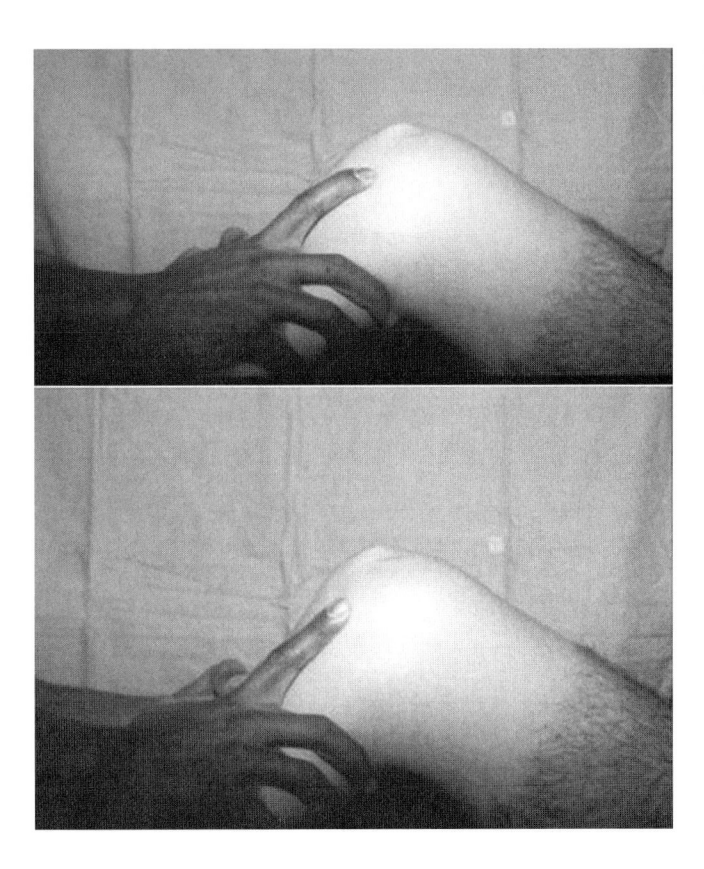

Fig. 6.7. Clinical example of posterior drawer test. (See color plate.)

drawer, the damaged PCL is not reconstructed. Management of grade II posterior laxity is a subject of debate, and surgical decision making is multifactorial.

PCL grading terminology can be somewhat confusing because some authors correlate the amount of posterior sag with the grade of PCL tear. Classically, a grade I, II, or III ligament tear refers to partial, moderate, or complete damage to the ligament, respectively. However, complete disruption of the posterior cruciate ligament does not necessarily correlate with grade III posterior laxity as described earlier. Grade III tearing of the posterior cruciate ligament, such as may occur in a knee hyperflexion injury, does not necessarily result in grade III posterior drawer. It is generally agreed that damage to other posterior structures in the knee are required to produce grade III posterior drawer. Decision making in regard to PCL reconstruc-

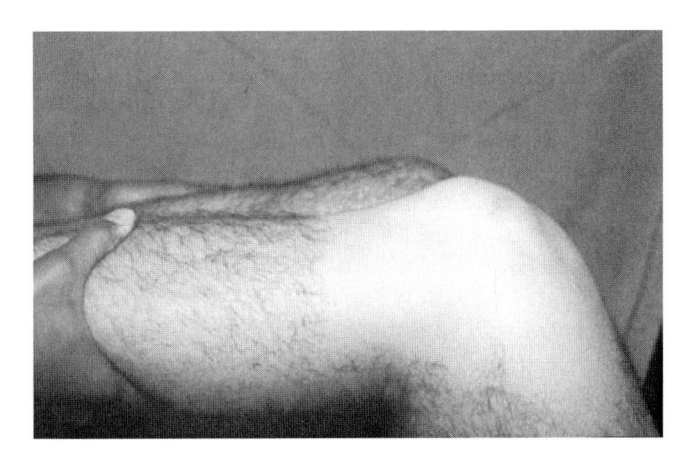

Fig. 6.8. Godfrey posterior sag sign.

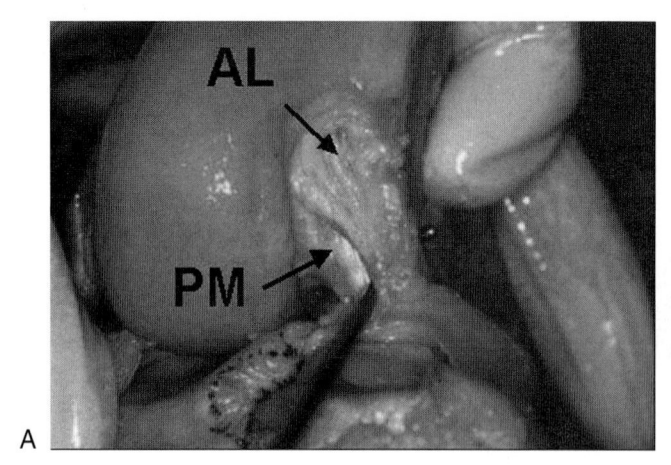

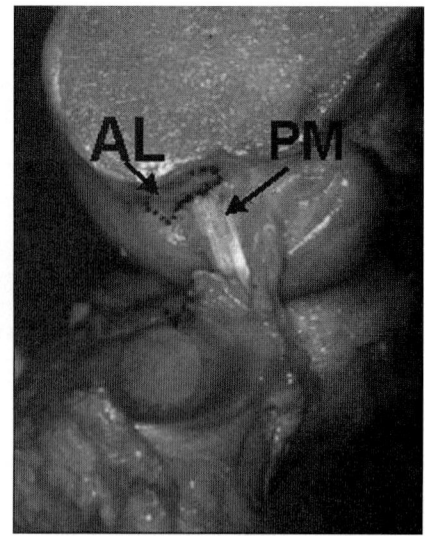

Fig. 6.9. Cadaveric dissection of anterolateral (AL) and posteromedial (PM) components of the PCL in the (A) coronal and (B) sagittal planes. (See color plate.)

tion depends not on the grade of PCL tear but on the grade of the posterior drawer. While the PCL is the primary posterior stabilizer, there are important secondary stabilizers, such as the meniscal femoral ligaments of Humphrey and Wrisberg. Cadaveric dissection has demonstrated that at least one of these ligaments is always present, with both present in 46% of knees examined.[27] In addition, the posterior horns of the menisci, the posterior capsule, and the posterolateral corner are important secondary stabilizers to the knee. The posterolateral corner can be assessed by comparing the tibial external rotation with the contralateral knee at 30° of knee flexion. It is important to reduce the tibia when one is performing this exam. Increased external tibial rotation at 30° is clinically suggestive of damage to the posterolateral corner. Increased tibial external rotation at 90°, however, is indicative of damage to the posterior cruciate ligament. It is critical to assess the posterolateral corner for damage in the setting of the multiple ligament injured knee. While this is addressed in great detail in another chapter, it remains important to rule out a posterolateral corner injury even when there is significant medial side knee damage. When the surgeon reconstructs only the cruciate ligaments in the presence of significant involvement of the posterolateral corner, the PCL graft experiences increased forces, possibly resulting in failure.[28]

There are three main components to the posterior cruciate ligament complex based on tensioning.[29] These components consist of the anterolateral bundle, the posteromedial bundle, and the meniscofemoral ligaments (Figure 6.9; see color plate). The nomenclature for description of the PCL bundles refers to the anatomic femoral insertion first, followed by the tibial side insertion. The anterolateral and posteromedial components have differing tensioning patterns, depending on the knee flexion angle. The anterolateral bundle shows increasing tension with the knee flexed, while the posteromedial bundle is more tensioned with the knee in extension.[29] Regarding size, the anterolateral bundle has twice the cross-sectional area of the posteromedial component. The anterolateral bundle has approximately 150% of the stiffness and ultimate strength of the posteromedial component.[29] In performing a transtibial PCL reconstruction, our goal is, therefore, to reproduce the anterolateral component of the PCL.

There has been recent interest in reconstruction of both the posteromedial and anterolateral bundles of the PCL, and we have utilized this approach in performing transtibial PCL reconstructions. Technically, this approach is slightly more difficult. Double-bundle graft at present shows no proven functional advantage over conventional single-bundle techniques. Therefore, in the multiple ligament injured knee, our preference is to reproduce the anterolateral bundle of the PCL with a very large Achilles tendon graft.

Surgical Timing

Once the knee has been reduced, the physical examination has been performed, vascular integrity of the limb has been ensured, and the appropriate imaging studies have been obtained, the surgeon has 1 to 2 weeks to devise the surgical plan. Close observation for several days is warranted prior to proceeding with knee ligament surgery to assure adequate limb perfusion, allow the soft tissue swelling to decrease, and to ensure that there is no intimal endothelial damage to the vessels. The surgical repair/reconstruction can be performed within the first 10 to 14 days without compromising the end result. By delaying surgery for more than 2 weeks, one increases the risk of developing a fixed posterior subluxation, and decreases the opportunity for repair of avulsed structures.

Bracing Versus External Fixation

If the knee will remain located in a hinged brace, there is no need for external fixation when surgical reconstruction is planned. Bracing is preferable to casting or splinting to avoid circumferential compression of the limb. If external fixation is not performed, then a repeat radiograph in the brace should be obtained to assure maintenance of reduction. If immobilization in the brace does not maintain the tibia in a reduced position, then an external fixator should be applied, even if early reconstruction is planned. Pins should be placed far from the future surgical field. The pins should not compromise or coincide with future incisions or tunnels. If surgery is not planned within 10 to 14 days following the injury, then a knee-spanning external fixator should be applied for 4 to 6 weeks to maintain a reduced knee and allow soft tissue scarring. External fixator removal is optimally performed in the operating room to allow irrigation and debridement of the pin sites and a repeat examination under anesthesia, as well as manipulation under anesthesia to assist with regaining knee flexion. The knee is then placed in a hinged brace, and repeat radiographs are required to ensure that the knee remains located.

If acute surgery is not planned, then consideration should be made for placing a hinged knee-spanning external fixator (Figure 6.10). The hinged external fixator allows for knee range of motion, particularly from 0 to 90°, and will decrease the likelihood for significant postinjury stiffness. In placing a hinged external fixator, it is important to identify the main axis of tibiofemoral rotation (Figure 6.11).

Surgery and Surgical Preparation

Positioning and Preoperative Preparation

During surgical repair and reconstruction of the dislocated knee, the surgeon must have access to the entire lower extremity. The patient is placed in the supine position; a kidney rest or post can be placed against the greater trochanter so that the knee can remain flexed without mechanical support. A tourniquet is placed over the proximal thigh; however, it is not usually

Fig. 6.10. Clinical photograph of hinged external fixation.

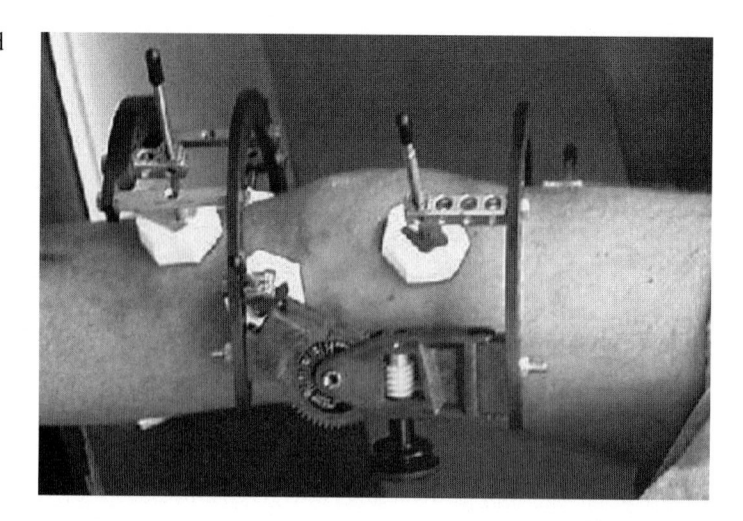

elevated during this procedure. Certainly, the tourniquet should not be used if concerns regarding the vascular status remain or if massive soft tissue swelling is present. Use of the tourniquet should also be avoided if a vascular reconstruction was performed within a few weeks prior to ligament reconstruction.

The patient is provided with antibiotics intravenously for prophylactic antibiotic coverage. After the patient has been placed in a supine position, a sandbag is placed at the foot of the bed so that the injured knee can rest comfortably against the kidney at approximately 75 to 90° of flexion. A Foley catheter is inserted. After bilateral knee examinations under anesthesia, the nonoperative limb is placed in extension with the posterior portion well padded. Care is taken to ensure that there are no areas of compression, particularly in the region of the superficial peroneal nerve.

Examination Under Anesthesia

It is vital to perform a thorough and comprehensive knee examination under anesthesia, with the contralateral knee assessed as the standard. The surgical exposure and plan will be dictated by the pattern of instability found

Fig. 6.11. Radiograph of hinged external fixation.

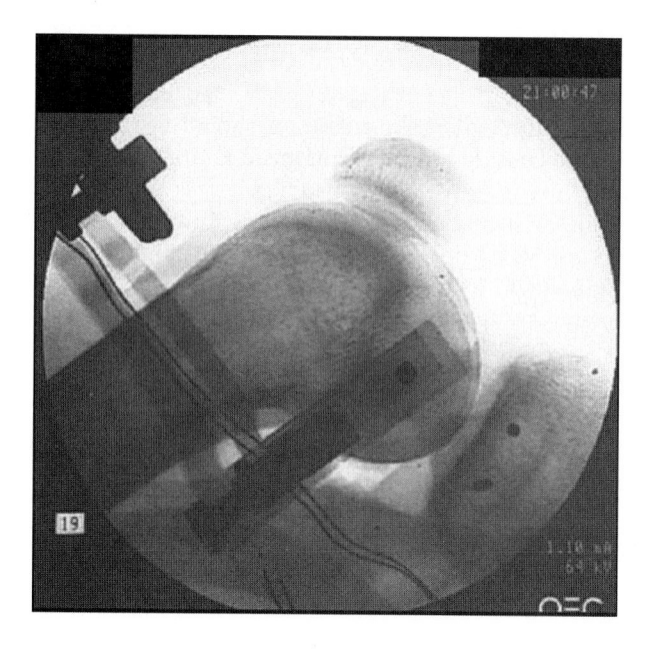

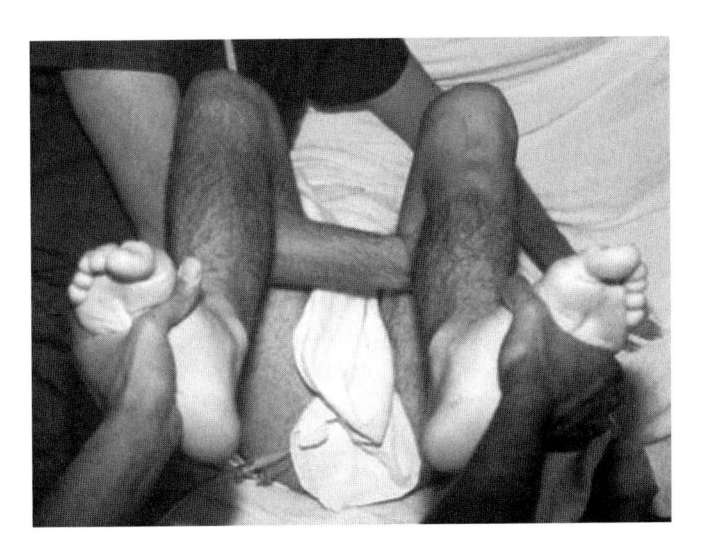

Fig. 6.12. The dial external rotation test at 90° of knee flexion.

during the exam. This is particularly true in assessing the posterior injury and deciding whether to perform PCL reconstruction. The comprehensive examination includes the anterior drawer, the posterior drawer, varus and valgus stress testing at extension and at 25° of flexion, and assessment of the relative tibial external rotation, at both 30 and 90° of knee flexion (Figure 6.12). Care must be taken when one is performing pivot shift or reverse pivot shift maneuvers. The knee is frequently quite unstable, and an iatrogenic vascular injury can result if these tests are performed too vigorously.

Vascular Examination

The dorsalis pedis and posterior tibial pulses need to be assessed, both by palpation and by Doppler signal, to help assess adequate limb perfusion. This is particularly important when vascular surgery was performed prior to the ligamentous repair/reconstruction. At the conclusion of the procedure, a repeat vascular examination should be carried out.

Arthroscopy

The joint capsule may be widely disrupted, and during arthroscopy, one must ensure that fluid extravasation into the calf and the knee tissues does not induce a compartment syndrome. Arthroscopic evaluation can provide additional information, such as an assessment of chondral damage and posterior meniscal root injuries. Gravity flow is recommended to minimize the pressure inside the joint. If pump flow is used, the pump pressure must be maintained in the 40 mmHg range. Arthroscopy should be used in a dry setting as much as possible to allow for direct and improved visualization of the knee structures without the risk of increased fluid pressure in the knee (Figure 6.13; see color plate). The calf should be assessed frequently during the procedure. To assist in reduction of pressure, a small arthrotomy can be made, or the anterior tibial incision, later needed for drilling the ACL and PCL tunnels, can be made.

Incisions

The topographical anatomy should be drawn on the knee with a sterile marking pen (Figure 6.14; see color plate). When there is significant deep MCL and medial retinaculum injury, and when there is a large avulsion of the proximal portion of the MCL, the medial utility incision will

Fig. 6.13. Dry arthroscopic image demonstrating an ACL and PCL tear in the femoral notch. (See color plate.)

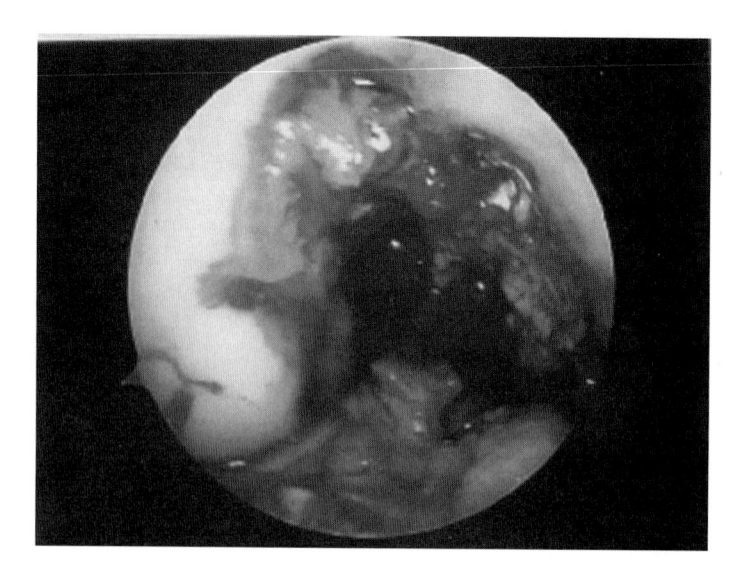

likely be needed. When one is performing multiple ligament reconstruction through this open incision, the arthroscope is still used, in a dry setting, for visualization.

If the deep MCL and medial capsule are not disrupted and there is no excessive capsular damage, then the cruciate reconstruction can be performed completely arthroscopically. The incisions required include the standard anteromedial and anterolateral inferior portal incisions. A posteromedial portal is then made above the joint line with the knee flexed at 90°. The use of a curette or the surgeon's finger protects the neurovascular structures while the transtibial PCL tunnel is being drilled.

Fig. 6.14. Topographical landmarks (incision, joint line, patella, and tibial tubercle) for the MCL reconstruction. (See color plate.)

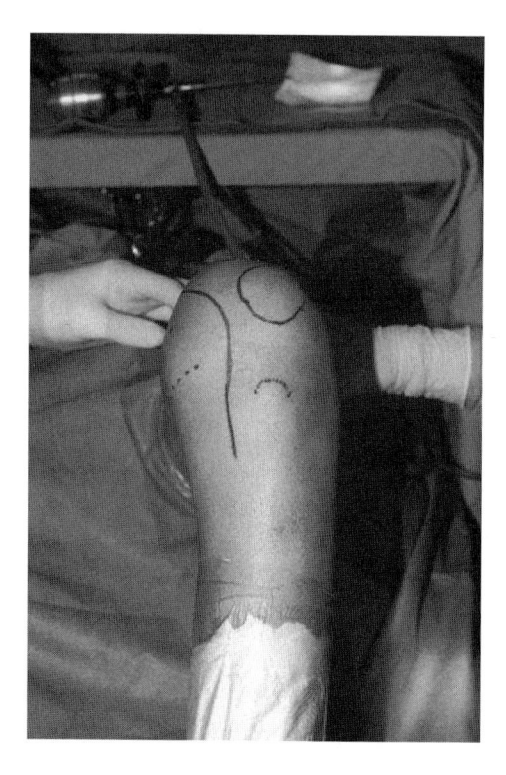

Arthroscopically Assisted Evaluation and Preparation

A thorough arthroscopic evaluation of the knee is performed. The articular cartilage is assessed for damage, and the menisci are thoroughly evaluated and probed. If the decision has been made to reconstruct both the anterior and posterior cruciate ligaments, then a thorough notch debridement is performed. The footprints of the ACL on the tibial side and the anterolateral bundle of the PCL on the femoral side should be maintained to assist with tunnel placement. In the ACL/PCL/medial side knee injury, there is frequently a medial drive-through sign analogous to an unstable shoulder. With valgus stress, the medial capsular damage can be assessed and a floating medial meniscus may also be visualized (Figure 6.6B; see color plate). After a comprehensive assessment of the knee has been made arthroscopically, any chondral or meniscal damage can be addressed.

Operative Management: Cruciate Ligament Reconstruction

PCL Surgery

One indication for PCL reconstruction is a grade III posterior drawer in the acute setting; symptomatic, chronic, grade II posterior instability is also indicative. PCL reconstruction graft options include allograft Achilles, allograft or autograft bone–patellar tendon–bone, and allograft tibialis anterior. There are various reconstruction techniques for both the femoral and tibial side. Tibial side fixation can be achieved by a posterior inlay approach or by a transtibial tunnel with anterior side fixation. Regarding the femoral side, the fixation can be performed via an outside-in or inside-out approach. Finally, it must be decided whether to reconstruct just the anterolateral bundle or both the anterolateral and posteromedial bundles of the PCL (Table 6.2).

Transtibial PCL Reconstruction: Graft Choice and Graft Position

If posterior cruciate ligament reconstruction is chosen, various PCL techniques and graft choices are at the surgeon's disposal. In the case of the multiple ligament injured knee with a midsubstance PCL tear, we prefer a transtibial PCL tunnel reconstruction with the use of an Achilles tendon allograft. Use of allograft tissue minimizes the surgical time as well as the iatrogenic trauma from graft.[30]

Table 6.2. Variables of PCL Reconstruction

Approach	Graft choice	Graft placement
Arthroscopic	Autologous	Femoral
Open with arthroscopic assistance	BPTB	Isometric
	Hamstring	Anatomic
Femoral side	Quadriceps tendon	Tibial
Outside-in	Allograft	Tibial tunnel
Inside-out	Achilles tendon	Direct fixation
Single/double bundle	BPTB	
Tibial side	Tibialis anterior	
Transtibial		
Posterior inlay		

Fig. 6.15. PCL reconstruction guides (left guide for femoral tunnel, center guide for tibial tunnel).

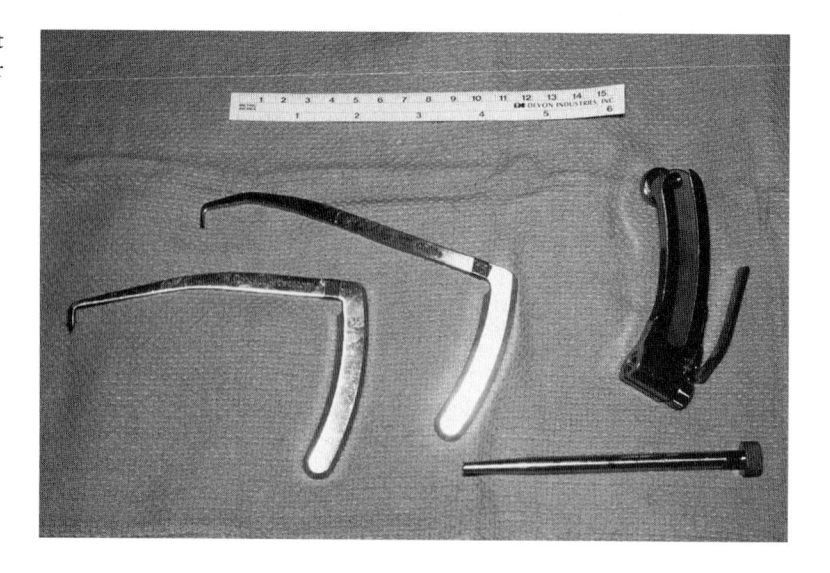

An Achilles tendon allograft provides a large amount of collagen that can fill the bone tunnels, completely. Additionally, the soft tissue end of the graft makes it easy to pass the graft through the bone tunnels, and bony fixation can be achieved on the femoral side by use of the calcaneal bone plug. When reconstructing the PCL through this technique, the goal is to reproduce the anterolateral component of the PCL.

PCL Transtibial Technique (Figure 6.15)

To reproduce the anterolateral bundle, the anterior tibia is exposed and a posterior cruciate ligament guide is placed such that the entry point, on the anterior tibia, is just medial to the anterior spine and a few centimeters below the level of the tibial tubercle. The angle is approximately 60°. At the posterior portion of the tibia, the guide is placed at the lateral border of the PCL tibial fossa. The guide is placed approximately 1 cm distal to the joint line (Figure 6.16).

Following guide positioning, a curette is placed through the posteromedial portal to protect the neurovascular structures. A transtibial guide pin

Fig. 6.16. Intraoperative placement of the PCL tibial guide.

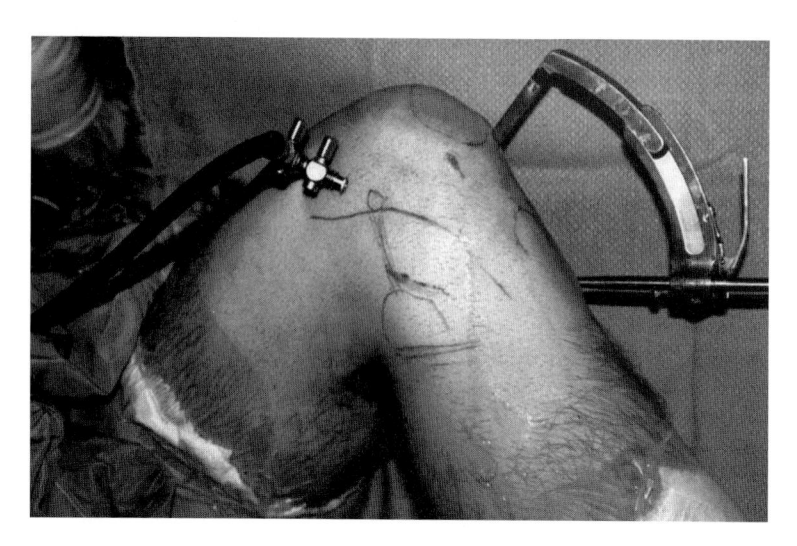

6. Surgery for ACL/PCL/Medial Side Knee Injuries

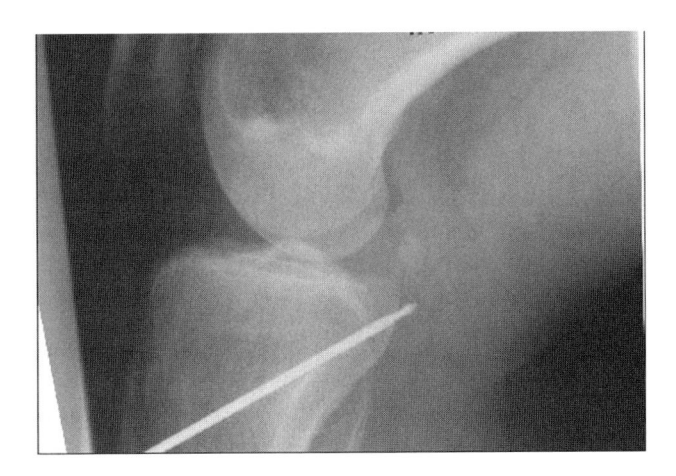

Fig. 6.17. Appropriate positioning of PCL guide pin.

is then drilled under direct arthroscopic visualization. An intraoperative radiograph is very helpful in confirming the correct placement of the tibial guide pin. On the lateral x-ray, the pins should be located in the inferior third of the posterolateral tibial fossa. A surgeon who uses arthroscopic landmarks only can be fooled, particularly when there is an extensive amount of scarring within the posterior aspect of the knee. When reconstructing both PCL and ACL, the lateral radiograph is obtained after the ACL guide pin has been positioned. Alternatively, a C-arm can be used to assess pin position (Figures 6.17, 6.18, and 6.19).

Once the ACL and PCL guide pins have been appropriately positioned, the PCL tibial tunnel is drilled. An 11 or 12 mm transtibial PCL tunnel is drilled, based on the patient's size. A cannulated drill bit is placed over the guide pin at the anterior tibia, and the initial drilling is done with power. A curette is placed on the posterior tibia to ensure protection of the posterior neurovascular structures. When the second cortex is approached, the drilling should be completed by hand, leaving the chuck attached to the drill bit. This decreases the risk of overpenetration. As an additional precautionary measure, the guide pin is removed just before completion of the drilling of the second cortex (Figure 6.20). Once the PCL tibial tunnel has been drilled, the ACL tibial tunnel is drilled with a 10 mm drill bit.

Regarding the femoral side for the PCL, the femoral tunnel is placed through the footprint of the anterolateral bundle of the PCL. This is in the anterior aspect of the medial femoral condyle near the 11 o'clock position, just under the subchondral bone. This PCL femoral side tunnel can be made by either an outside-in or an inside-out technique. With the outside-in technique, a PCL femoral guide is placed so that the bullet rests on the outer margin of the medial femur, approximately 6 mm from the cortical margin. The tip of the PCL guide is placed at either the 1 or the 11 o'clock position of the anterior medial femur within the femoral notch. The guide pin is then drilled from the outside in, exiting at the insertion of the anterolateral bundle within the femoral notch. Then a cannulated drill bit is used to drill the 11 mm femoral tunnel from the outside in.

For an all-inside or endoscopic technique, the guide pin is placed through the inferior lateral portal. The pin is placed at the 1 or 11 o'clock position; with the knee flexed at approximately 120°, the pin is then drilled 3 cm into the medial femur. It is then overdrilled using an 11 mm cannulated drill bit. This is analogous to arthroscopic drilling for the femoral side of the ACL.

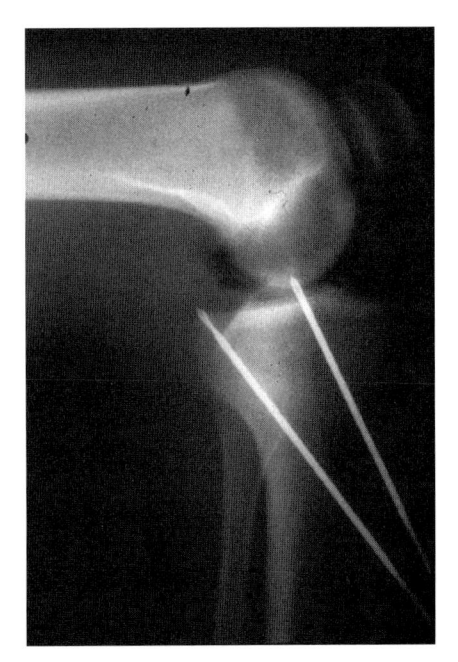

Fig. 6.18. Appropriate positioning of PCL guide and ACL guide pin, with knee in flexion.

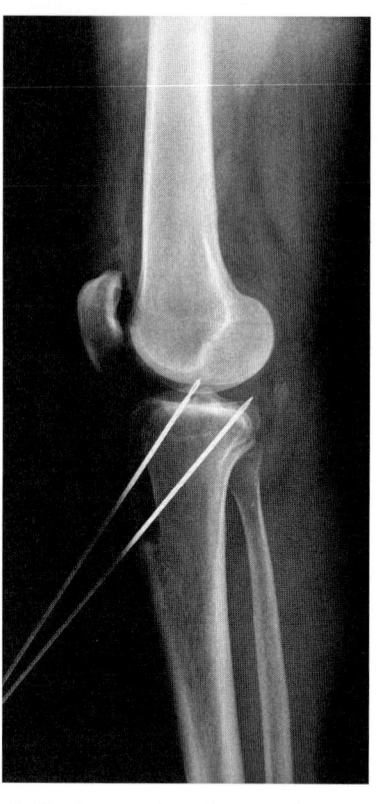

Fig. 6.19. Appropriate ACL guide pin position (with knee in full extension) immediately posterior and parallel to Blumensaat's line. The PCL guide pin is too anterior and was revised.

Fig. 6.20. Line drawing of position for tibial transtibial drilling.

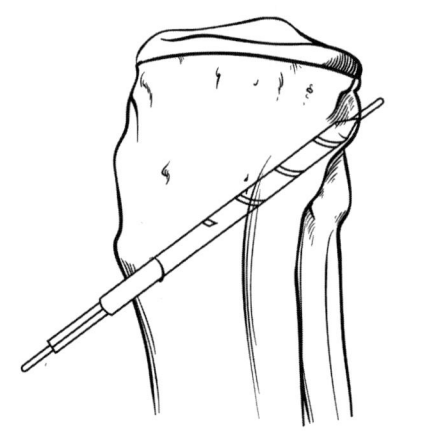

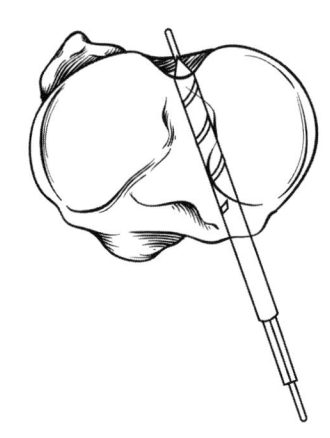

Achilles Tendon Graft Preparation

The Achilles tendon graft is thawed, and the bone portion is tubalized into an 11 mm plug approximately 25 mm long. The tendinous portion is tubalized and whipstitched to either 11 or 12 mm (Figure 6.21; see color plate). It is important to leave the most distal portion of the Achilles tendinous portion quite thin and well tubalized to facilitate graft passage. This distal portion will exit the transtibial tunnel, and there is no need for the distal portion to be excessively thick. A bulbous distal graft will impede passage through the tibial tunnel.

PCL Graft Passage: Outside-In Technique

An 18-gauge malleable wire is then passed in retrograde fashion through the transtibial tunnel. The wire is pulled within the femoral notch, and the curved end of the wire is brought through the femoral tunnel, exiting the anteromedial aspect of the knee (Figure 6.22; see color plate). The tendinous portion of the Achilles tendon graft is then brought from outside the knee into the PCL femoral tunnel, into the notch, into the posterior portion of the PCL tibial tunnel, and finally, through the tibial tunnel to the anterior aspect of the tibia. The graft is pulled through the anterior portion of the tibia until the calcaneal bone plug is flush with the surface of the medial femur. The femoral side of the graft is then secured by means of a metal interference screw placed from the outside in (Figure 6.23).

PCL Graft Passage with the Endoscopic Technique

When the femoral tunnel for the PCL has been made by an inside-out technique, the PCL graft passage is modified. The 18-gauge wire again is brought in retrograde fashion through the tibial tunnel into the notch and then through the anterolateral portal. The tendinous portion of the Achilles graft is then brought through the loop of the 18-gauge wire with assistance of the whipstitch. The tendinous portion of the graft is then brought into the femoral notch and through the transtibial tunnel and then out the anterior portion of the tibia. The bone plug is brought to the edge of the inferior portal. A Beath pin is then placed through the inferior–lateral portal and then through the PCL femoral tunnel, exiting the anterior–medial aspect of the thigh. A suture that is placed through the calcaneal bone plug is passed through the Beath pin. The pin and the calcaneal bone plug are then brought into the notch and into the femoral PCL tunnel. Fixation is achieved with the use of a metal interference screw. Attention is then turned to passage and fixation of the anterior cruciate ligament graft.

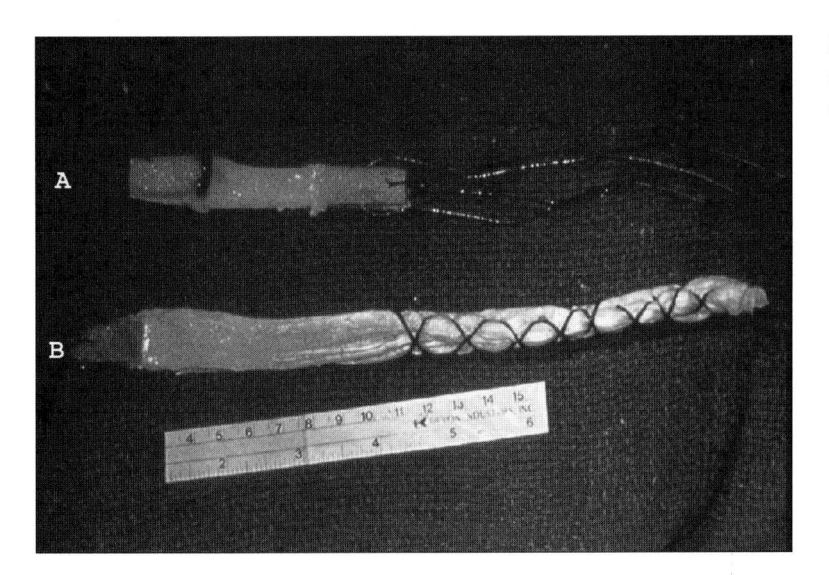

6. Surgery for ACL/PCL/Medial Side Knee Injuries 83

Fig. 6.21. Graft choices: (A) BPTB allograft and (B) Achilles allograft (with whipstitch). (See color plate.)

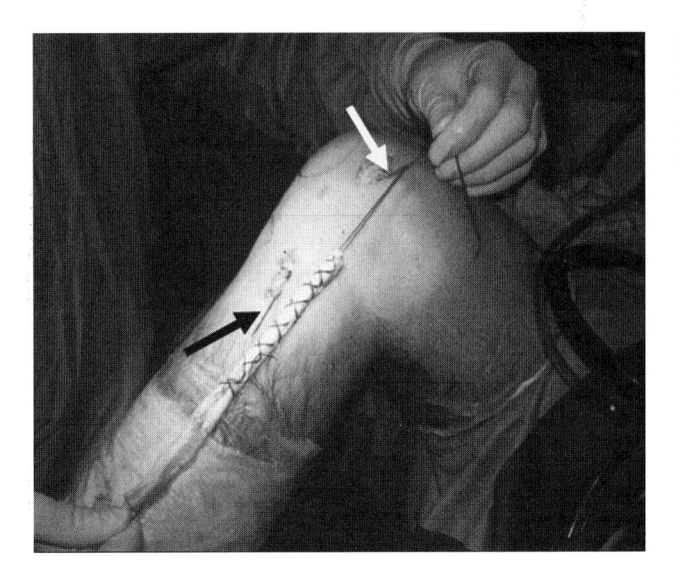

Fig. 6.22. Prepared Achilles graft prior to being passed from the outside in, utilizing an 18-gauge wire. Wire is visualized traversing both tibial and femoral tunnels (arrows). (See color plate.)

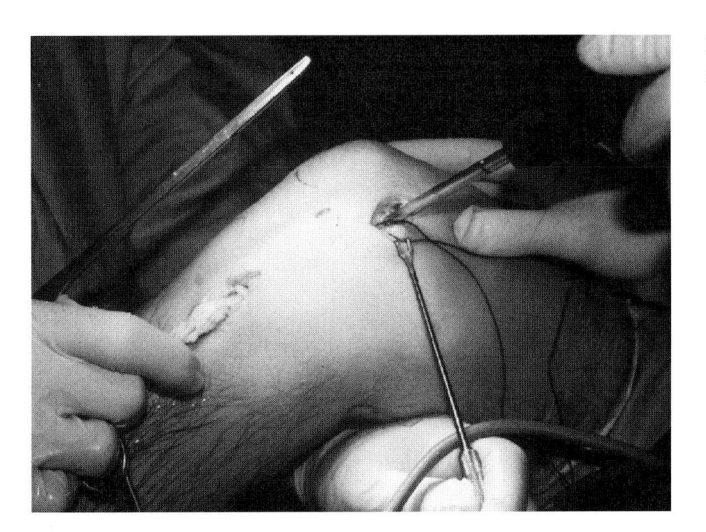

Fig. 6.23. Outside-in PCL femoral graft fixation using an interference screw.

PCL Reconstruction Alternative Techniques

Double-Bundle PCL Technique

In addition to the transtibial anterolateral bundle PCL reconstruction, the PCL can be reconstructed by means of a two-bundle technique. With this technique both the anterolateral and posteromedial bundles of the PCL are reconstructed. Two separate endoscopic femoral side PCL tunnels are drilled, one at the 1 o'clock position and one at the 3 o'clock position. The anterolateral bundle reconstruction is as described earlier; however, a smaller femoral tunnel, usually 9 mm, is utilized. Another allograft Achilles graft or allograft semitendinosus or allograft tibialis anterior can be used for the posterior medial bundle. With ACL, PCL, and medial side injury to the knee, the medial hamstring tendons are not used for the posterior medial bundle. The posterior medial graft is passed separately from the anterolateral graft. Femoral side fixation is secured by using an endoscopic technique as described earlier. Fixation for the posteromedial graft can be achieved by a bioabsorbable screw or a sterile button placed outside the anteromedial femoral cortex. The diameter of the anteromedial graft and femoral tunnel is 7 or 8 mm.

On the tibial side, a single transtibial tunnel is drilled. Both the anterolateral and posteromedial grafts are brought through this tunnel. The anterolateral bundle is secured via a bicortical screw and washer or a bone staple. The anterolateral graft is fixed with the knee flexed at 90°, and an anterior drawer is applied. Following fixation of the anterolateral graft, the posteromedial graft is secured by means of a bioabsorbable screw and possibly an additional post and washer or staple. The posteromedial graft is tensioned with the knee at 30° of flexion.

Posterior Inlay

In addition to the double-bundle reconstruction for the PCL, a posterior tibial inlay approach can be carried out. A transverse incision is made in the popliteal fossa, the medial head of the gastrocnemius is moved laterally, and the posterior capsule and posterior tibial plateau are exposed. The neurovascular structures are protected by the medial gastrocnemius. Steinmann pins are placed into the posterior tibia adjacent to the medial gastrocnemius, thus maintaining the lateral displacement of the medial gastrocnemius and protecting the neurovascular structures. A trough is then made in the tibial PCL fossa and a bone–patellar tendon–bone graft is secured in the fossa and fixed with a bone staple or a bicortical screw. With the knee flexed at 90°, the femoral side of the graft is then secured within the PCL femoral tunnel as an anterior drawer is applied to the tibia. To assist with working on both the posterior and anterior aspects of the knee when one is using this approach to perform a PCL reconstruction, the patient can be placed in a supine position. The hip can be internally and externally rotated to assist with visualizing the anterior aspect (hip external rotation) and posterior aspect (hip internal rotation) of the knee (Figure 6.24).

Repair of PCL Avulsion Injuries

PCL avulsion injuries without midsubstance tears can be successfully repaired. The MRI exam is very helpful in regard to making this diagnosis. Bony tibial side PCL avulsion injuries can be treated with screw fixation through a posterior approach and occasionally with sutures brought through a small transtibial tunnel. Tibial side avulsion injuries without a bony fragment can be treated in a similar manner, but with less reliable

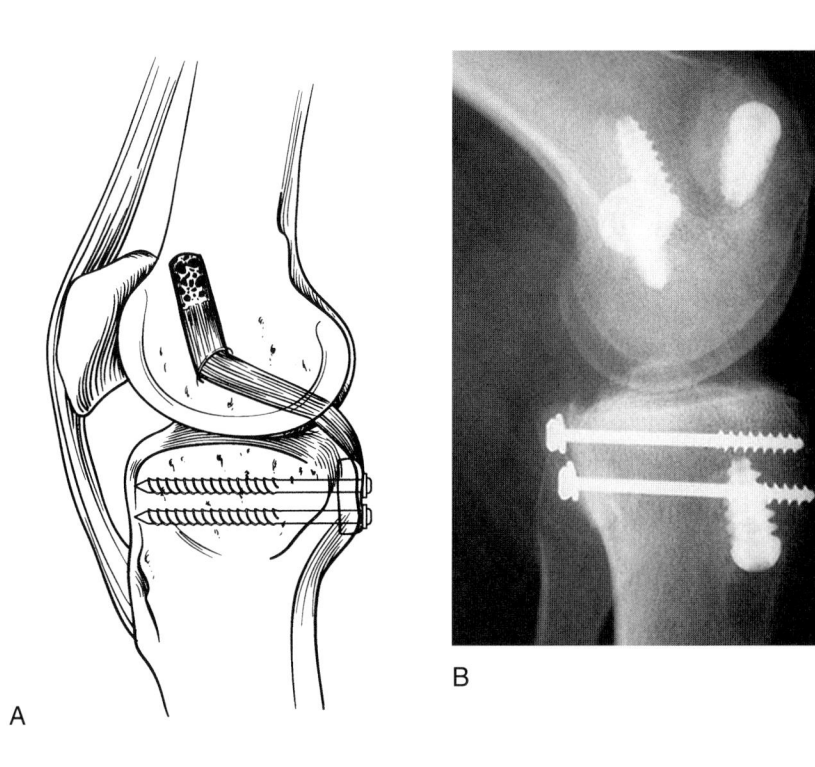

Fig. 6.24. Posterior tibial inlay technique: (A) schematic drawing and (B) radiograph.

results. Femoral side PCL peel-off injuries can be repaired successfully by using a bony bridge to suture the PCL (Figure 6.25; see color plate for parts C and F).

Anterior Cruciate Ligament Reconstruction

In performing a combined ACL–PCL reconstruction, the authors' graft of choice for the anterior cruciate ligament reconstruction is allograft bone–patellar tendon–bone (Figure 6.22A). Autograft bone–patellar tendon–bone is also a viable option, particularly for transtibial PCL techniques performed using an Achilles allograft. Autograft hamstring is not recommended for the combined ACL, PCL, medial side knee injury. Use of the medial hamstrings removes a secondary medial stabilizer to the knee. In addition, the medial hamstrings may be needed for augmentation of the medial collateral ligament. As with an isolated ACL reconstruction, the recommendation is to use a single-incision, arthroscopically assisted ACL reconstruction.[31]

An ACL transtibial guide pin is placed, using the same anterior medial tibial incision that served for placement of the PCL transtibial guide pin. The anterior tibial entry point for the ACL guide pin is approximately 2 cm superior and medial to the entry point for the PCL guide pin. The angle for the ACL guide is set at 45°. This maintains a bridge of cortical bone between the anterior portions of the anterior cruciate ligament and the posterior cruciate ligament tibial tunnels. The entry point for the anterior tibial tunnel is midway between the anterior border and the posterior medial border of the anterior tibia (Figure 6.26; see color plate).

Within the femoral notch, the ACL guide pin is brought to the central portion or the posterior–central portion of the ACL tibial footprint. The guide pin is aimed toward the 10 and 2 o'clock positions on the femur. After the ACL and PCL transtibial guide pins have been placed, a lateral radiograph is obtained. With the knee in full extension, the ACL guide pin should be parallel and just posterior to an extension of Blumensaat's line (Figure

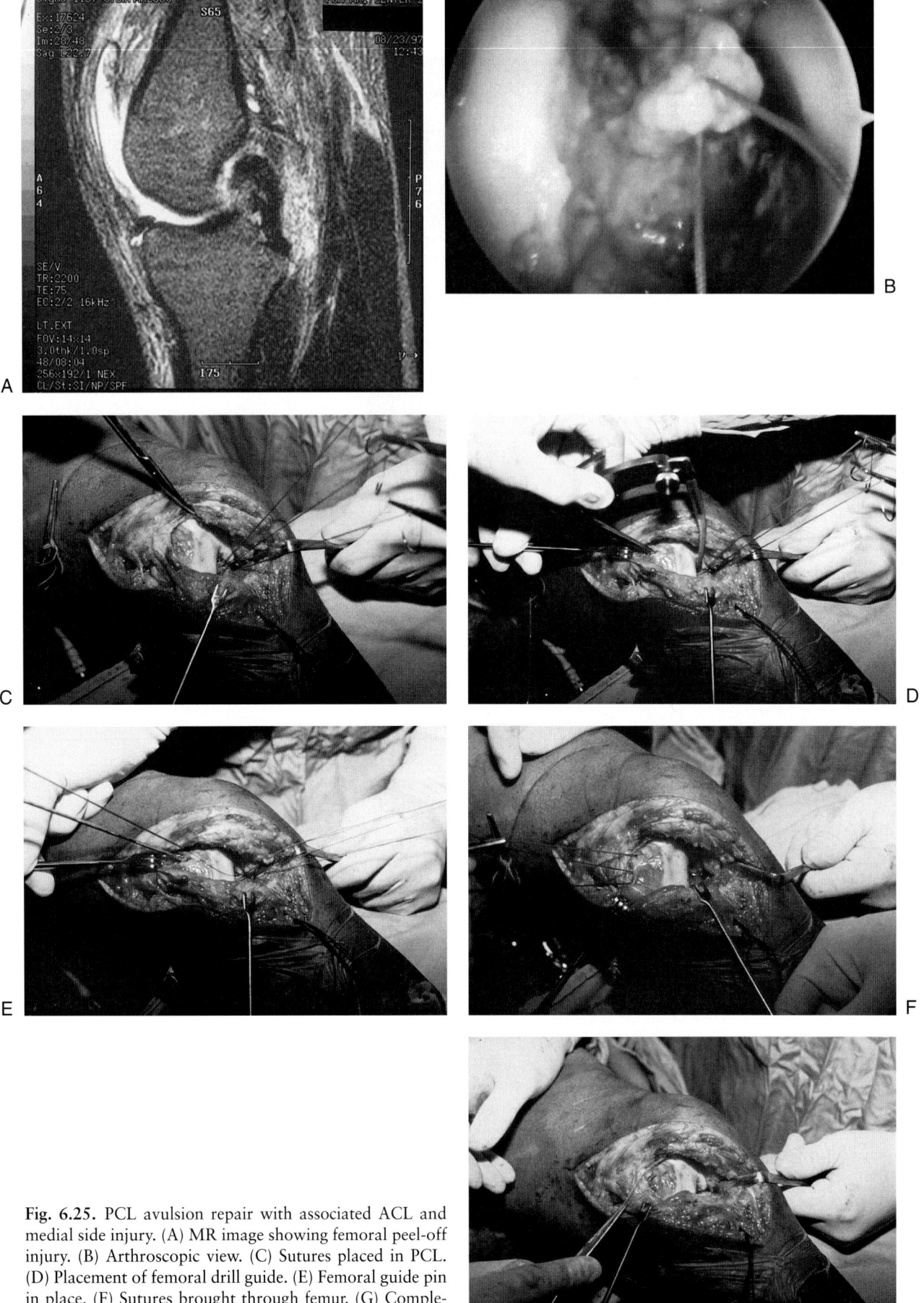

Fig. 6.25. PCL avulsion repair with associated ACL and medial side injury. (A) MR image showing femoral peel-off injury. (B) Arthroscopic view. (C) Sutures placed in PCL. (D) Placement of femoral drill guide. (E) Femoral guide pin in place. (F) Sutures brought through femur. (G) Completion of PCL repair. (See color plate.)

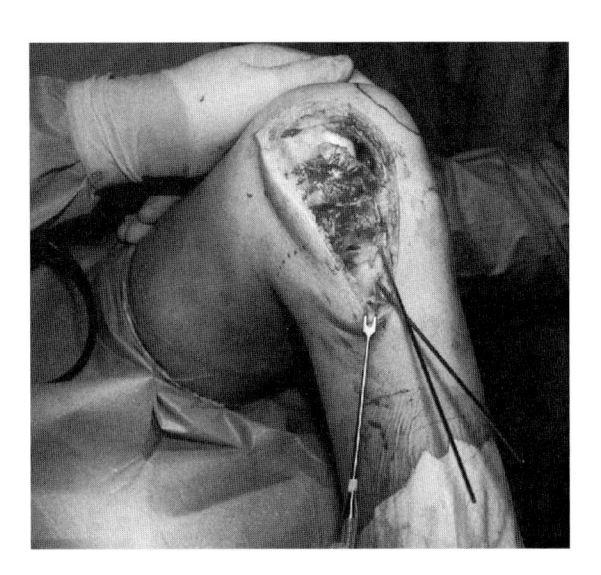

Fig. 6.26. Intraoperative photograph of ACL and PCL guide pin placement. (See color plate.)

6.18). In the significantly traumatized knee, there may be no clear ACL tibial footprint. Additional reference sources include the tibial spines. Within the notch, the ACL guide pin should be immediately adjacent to the lateral border of the medial tibial spine. Additionally, the anterior horn of the lateral meniscus can be used as a reference point. The ACL guide pin should lie approximately 5 mm medial and 5 mm posterior to the insertion of the anterior horn of the lateral meniscus.

A 10 mm transtibial ACL tunnel is drilled once appropriate pin position has been verified. A 7 mm over-the-top guide is placed at the posterior lateral portion of the femur at the 10 or the 2 o'clock position. A femoral guide pin is then placed, followed by drilling a 30 mm femoral tunnel by means of a 10 mm cannulated drill bit.

Once the PCL graft has been secured on the femoral side, the ACL graft is passed by means of a Beath pin or a two-pin passer. The femoral side of the ACL bone–patellar tendon–bone graft is secured by using a metal interference screw.

Tibial Side Fixation of the PCL and ACL Grafts

Following femoral fixation of the PCL and the ACL grafts, attention may be turned to the medial aspect of the knee. The details of medial side knee surgery will be discussed in the following section. If the need for medial side knee surgery is equivocal, or if the procedure has been determined to be unnecessary based on the examination under anesthesia, tibial side ACL and PCL fixation can be carried out. Occasionally, the decision to operate or not operate on the medial side of the knee is based on the assessment of the valgus laxity following fixation of the PCL and the ACL on the tibial side.

Tibial Side PCL Fixation

Tibial side PCL fixation can be achieved by a bicortical screw and a spiked washer, bone staples, and/or bioabsorbable interference screws. The authors' preference is to place a bioabsorbable screw in retrograde fashion so that its tip is near the joint line at the posterior aspect of the tibia. Supplemental fixation is achieved by either a spiked screw and washer or a Richard's bone staple. The knee is flexed to 90° and the anterior medial tibial step-off is recreated by placing an anterior drawer on the tibia. Prior to fixing the graft, the knee is cycled, with tension placed on the tibial side

Fig. 6.27. Arthroscopic view of ACL and double-bundle PCL reconstruction. (See color plate.)

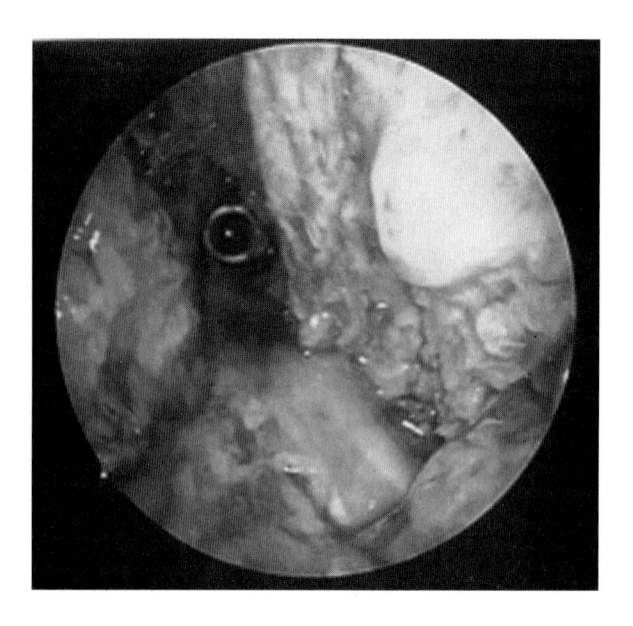

of the graft to remove the creep from the graft. Tibial side PCL fixation can be carried out with the knee in more extension than 90°. When the tibial side of the PCL is fixed at less than 90° of flexion, however, care must be taken to ensure that knee flexion has not been sacrificed. With the hip at 90° of flexion and gravity pulling on the tibia, the knee should flex to at least 120°.

Tibial Side ACL Fixation

It can be difficult to assess the center of rotation of a multiple ligament injured knee. For this reason, our preference is to utilize the knee's screw home mechanism, which exists in full extension, to secure the tibial side of the ACL. An axial load is placed on the knee, and no posterior drawer is applied. With tension placed on the tibial side of the ACL graft, the graft is secured by means of a metal interference screw.

Following ACL and PCL tibial side fixation, the posterior drawer and anterior drawer are assessed, and Lachman's test is performed. Valgus stress is applied at both 25° of knee flexion and full extension to determine the magnitude of the medial collateral ligament injury and laxity (Figure 6.27; see color plate).

Medial Side Knee Surgery

After the central pivot has been addressed, attention is turned to the medial side knee injury. In the acute setting, the preoperative examination under anesthesia, as well as the MRI findings, determine whether the medial side of the knee needs to be surgically addressed and the likely surgical approach (Table 6.3). Most commonly, posteromedial surgery is performed through a medial hockey stick incision. The anteromedial incision used for reconstruction of the ACL and PCL can be extended proximally. The superficial medial collateral ligament is exposed, and an incision is made just posterior to the posterior border of the MCL. After development of the interval between the medial meniscus and the posteromedial capsule, the posteromedial capsule is shifted anteriorly and superiorly. The stability of the medial meniscus is then assessed. Meniscal surgery is carried out in the stan-

6. Surgery for ACL/PCL/Medial Side Knee Injuries

Table 6.3. Variables of Medial Side Reconstruction

Acute	Chronic
Direct repair	Reconstruction
Avulsion fixation	Autologous semitendinosus
Staple	Free graft
Suture anchor	Tibial insertion left intact
Screw and washer	Allograft
Augmentation	Achilles
Reconstruction if repair inadequate	BPTB
Posteromedial capsular advancement	Posteromedial capsular advancement

dard fashion with peripheral red-zone tears being repaired and white-zone tears that are not amenable to repair appropriately debrided. If there is extensive medial capsular damage, the meniscal capsular region needs to be repaired. This can be done with suture anchors placed just below the joint line for outside-in meniscal repair.

Mitek suture anchors are placed along the rim of the proximal medial tibia just below the joint line. The sutures from these anchors are used to secure the medial edge of the medial meniscus and the deep medial capsule to the tibial plateau (Figures 6.28 and 6.29; see color plate for 6.29A). After the posterior medial capsule has been shifted anteriorly and superiorly, these sutures are tied to the capsule. Following repair of the deep capsule and the medial meniscus, the superficial medial collateral ligament may need to be addressed. If there is not extensive medial capsular damage, then the meniscus can be repaired through a standard inside-out technique. Our preference is to use 2-0 Tycron vertical mattress sutures.

MCL avulsion off the femoral or the tibial side may be repaired via use of suture anchors, bone staples, or a screw with a spiked washer. The medial collateral ligament is reattached at its point of origin. The ligament can be reassesed to increase tension, since there can be some intersubstance stretching of the ligament in addition to the avulsion injury. The MCL avulsion injury is repaired with the knee in 30° of flexion and with a varus stress applied to the knee and the knee in a figure-of-four position. In acute cases with significant intersubstance tearing of the superficial and deep MCL, direct repair is made by means of nonabsorbable suture. A posteromedial

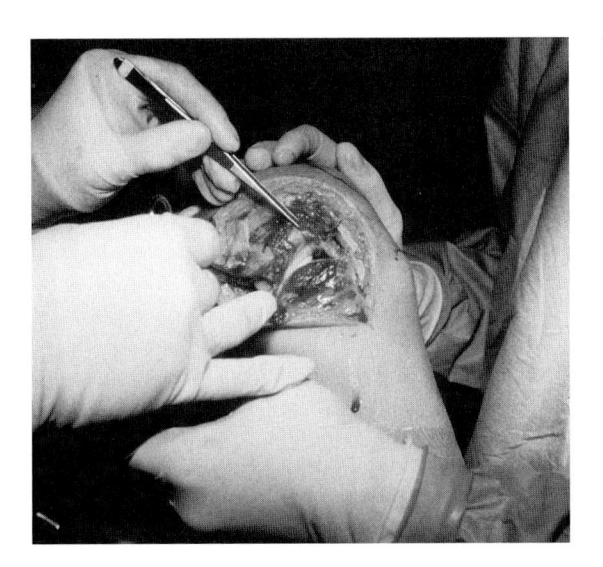

Fig. 6.28. Exposure of medial side injury.

Fig. 6.29. Repair of medial side injury with associated ACL/PCL injury showing suture anchors in medial tibia to secure medial meniscus and deep medial capsule (A), PCL tibial tunnel and graft (B), ACL tibial tunnel and graft (C), and femoral PCL tunnel and bone plug (D), (E,F) AP and lateral x-rays. (See color plate.)

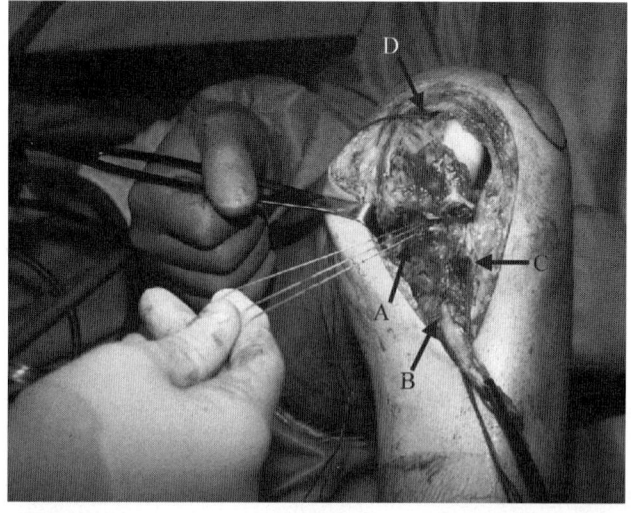

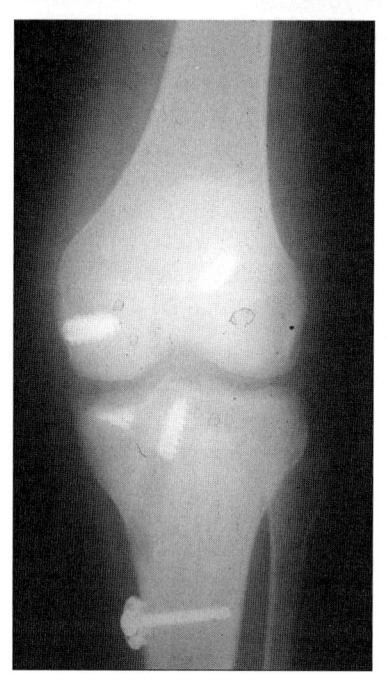

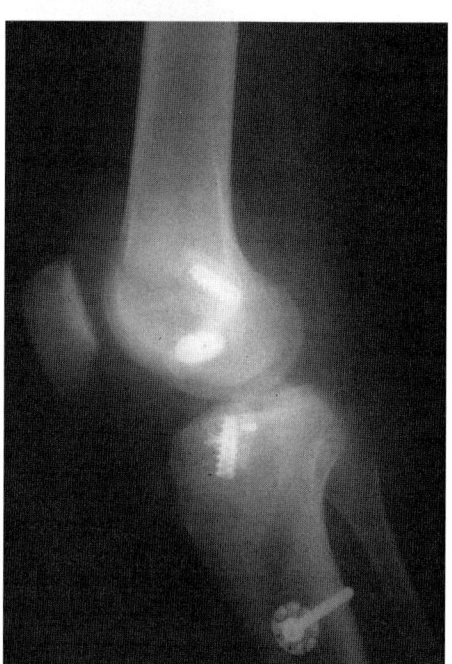

capsular advancement is also performed and sewn into the repaired MCL. The results of midsubstance repair can be less favorable. Following the repair, valgus laxity is reassessed at full extension and at 25° of knee flexion. If there is still excess laxity despite the posteromedial capsular advancement and the medial collateral ligament repair, medial collateral ligament reconstruction, as described next, may be considered even in this acute setting.

Treatment of Chronic Medial Side Laxity

Chronic medial knee instability is one of the more difficult knee problems to treat, particularly in the face of chronic instability of the central pivot. During the performance of a simultaneous cruciate ligament reconstruction, the chronically unstable medial side can be treated by advancement of the posterior medial capsule anteriorly and superiorly. This is particularly helpful when the instability is posterior and medial. Chronic posteromedial

6. Surgery for ACL/PCL/Medial Side Knee Injuries

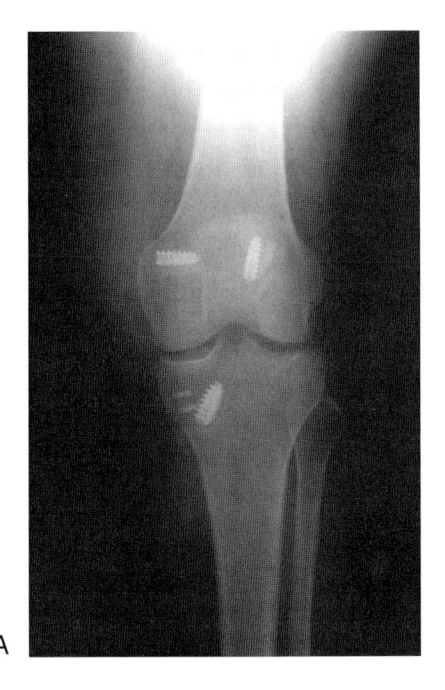

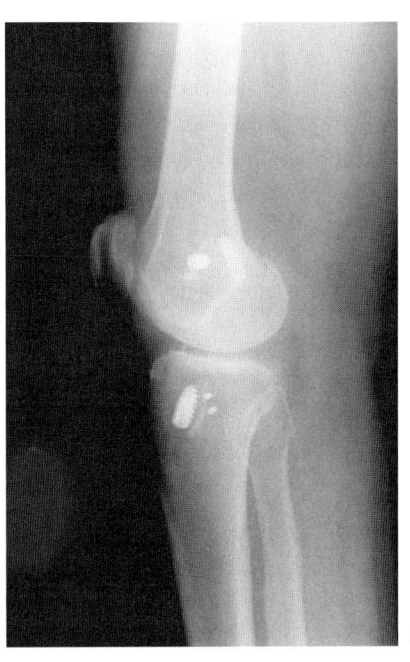

Fig. 6.30. Radiographs (A) AP and (B) lateral of combined ACL/medial side reconstruction/repair.

instability can be assessed by increasing the tibial internal rotation in comparison to the contralateral side with the knee at 30° of flexion.

An Achilles tendon allograft can be used to reconstruct the medial collateral ligament. The calcaneal bone plug is inserted via a closed-end tunnel into the medial femoral epicondyle. Tibial side fixation can be achieved via a spiked screw and washer or a bone staple. When there is a healthy remnant of MCL attached on the tibial side, the Achilles allograft can be sutured to the remaining tibial side MCL and then secured on the femoral side as described earlier, using the calcaneal bone plug and a closed-end tunnel (Figure 6.30). A bone–patellar tendon–bone allograft can also be utilized. A closed-end tunnel is placed into the femoral epicondyle, and tibial side fixation can be achieved by means of a bony trough, using a bone staple analogous to the type of tibial side fixation used to secure a bone–patellar tendon–bone ACL graft that is exiting a tibial tunnel (Figure 6.31; see color plate).

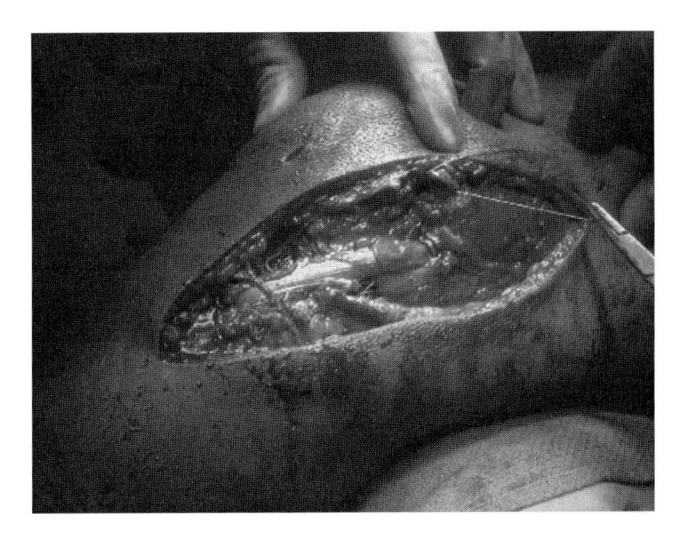

Fig. 6.31. Medial side repair using bone staples for fixation. (See color plate.)

Fig. 6.32. X-rays: (A) AP and (B) lateral opening wedge high tibial osteotomy.

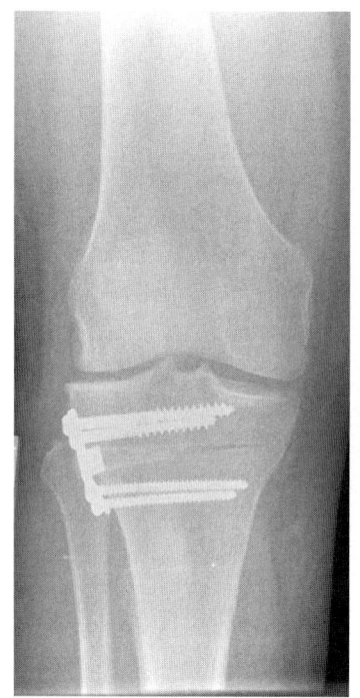

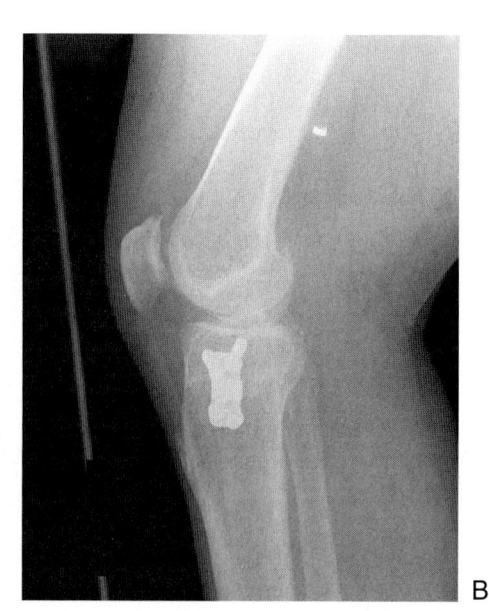

An alternative choice to allograft tissue for the reconstruction of the medial collateral ligament is the semitendinosus and, in cases of significant instability, the gracilis as well. A medial hamstring tendon is harvested by means of a corkscrew tendon stripper. The tibial side attachment of the hamstring is maintained. The tendon is then secured to the medial femoral epicondyle by means of a cortical screw and a spiked washer. Extra tendon is sutured back to itself and also to the deep medial capsule.

For graft tensioning and knee position with either allograft or autograft hamstring medial collateral ligament reconstruction, the knee is placed at 30° of flexion. A varus stress is applied to the knee, and the leg is placed in a figure-of-four position. Care must be taken to ensure that the femoral side of the graft is secured in the appropriate position. If the graft is placed too anteriorly, there can be difficulty obtaining knee flexion. The remnant of the proximal portion of the MCL should be palpable at the medial epicondyle. In cases of significant injury with the femoral side of the MCL not visible or palpable, a lateral radiograph or fluoroscopic image can be used to determine the appropriate position of the graft in the sagittal plane. In addition, the relative isometry of the graft can be assessed by tentatively fixing the femoral side of the graft with use of a k-wire and flexing and extending the knee to assess the variable graft excursion. The graft should be fixed at the insertion point that produces the least excursion.

For patients with chronic medial laxity and valgus alignment, an osteotomy to produce a more varus alignment should be considered. A lateral proximal tibial opening wedge high tibial osteotomy can produce a more varus limb, decreasing the overall medial side stress on the knee. In addition, a biplanar osteotomy can be used to increase the posterior tibial slope in cases of moderate PCL laxity. For moderate anterior cruciate ligament laxity, the posterior tibial slope can be decreased (Figure 6.32).

Rehabilitation

Rehabilitation guidelines following reconstruction of the ACL, PCL, and medial side knee injury are evolving. These guidelines take into account the surgical technique, the magnitude of soft tissue swelling in the limb, the surgeon's satisfaction with the repair/reconstruction of the medial side injury, and the patient's weight and body habitus. General principles include an 8-week maximum protection phase. It takes approximately 8 weeks for significant graft-to-bone healing. Care is taken to avoid posterior tibial translation. This includes no kinetic open-chain hamstring exercises. All range-of-motion exercises for the first month are therapy assisted, with the therapist applying an anterior drawer to the tibia to prevent posterior tibial sagging. Physical therapy can be broken up into four phases, with phase one occurring in the first month following surgery; phase two in the second and third months following surgery; phase three in the third to ninth months following surgery; and phase four, 9 months to a year postoperatively.

During phase one, the emphasis is on protecting the medial side and posterior cruciate ligament repair. The brace is locked in extension for the first week, and then therapy-assisted range-of-motion exercises are initiated with an anterior drawer applied to the tibia and varus stress applied to the limb. The knee is ranged with the assistance of the athletic trainer or physical therapist. Patients maintain touch-down weight bearing with their brace locked in extension for the first month. Therapy exercises include quad sets, hip abduction and adduction, ankle range of motion, calf and hamstring stretching, and calf presses with Thera-Band resistance. If quadriceps tone is poor, adjuvant functional electrical stimulation can be initiated.

Phase two begins one month postoperatively and extends until the end of the third month. Expectations include maintaining full knee extension, decreasing the inflammation in the knee, obtaining 90° of knee flexion by 8 weeks, and maintaining full knee extension. Patients may begin weight bearing, except in cases of excessive lower extremity valgus. A brace is maintained in full extension for weight bearing. After 8 weeks, the patients may discontinue their crutches if there is no quadriceps lag with straight leg raise testing and if the knee can be comfortably flexed to 90°.

Approximately 3 months after surgery, phase three begins. The patient may discontinue the protective brace. Range-of-motion exercises are progressed. Stationary bicycle and closed-chain exercises with stair-stepping machines are performed. Proprioceptive training is advanced, and gait training is addressed. At the end of phase three, patients can begin jogging in a pool with a wet vest or belt.

Phase four begins 9 months postoperatively and extends until the patient has returned to work or the desired activity. Return to athletic participation is variable.

References

1. Green NE, Allen BL. Vascular injuries associated with dislocation of the knee. J Bone Joint Surg Am 1977; 59(2):236–239.
2. Quinlan AG, Sharrard WJW. Postero-lateral dislocation of the knee with capsular interposition. J Bone Joint Surg Br 1958; 40:660–663.
3. Good L, Johnson RJ. The dislocated knee. J Am Acad Orthop Surg 1995; 3(5):284–292.
4. Almekinders LC. Results following treatment of traumatic dislocations of the knee joint. Clin Orthop 1992; (284):203–207.
5. Sisto DJ, Warren RF. Complete knee dislocation: a follow-up study of operative treatment. Clin Orthop 1985; 198:94–101.

6. McCoy GF. Vascular injury associated with low-velocity dislocations of the knee. J Bone Joint Surg Br 1987; 69(2):285–287.
7. Shields L, Mital M, Cave EF. Complete dislocation of the knee: experience at the Massachusetts General Hospital. J Trauma 1969; 6:192–212.
8. Meyers MH, Moore TM, Harvey JP. Traumatic dislocation of the knee joint. J Bone Joint Surg Am 1975; 57(3):430–433.
9. Taylor AR, Williams E. Traumatic dislocation of the knee. A report of forty-three cases with special reference to conservative treatment. J Bone Joint Surg Br 1972; 54(1):96–102.
10. Frassica FJ, Sim FH, Staeheli JW, Pairolero PC. Dislocation of the knee. Clin Orthop 1991; (263):200–205.
11. Meyers MH. Traumatic dislocation of the knee joint. A study of eighteen cases. J Bone Joint Surg 1971; 53(1):16–29.
12. Shelbourne KD, et al. Low-velocity knee dislocation. Orthop Rev 1991; 20(11):995–1004.
13. Shapiro MS, Freedman EL. Allograft reconstruction of the anterior and posterior cruciate ligaments after traumatic knee dislocation. Am J Sports Med 1995; 23(5):580–587.
14. Fanelli GC, et al. Arthroscopically assisted combined anterior and posterior cruciate ligament reconstruction. Arthroscopy 1996; 12(1):5–14.
15. Noyes FR. Reconstruction of the anterior and posterior cruciate ligaments after knee dislocation. Use of early protected postoperative motion to decrease arthrofibrosis. Am J Sports Med 1997; 25(5):626–634.
16. Wascher DC, et al. Reconstruction of the anterior and posterior cruciate ligaments after knee dislocation. Results using fresh-frozen nonirradiated allografts. Am J Sports Med 1999; 27(2):189–196.
17. Yeh WL, et al. Knee dislocation: treatment of high-velocity knee dislocation. J Trauma Inj Infect Cri Care 1999; 46(4):693–701.
18. Arnoczky SP. Replacement of the anterior cruciate ligament using a patellar tendon allograft. An experimental study. J Bone Joint Surg 1986; 68(3):376–385.
19. Jackson DW. Biologic incorporation of allograft anterior cruciate ligament replacements. Clin Orthop 1996; (324):126–133.
20. Harner CD. Allograft versus autograft anterior cruciate ligament reconstruction: 3- to 5-year outcome. Clin Orthop 1996; (324):134–144.
21. Indelicato PA. Clinical comparison of freeze-dried and fresh frozen patellar tendon allografts for anterior cruciate ligament reconstruction of the knee. Am J Sports Med 1990; 18(4):335–342.
22. Indelicato PA. The results of fresh-frozen patellar tendon allografts for chronic anterior cruciate ligament deficiency of the knee. Am J Sports Med 1992; 20(2):118–121.
23. Noyes FR. Reconstruction of the anterior cruciate ligament with human allograft. Comparison of early and later results. J Bone Joint Surg 1996; 78(4):524–537.
24. Shino K, Inoue M, Horibe S, Hamada M, Ono K. Am J Sports Med 1990; 18(5):457–465.
25. Harner CD, Hoher J, Vogrin TM. The effect of sectioning of the posterolateral structures on the in situ forces in the human posterior cruciate ligament. Trans Orthop Res Soc 1998; 23:47.
26. Clancy WG Jr. Treatment of knee joint instability secondary to rupture of the posterior cruciate ligament. Report of a new procedure. J Bone Joint Surg 1983; 65(3):310–322.
27. Kusayama T, Harner CD, Carlin GJ, Xerogeanes JW, Smith BA. Anatomical and biomechanical characteristics of human meniscofemoral ligaments. Knee Surg Sports Traumatol Arthros 1994; 2(4):234–237.
28. Harner CD. Evaluation and treatment of posterior cruciate ligament injuries. Am J Sports Med 1998; 26(3):471–482.
29. Harner CD. The human posterior cruciate ligament complex: an interdisciplinary study. Ligament morphology and biomechanical evaluation. Am J Sports Med 1995; 23(6):736–745.
30. Bullis DW. Reconstruction of the posterior cruciate ligament with allograft. Clin Sports Med 1994; 13(3):581–597.
31. Fu FH, Bennett CH, Latterman C, Ma CB. Current trends in anterior cruciate ligament reconstruction. 1: Biology and biomechanics of reconstruction. Am J Sports Med 1999; 27(6):821–830.

Chapter Seven

Surgical Treatment of Acute and Chronic ACL/PCL/Lateral Side Injuries of the Knee

Daniel C. Wascher

Dislocation of the knee usually involves injury to both the anterior and posterior cruciate ligaments; associated collateral ligament injuries are common. Knee dislocations with injury to the posterolateral structures are among the most challenging problems that orthopaedic surgeons will encounter. In the acute setting, these injuries can present as frank dislocations or after spontaneous reduction. Late presentation involves chronic complex instability patterns in nonoperatively treated patients or following failed surgical treatment. Knee dislocations can be classified based on the anatomic injury pattern.[1] This chapter addresses the management of injuries classified as KDIIIL (see Chapter 3, Table 3.1), with the focus on evaluation and management of the posterolateral injury.

Anatomy

A thorough understanding of the posterolateral knee anatomy is essential to diagnosing and treating posterolateral injuries. The posterolateral anatomy is complex and variable. To make matters worse, different nomenclature has been applied to the structures of the posterolateral corner. The posterolateral structures have been divided into three layers.[2] Layer I consists of the iliotibial tract with its anterior expansion, and the superficial portion of the biceps femoris tendon and its expansion posteriorly. Layer II includes the quadriceps retinaculum anteriorly; posteriorly layer II is incomplete and is represented by the two patellofemoral ligaments and the patellomeniscal ligament. Layer III includes the lateral or fibular collateral ligament (LCL), the popliteofibular ligament, and the posterolateral capsule, which includes the arcuate ligament and the fabellofibular ligament (Figure 7.1). The LCL is the smallest of the four major knee ligaments. It arises from a fovea located immediately posterior to the ridge of the lateral epicondyle and inserts onto a superiorly and laterally facing V-shaped plateau on the fibular head.[3] In cross section, it is elliptically shaped, with the major diameter in the anterior-to-posterior direction averaging 3.4 mm and an average medial–lateral diameter of 2.3 mm.[3] The popliteofibular ligament shares a femoral origin with the popliteus tendon anterior to the LCL insertion on the epicondyle; however, it attaches posterior to the LCL on the fibular head.[4] In cross-sectional area, the popliteofibular ligament is only slightly smaller than the LCL.[4] The posterolateral capsule attaches to the tibia and femur circumferentially in horizontal planes. Posteriorly, the capsule divides into two laminae.[2] The superficial lamina encompasses the

Fig. 7.1. Oblique view of the posterolateral structures of the knee. Layers I and II have been removed. The components of layer III can be seen. (From Chen et al. © 2000, American Academy of Orthopaedic Surgeons. Reprinted from J Am Acad Orthop Surg 2000, Volume 8(2) pp. 97–110 with permission.)

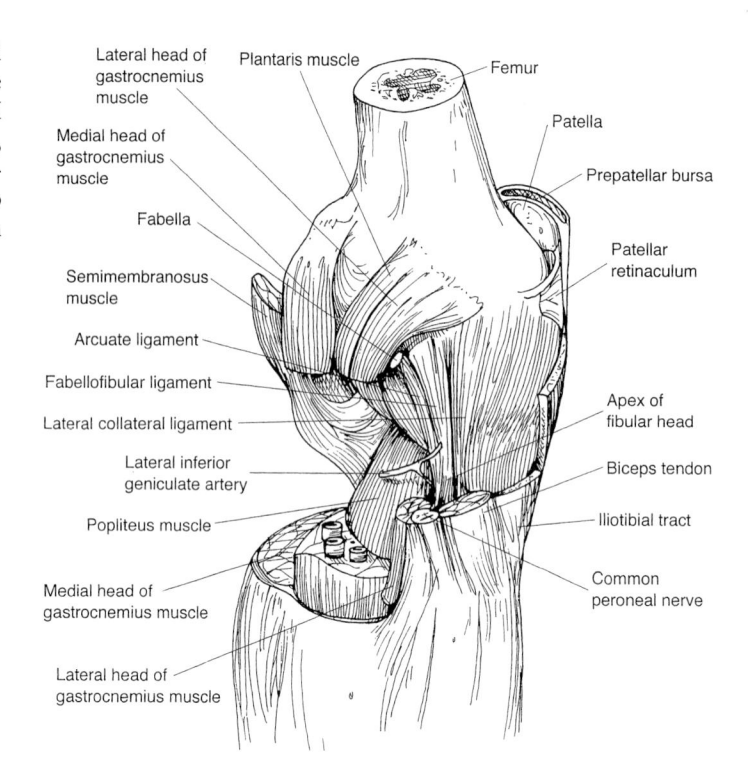

LCL; its posterior margin is an expansion known as the fabellofibular ligament. The deep lamina of layer III forms the coronary ligament, the capsular attachment to the outer edge of the lateral meniscus. The popliteus tendon courses through a hiatus in the coronary ligament to reach its femoral attachment. The deep lamina ends posteriorly at the arcuate ligament, a Y-shaped ligament that courses from the fibular styloid process and popliteus muscle to the posterolateral femur. Both the arcuate ligament and fabellofibular ligament are present in 67% of knee specimens; however, when a large fabella is present, the arcuate ligament tends to be absent and a large fabellofibular ligament is present. Conversely, if the fabella is absent, the fabellofibular ligament is absent and only the arcuate ligament is present.

The musculotendinous units on the lateral side of the knee include the iliotibial band, the biceps femoris tendon, and the popliteus tendon. The iliotibial band forms the superficial layer anterior to the intermuscular septum and inserts distally on the anterolateral tibia at Gerdy's tubercle. The biceps femoris tendon is also located in layer I but is posterior to the intermuscular septum; its insertion is primarily into the posterolateral edge of the fibular head, but it has additional attachments to the tibia, capsule, iliotibial tract, and lateral collateral ligament.[5] The popliteus muscle arises from the posterior aspect of the proximal tibia and courses around the lateral side of the knee. Its tendon travels through the popliteus hiatus of the lateral meniscus, deep to the LCL to insert anterior to the lateral epicondyle. Injuries to any or all of these musculotendinous structures can occur in dislocated knees with posterolateral ligament injuries.

Biomechanics

The functions of the posterolateral complex of the knee have been well described by several authors.[4,6–8] Isolated sectioning of all posterolateral structures causes increased varus and external rotation laxity that is greatest at 30° flexion. A small increase in posterior translation is seen. A coupled external rotation with posterior translation also occurs after isolated posterolateral sectioning. Additional cutting of the posterior cruciate ligament causes a further increase in varus and external rotation laxity and a marked increase in posterior translation. Combined sectioning of the anterior cruciate ligament (ACL) and the posterolateral corner causes increased internal rotation laxity at 30 and 60°. The popliteofibular ligament has a load to failure of 425 N compared with 750 N for the LCL.[4] However, the popliteofibular ligament does play an important role in resisting posterior translation, varus bending, and external rotation forces.[9,10] In situ forces in the posterolateral structures resulting from posterior tibial loading are greatest at full extension; sectioning of the posterior cruciate ligament (PCL) increased posterolateral forces at all angles of knee flexion.[11] Complete sectioning of the posterolateral structures increases the forces seen by the native cruciate ligaments and on ACL and PCL grafts.[12–14] Unrecognized or inadequately treated posterolateral corner injury in the dislocated knee can lead to failure of cruciate ligament reconstructions.

History

Knee dislocations with posterolateral injuries are usually caused by severe hyperextension, a severe varus bending moment, or a severe external rotation torque.[15–17] Knee dislocations with associated posterolateral injuries are more commonly high energy dislocations but can result from lower energy mechanisms.[18] Patients present acutely with severe pain, swelling, and instability. Patients usually describe gross deformity of the knee, although 50% of dislocated knees initially present reduced.[18] Peroneal nerve injuries occur more commonly in KDIIIL and KDIV injuries, and a history of numbness or foot drop should be sought. The associated trauma in patients with high energy dislocations may preclude a detailed history. The physician should maintain a high index of suspicion of knee ligament injury in trauma patients. Patients with chronic combined cruciate and posterolateral laxity usually are unable to perform sporting activities and frequently describe knee instability with activities of daily living.

Physical Examination

All patients with high energy dislocations should undergo a thorough physical examination to identify associated injuries. A careful neurovascular exam including ankle–brachial indices (ABI) should be performed on all dislocated knees at initial presentation and after reduction. Patients with absent or diminished pedal pulses should have immediate vascular consultation and/or arteriography. Arteriography should not excessively delay surgical exploration. Since intact pulses do not preclude delayed vascular compromise, patients with intact pulses should undergo frequent serial examinations for 48 h. Arteriography should be performed in all patients with ABIs below 0.8, neurologic injury, or associated trauma that prevents serial examinations.[19–21] Motor and sensory examination of the peroneal and tibial nerves should be documented pre- and postreduction. The physician should have a low threshold for measuring compartment pressures in dislocated knees.

Examination of the dislocated knee should include evaluation of the skin to identify open dislocations that require immediate debridement and

Fig. 7.2. Spin test. The patient is placed prone with the knee flexed at 30°. The feet are externally rotated by the examiner. The thigh–foot axis is measured, and the injured side is compared with the uninjured side. The spin test is considered to be positive if external rotation on the injured side is 10° or more greater than that on the normal side. The test can also be performed at 90° of knee flexion to detect combined posterior cruciate ligament and posterolateral corner injuries. [From Veltri and Warren[22] © 1993, American Academy of Orthopaedic Surgeons. Reprinted from J Am Acad Orthop Surg 1993, Volume 1 (2) pp. 67–75 with permission.]

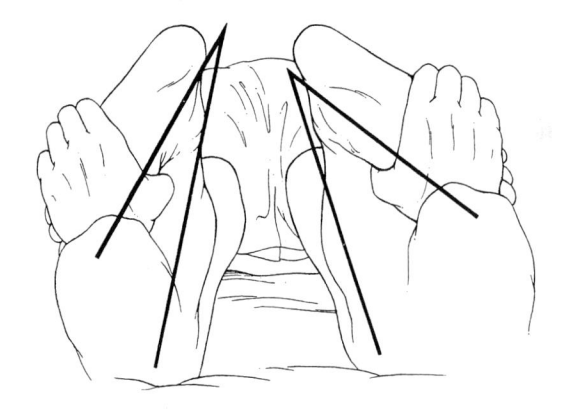

compromised skin that may necessitate a delay in surgical treatment of the ligament injury. The examiner should record active and passive range of motion and carefully look for avulsions of the biceps femoris tendon and iliotibial band. Finally, a careful examination of all knee ligaments should be performed after reduction has been achieved. A Lachman test and posterior drawer are used to assess the ACL and PCL, respectively. Large posterior displacements or coupled external rotation with posterior drawer forces should alert the examiner to the possibility of a posterolateral corner injury. Varus and valgus stress test at 30° flexion will assess the laxity of the posterolateral complex and the medial collateral ligament (MCL), respectively. Increased external rotation laxity in isolated posterolateral corner injuries is assessed by the spin test at 30° (Figure 7.2).[22] Increased external rotation laxity at 90° is indicative of combined posterior cruciate and posterolateral corner injuries. The external rotation recurvatum test identifies combined ACL and posterolateral corner injuries.[23] This test is performed by grasping the great toes of the supine patient and gently lifting the feet. In a positive test, the injured knee will go into hyperextension and the tibia will simultaneously externally rotate. The reverse pivot shift occurs when there is reduction of the lateral tibial plateau when the flexed, externally rotated knee is extended with a valgus load.[24] A positive reverse pivot shift indicates injury to the posterolateral corner. Lower extremity alignment and gait should be assessed in patients with chronic posterolateral injuries to detect the presence of varus alignment, a varus thrust, or a hyperextension gait pattern.[25]

Imaging Studies

Anterior–posterior (AP) and lateral radiographs of the knee should be made on all patients with knee dislocations. Radiographs made prior to reduction have a higher chance of demonstrating bony avulsions; however, the availability of radiographs should not cause undue delay in reducing a dislocated knee. After reduction, AP, lateral, oblique, and patellofemoral views should be obtained to again look for bony avulsions and to confirm adequate reduction. Radiographic signs of posterolateral corner injuries include fibular head avulsions and lateral joint opening (Figure 7.3). Fibular head avulsions can involve the attachments of the lateral collateral ligament, the popliteo-

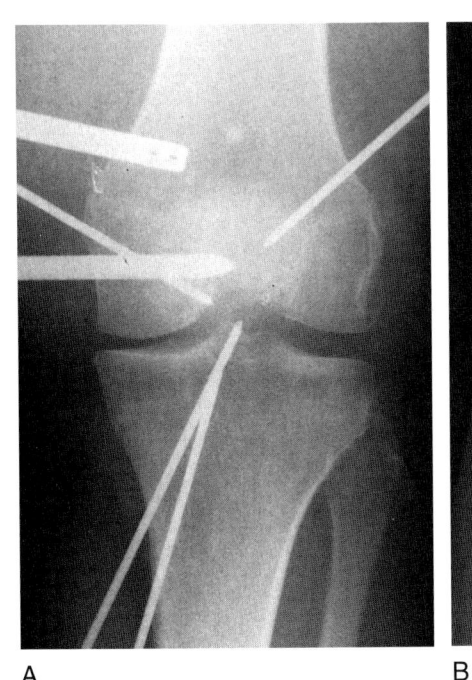

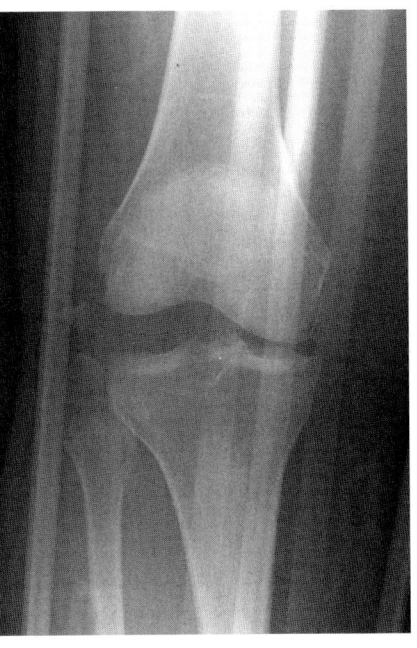

Fig. 7.3. Anteroposterior radiographs of a 49-year-old man who tripped and fell in his bedroom. (A) Prereduction x-rays show a medial knee dislocation. Bony fragments can be seen off the fibular head. (B) Postreduction x-rays show a marked varus opening of the joint and several large bony fragments on the fibular head, which represents avulsion of the lateral collateral ligament and the biceps femoris tendon.

fibular ligament, and/or the biceps femoris tendon. Avulsion of Gerdy's tubercle indicates injury to the iliotibial band insertion.

Magnetic resonance imaging (MRI) can assist the surgeon in preoperative planning and should be obtained in all patients with knee dislocations.[26–29] MRI can identify PCL peel-off injuries that may be amenable to repair rather then reconstruction. MR images can also identify the location of the lateral collateral ligament tear, the presence of biceps tendon, popliteal tendon, or iliotibial band tears, and the presence of meniscal tears. The accuracy of MRI has been shown to be high (>85%) for lateral collateral ligament, posterolateral capsule, and tendon injuries but less accurate for diagnosing popliteofibular ligament injuries (68%).[26] Secondary signs of posterolateral injury include separation of the coronary ligaments of the lateral meniscus and a bony contusion on the anteromedial femoral condyle or medial tibial plateau (Figure 7.4).[28]

Stress radiographs are useful in evaluating patients with chronic posterolateral injuries. Varus and valgus stress should be applied at 30° flexion; comparison views can also be obtained. Smaller amounts of lateral joint opening indicate partially functioning posterolateral ligaments. Gross lateral joint opening indicates nonfunctional posterolateral structures (Figure 7.5). Medial compartment narrowing from accelerated chondral wear can also be identified. Long-leg alignment films should be obtained in patients with chronic posterolateral injuries. A varus mechanical axis can cause increased stress on the posterolateral structures and ultimately failure of a posterolateral reconstruction.

Initial Management

Patients with high energy knee dislocations may have remote injuries that take precedence over the knee dislocation: aggressive treatment of the extremity is required to prevent amputation and to allow the best chance for functional recovery of the injured knee. Patients with frank dislocation

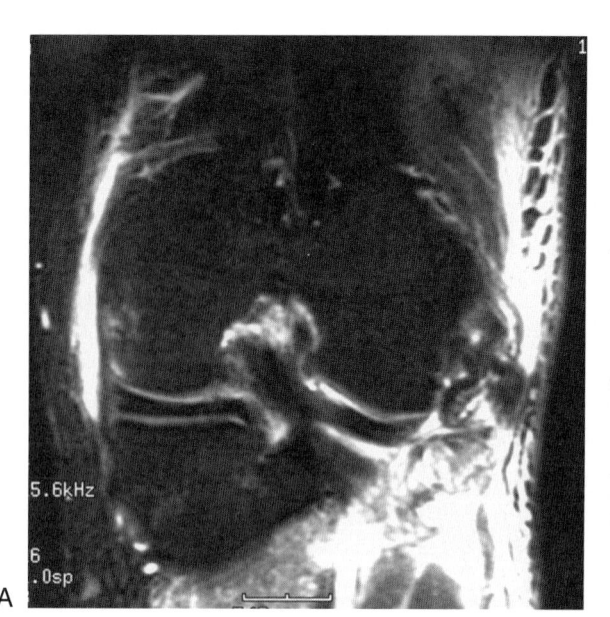

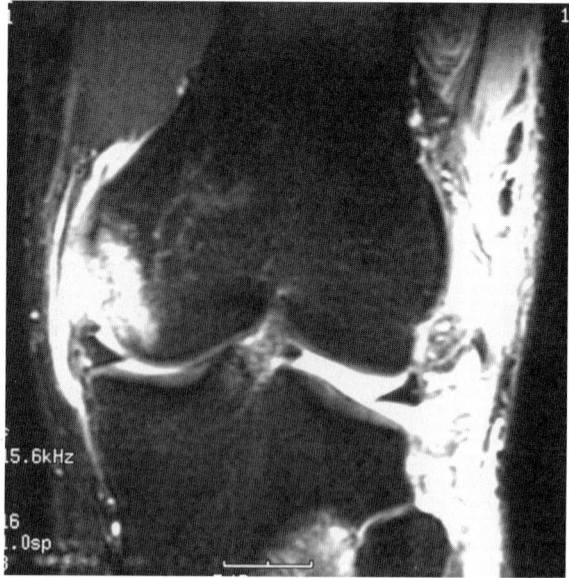

Fig. 7.4. STIR [short-term tau inversion recovery] MR coronal images of a 29-year-old male who sustained a severe varus injury in a mountain bike accident. (A) Complete disruption of the lateral collateral ligament and popliteus tendon. (B) Separation of the coronary ligaments and a contusion on the anterior medial femoral condyle, secondary signs of posterolateral corner injury.

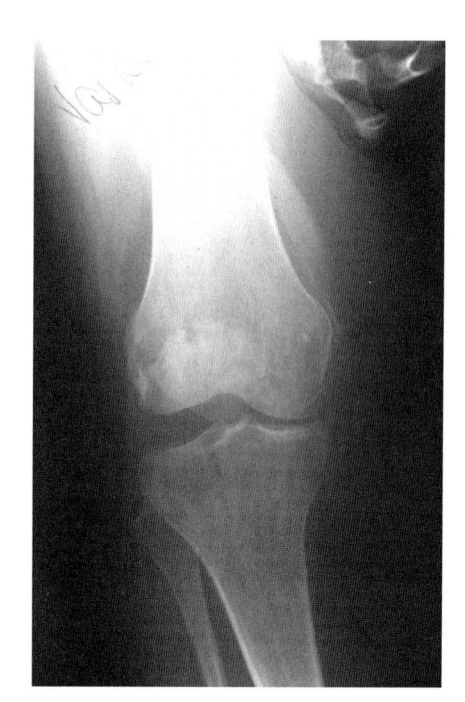

Fig. 7.5. Varus stress x-ray of a 49-year-old woman who had received nonoperative treatment for a severe knee injury in a motor vehicle accident 1 year. The varus stress x-ray demonstrates 14mm of lateral joint opening, indicating deficiency of the posterolateral structures. The patient was also found to have complete tears of both the anterior and posterior cruciate ligaments. At the time of injury, she also had a medial collateral ligament tear, which had healed with nonoperative treatment; there is a Pelligrini–Stieda lesion of the medial epicondyle.

of the knee should have urgent reduction of the joint. If the physician is unable to achieve a reduction, a closed or open reduction under anesthesia should be performed at the earliest opportunity. All vascular injuries need to be promptly identified and blood flow restored to the limb within 8h of injury.[30] Any suspicious leg compartments should have compartment pressures measured and, if indicated, fasciotomies performed. Open injuries require urgent irrigation and debridement. An external fixator that spans the knee joint is applied in patients with severe polytrauma, vascular repair, open dislocations, or dislocations that are grossly unstable after reduction. Otherwise the knee can be braced or splinted in 20° flexion. Serial radiographs should be obtained after splinting or external fixator placement to ensure that reduction is maintained.

Timing of Surgery

Patients treated nonoperatively usually have severe instability and functional disability; however, surgical treatment of the knee ligament injuries should be delayed until conditions are optimal for the patient and the surgeon. Patients with high energy dislocations should not undergo extensive knee surgery until they are able to participate in a rehabilitation program. MR imaging will help plan the operative approach. Allograft tissue should be available for cruciate ligament reconstruction. The surgical team should be experienced in knee ligament reconstruction and well rested when the procedure is begun.

If there are no contraindications, knee dislocations with posterolateral injuries are best treated within 7 days of injury. Bony avulsions are best repaired early and can yield very good results if anatomic reduction and internal fixation are obtained. Surgical dissection of the posterolateral structures becomes increasingly difficult more than 2 weeks postinjury, and eventually primary repair of the posterolateral ligaments is not possible.[31] The results of early surgery of the dislocated knee and posterolateral corner injuries are superior to those of late reconstructive procedures.[16,31–34]

Sometimes the condition of the patient or the affected extremity prohibits early knee ligament surgery. In these cases, external fixation or bracing can maintain the overall alignment of the knee joint during the waiting period. To minimize the risk of arthrofibrosis, an external fixator that spans the knee joint should not be used longer than 6 weeks. An attempt should be made to achieve full range of motion prior to reconstruction of chronic posterolateral instability. Knee hyperextension gait abnormalities should be corrected prior to surgery.[25] In patients with chronic PLC injuries, advancement or reconstruction of the posterolateral structures must be performed. The integrity of the semitendinosus and biceps femoris tendons must be assessed if these autografts are being considered for posterolateral reconstruction. Despite many difficulties, late surgery for chronic instability can improve objective stability and the functional status of most patients.[31,35–37]

Treatment Principles

When surgery is undertaken, the surgeon should repair or reconstruct all injured knee ligaments.[38,39] Failure to address all ligament deficiencies at the index procedure causes increased loads on the repaired/reconstructed ligaments.[12,13] A careful examination under anesthesia should be performed to accurately assess the knee laxity patterns. A diagnostic arthroscopy should be performed prior to any open procedures. Arthroscopy yields additional information about the cruciate and posterolateral injuries and allows treatment of meniscal and chondral pathology.[37,40] Because multiple grafts must be obtained in these knees that have already sustained severe trauma, allografts should be utilized for reconstruction of the ACL and PCL.[39,41–43] The surgeon can use two Achilles tendon allografts, a whole patellar tendon allograft divided into two bone–patellar tendon–bone (BPTB) grafts, or one Achilles tendon and one hemipatellar tendon allograft. Using an Achilles tendon allograft facilitates arthroscopic passage of the PCL graft; a patellar tendon allograft offers the advantage of interference fixation on both ends of the graft. A two-tunnel technique for the PCL reconstruction will minimize the need for additional surgical dissection. Autograft (biceps femoris or semitendinosus tendon) or allograft can be used if reconstruction of the LCL is necessary. A tourniquet should be utilized to minimize blood loss and to facilitate surgical dissection. Patients who have undergone vascular repair or have evidence of an intimal flap tear should receive a 5000-unit bolus of heparin prior to tourniquet inflation.

A surgical approach to the posterolateral structures has been described that provides access to all potentially injured posterolateral structures.[44] An extended curvilinear incision is made that overlies the lateral epicondyle and is centered distally between Gerdy's tubercle and the anterior aspect of the fibular head. This exposes the superficial fascia of the iliotibial tract and the biceps femoris. Three fascial incisions are then made. The first is along the posterior aspect of the biceps femoris muscle and tendon parallel to the peroneal nerve. The peroneal nerve is identified, mobilized, and marked with vessel loops to allow retraction and prevent iatrogenic injury. This incision then allows access to the popliteus muscle, the tibial attachments of the posterolateral capsule, and the lateral gastrocnemius muscle. A second fascial incision is made in the interval between the superior aspect of the biceps femoris and the posterior aspect of the iliotibial tract. Dissection in this interval gives exposure to the distal attachments of the LCL and popliteofibular ligaments and the posterolateral capsule. The third fascial incision splits the iliotibial tract over the lateral epicondyle and is extended to Gerdy's tubercle. This provides assess to the proximal attachments of the

LCL and popliteofibular ligament as well as the femoral attachments of the posterolateral capsule. If needed, a capsular incision is made parallel to the LCL at the anterior aspect of the fibular head to allow inspection of the anterolateral capsule, lateral meniscus, and proximal popliteal tendon. Following repair or reconstruction, the capsular and fascial incisions are closed.

Acute Repairs/Reconstruction

After an initial diagnostic arthroscopy, an open approach is utilized in acute repair/reconstructions. Arthroscopic surgery for the cruciate ligaments can be lengthy, and there is often fluid extravasation through the posterolateral capsule injury. The cruciate ligaments are approached via an anteromedial arthrotomy. Avulsions of the cruciate ligaments can be repaired with sutures through bony tunnels or, in the case of large bony fragments, with a compression screw. Most commonly, the cruciate ligament injuries are midsubstance, and the surgeon must perform ACL and PCL reconstructions. The ACL and PCL stumps are debrided and a notchplasty performed. Guide pins for the cruciate tunnels are drilled in the following order: PCL tibial tunnel, ACL tibial tunnel, ACL femoral tunnel, and PCL femoral tunnel. Since the ACL and PCL tibial tunnels are divergent, both can be located on the anteromedial tibial surface; a 1 cm bridge of bone should be between them. The PCL tibial insertion can be accessed through the posterolateral capsule tear to aid in guide pin placement. Intraoperative radiographs or fluoroscopy will confirm pin placement (Figure 7.6).

When proper pin placement has been achieved, the tunnels are drilled in the reverse order. Care must be taken to protect the popliteal artery by placing a curette over the tip of the PCL tibial pin prior to drilling. A Gore-Tex smoother helps chamfer the edges of the PCL tunnel and facilitates graft passage. The grafts are passed and fixed on the femoral side. Tibial fixation is achieved after dissection of the posterolateral structures. The PCL graft tibial fixation is performed with the knee in 90° flexion while reproducing

Fig. 7.6. Intraoperative radiographs after pin placement for combined anterior and posterior cruciate reconstruction. (A) Anteroposterior view. (B) Lateral view.

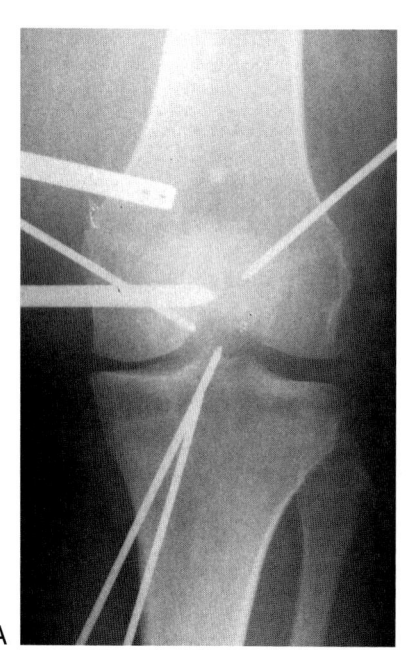

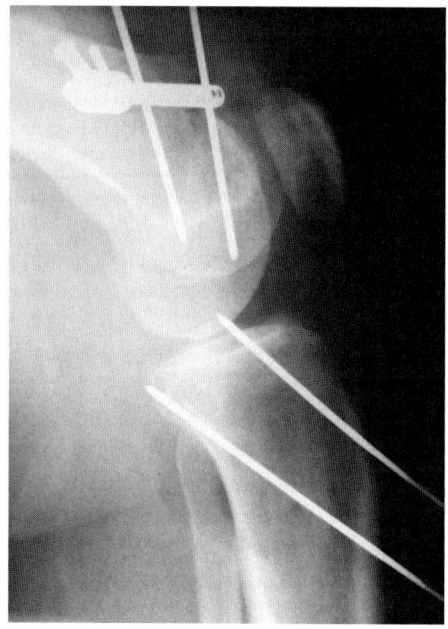

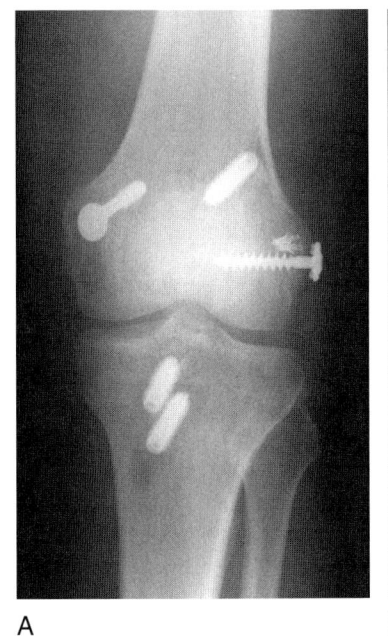

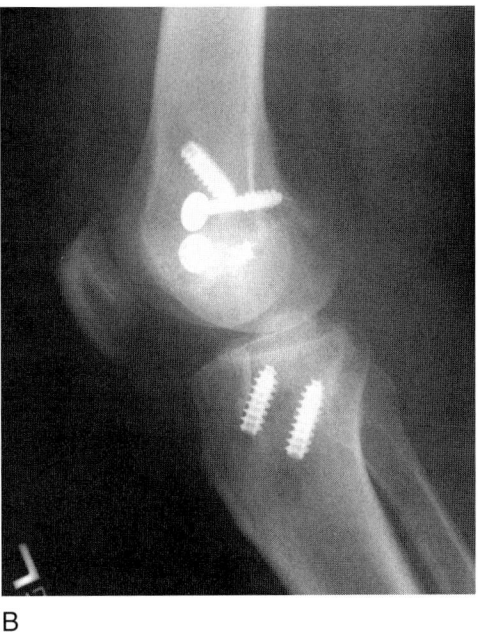

7. Surgery for ACL/PCL/Lateral Side Knee Injuries

Fig. 7.7. (A) Anteroposterior and (B) lateral radiographs of a 39-year-old man who was involved in a motor vehicle accident: Films taken 6 months after allograft reconstruction of the anterior and posterior cruciate ligaments and repair of the posterolateral corner. The patient had proximal avulsion of the lateral collateral ligament that was repaired with a soft tissue screw and washer. Avulsion of the posterolateral capsule off the femur was repaired with suture anchors.

the normal tibiofemoral step-off. The knee is brought into 10° flexion and the ACL graft fixed on the tibia.

The posterolateral structures are then approached as just outlined. The LCL and popliteofibular ligaments are frequently torn directly off the femur or the fibular head.[15,16,33] Dissection is begun at the intact attachment site as indicated by MRI. Proximal avulsions are best repaired with a screw and soft tissue washer (Figure 7.7). Fibular avulsions are repaired with sutures through drill holes or with suture anchors. Midsubstance ruptures are sutured end to end, but if the repair is not satisfactory they may require augmentation with a biceps tenodesis or allograft as outlined shortly. Large bony avulsions of the fibular head can be anatomically fixed with a screw (Figure 7.8). The posterolateral capsule is usually torn off as a sleeve of the femur or tibia. A series of suture anchors can be placed to reapproximate the capsule. Tendon avulsions are repaired using sutures through bone tunnels or suture anchors. Musculotendinous ruptures are primarily sutured. Final fixation of the posterolateral structures should be performed after fixation of the cruciate ligaments. The posterolateral repair is secured with the knee in 30° flexion with a valgus stress.

Published results of acute surgical treatment of ACL-PCL-LCL injuries are limited to small numbers usually grouped with other ligament injury patterns. In Baker's series on primary repair of acute combined PCL and posterolateral knee injuries, 8 of the 13 knees had associated ACL injuries.[32] Baker and his collaborators stated, "no knee can be rated as excellent following such extensive injury," but they reported good results in most knees. DeLee et al. reported a series of patients who underwent primary repair for ACL-PCL-LCL injuries, a condition they termed "acute straight lateral instability of the knee."[33] Of the 7 patients available for follow-up, results were as follows: 4 good, 2 fair, and 1 poor. In a series of patients with LCL injuries, Grana and Janssen included 5 patients with ACL-PCL-LCL injuries.[16] Only 2 patients treated with acute repair were available for follow-up, and both had satisfactory results. More recent studies have included patients undergoing combined allograft ACL/PCL reconstruction and posterolateral corner repair using techniques similar to that described

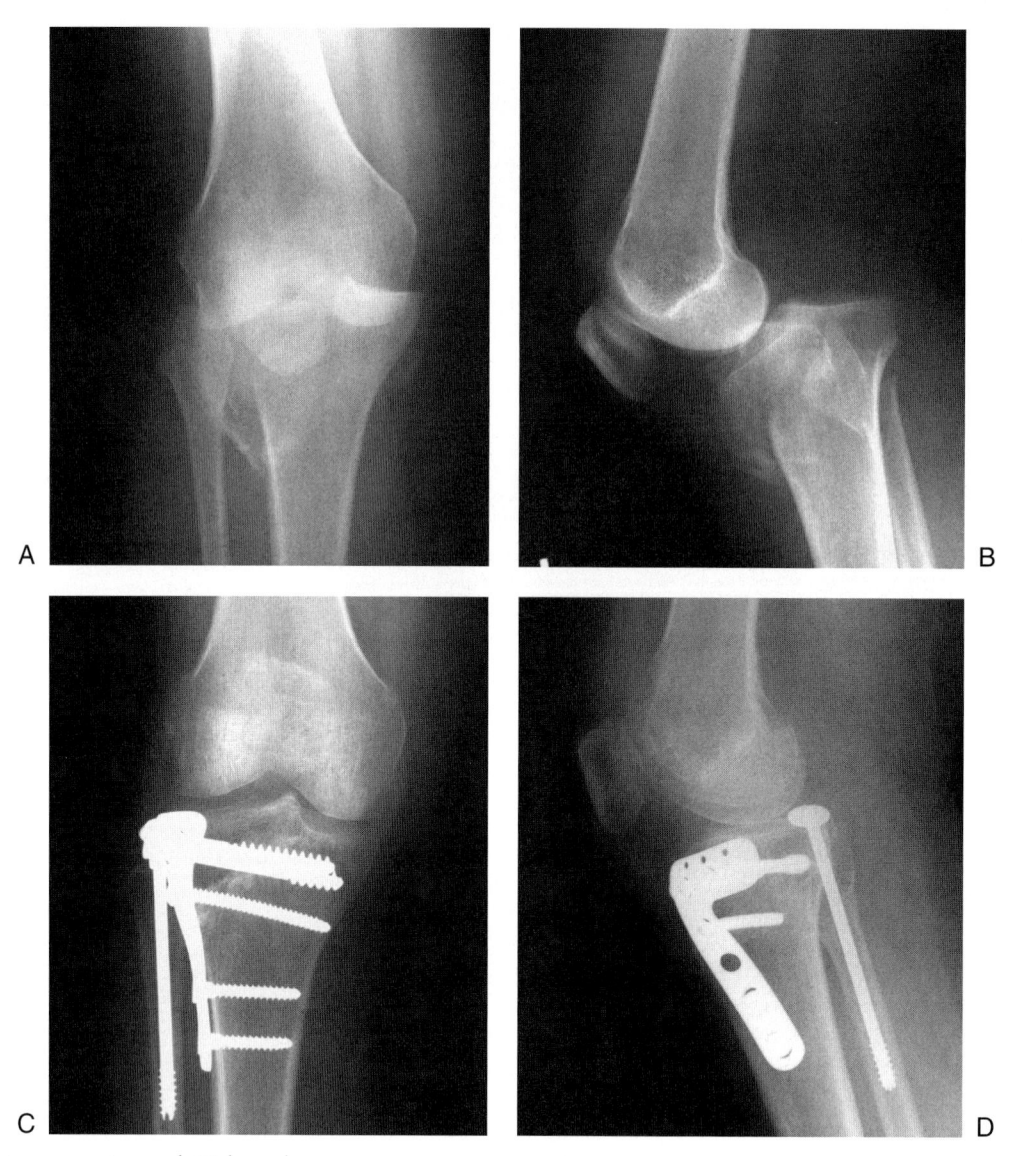

Fig. 7.8. (A) Anteroposterior and (B) lateral injury films of a 42-year-old female who was involved in a motor vehicle accident. The injury x-rays demonstrate a fracture dislocation of the knee (KDV). Note the fracture and displacement of the fibular head. (C) Anteroposterior and (D) lateral postoperative radiographs after fixation of the lateral tibial plateau and open reduction internal fixation of the fibular head with a 6.5 mm screw and washer.

earlier.[39,42,43] Of the 8 patients with acute ACL-PCL-LCL injuries described in these studies, 7 had no varus instability and 1 had 1+ laxity. Although sample sizes are small, acute primary repair of posterolateral structures in the dislocated knee appears to restore functional stability in the majority of patients.

Chronic Reconstructions

Patients with chronic posterolateral instability will occasionally have medial compartment degenerative changes that cause a varus mechanical alignment. These patients should have a high tibial osteotomy performed to correct the mechanical axis to slight valgus prior to any ligament reconstruction. Fixation of the osteotomy should be performed to avoid interfering with future cruciate tunnel placement. The osteotomy fixation may need to be removed prior to ligament surgery.

For chronic reconstructions, the cruciate ligaments are reconstructed as already described for acute injuries. Chronic injuries are more amenable to arthroscopic cruciate reconstruction because the lateral capsular injury has sealed. Allografts are still preferred because of the number of grafts needed for reconstruction. A variety of procedures have been described to address chronic posterolateral laxity. These included posterolateral advancement or posterolateral reconstruction by means of autograft or allograft.

If the posterolateral complex is structurally intact but lax, then a posterolateral advancement can be performed.[31,37] Hughston and Jacobson described advancing the femoral attachment of the LCL, popliteus complex, and lateral head of the gastrocnemius tendon.[31] An osteotome is used to create a bone flap from the lateral epicondyle, preserving the aforementioned soft tissue attachments. With the knee flexed 90°, this bone flap is advanced anteriorly and distally and is then fixed under tension to a prepared site on the femur by means of a Stone staple. Hughston and Jacobson reported 85% good results in 95 patients when this posterolateral advancement technique was used.[31] Noyes and Barber-Westin described a modification of the posterolateral advancement.[37] They also described the advance of a bony wafer containing the femoral attachments of the LCL, popliteus complex, and lateral half of the lateral gastrocnemius tendon. These authors recommended that the bony wafer be advanced in a proximal direction along the course of the LCL. They also recommended tensioning the posterolateral complex at 30° of flexion and ensuring that the inferior margin of the staple is at the anatomic attachment site of the LCL to restore normal length. Noyes and Barber-Westin reported on 21 patients who had undergone the posterolateral advancement in combination with ACL and/or PCL reconstruction.[37] The posterolateral complex was graded "functional" in 64%, "partially functional" in 27%, and "a failure" in 9%. Posterolateral advancement improves posterolateral laxity in the majority of patients with a structurally intact but lax posterolateral complex.

If the posterolateral structures are irreparable or deficient, a posterolateral reconstruction of the LCL and/or popliteofibular ligament must be performed by means of autograft[22,45,46] or allograft.[36,47] Clancy and Sutherland have described a reconstruction of the lateral collateral ligament in which the biceps femoris tendon is tenodesed to the lateral femoral epicondyle.[46] The use of the biceps tenodesis has been criticized for not reconstructing the popliteofibular ligament, but it has been shown to decrease varus and external rotation laxity in vitro and in vivo.[35,48] The technique involves mobilizing the biceps tendon and attaching it proximally to the lateral epicondyle with a screw and soft tissue washer. Tensioning and fixation is performed with the knee in 30° flexion, tibial internal rotation, and a valgus load applied to the knee. Although the original description entailed the entire biceps tendon, this completely removes an important dynamic stabilizer from the lateral side of the knee; therefore, the technique has been modified to use half or a central slip of the biceps tendon to perform the tenodesis.[22] Fanelli and his colleagues have reported on 11 patients who underwent a biceps tenodesis at the time of ACL and PCL reconstruction,[41] and 21 patients who underwent biceps tenodesis at the time of PCL reconstruction.[35] They noted that varus and external rotation laxity were corrected or overcorrected in all patients who underwent a biceps tenodesis.

Because of the concern that the biceps tenodesis may remove an important lateral dynamic stabilizer and because, on occasion, a biceps tendon avulsion renders this approach unavailable, several other posterolateral reconstructions have been described. Noyes and Barber-Westin reported on a technique that uses a circle allograft to reconstruct the LCL.[36] A strip of

Achilles tendon allograft 6 to 7 mm in diameter is prepared to a length of 20 cm. A drill hole is made through the fibular head, and a tunnel is fashioned beneath the LCL insertion on the lateral epicondyle. The allograft is passed through the tunnels forming a circle around the old LCL. With the knee in 30° flexion, the allograft is tensioned and then sutured to itself and the remaining lateral collateral ligament tissue. The authors reported a success rate of 76% for this procedure.

Latimer et al. described a lateral collateral ligament reconstruction using bone–patellar tendon–bone allograft.[47] A 9 mm graft is placed by means of fixation tunnels in the fibular head and at the isometric point on the femur. The allograft is secured with interference screws. The authors reported that 9 of 10 patients who underwent this procedure had correction of excessive external rotation at 30°. Six patients had no varus laxity, and 4 had mild residual varus laxity. The authors felt that in addition to replacing the LCL, the increased bulk of the reconstruction may have substituted for the popliteofibular and arcuate ligaments.

Other surgical techniques have focused on reconstruction of the popliteus complex. Albright and Brown described a posterolateral sling procedure that approximates the popliteus tendon to correct posterolateral instability.[45] The technique involves drilling a tibial guide pin beginning near Gerdy's tubercle and exiting 1 cm below the tibial articular surface and 1 cm medial to the proximal tibiofibular articulation. The guide pin is then reamed to create a tunnel 6 to 8 mm in diameter. An 18 cm long graft is fashioned by using iliotibial band autograft or Achilles or iliotibial band allograft. The graft is passed through the tibial tunnel in an anterior-to-posterior direction and then brought up to an isometric point slightly superior and anterior to the femoral attachment of the LCL. The graft is fixed to the anterior tibia and lateral femoral epicondyle by means of screws and soft tissue washers. Albright and Brown reported on the results of the posterolateral sling procedure in 30 patients. Twenty-nine patients underwent concomitant ACL reconstruction; 5 had PCL reconstruction, and 7 had LCL reconstruction. The sling procedure eliminated posterolateral instability in 87% of patients, although only 53% achieved knees that were stable in all directions. Veltri and Warren have also described a reconstruction of the popliteus complex.[22] This technique involves using a split graft in which both the popliteofibular ligament and the tibial attachment of the popliteus are reconstructed. The graft is attached proximally at the popliteus insertion on the lateral femoral epicondyle. One limb of the graft travels through a posterior-to-anterior tunnel in the fibular head; the other limb courses through a tibial tunnel similar to the posterolateral sling reconstruction. No clinical results on this procedure have been published.

I prefer a selective approach to patients with posterolateral instability. If the posterolateral structures are intact but lax, a posterolateral advancement is performed, using the technique described by Noyes and Barber-Westin. If the posterolateral structures are insufficient and the biceps tendon is intact, a biceps tenodesis is performed. Only half of the biceps tendon is used, to maintain the tendon's role as a dynamic stabilizer of the lateral aspect of the knee. This is a relatively easy procedure to perform, and, while it does not reconstruct the popliteofibular ligament, it eliminates posterolateral instability in the majority of patients. If the biceps tendon is injured, I prefer to reconstruct the LCL by using the circle allograft technique. Again, this technique is simpler than most other techniques and restores posterolateral stability in the majority of patients.

a new technique in combined ligament injuries. Am J Sports Med 1998; 26:656–662.
48. Wascher DC, Grauer JD, Markoff KL. Biceps tendon tenodesis for posterolateral instability of the knee. An in vitro study. Am J Sports Med 1993; 21:400–406.
49. Meyers MJ, Moore TM, Harvey JP Jr. Follow-up notes on articles previously published in the journal: traumatic dislocation of the knee joint. J Bone Joint Surg Am 1975; 57:430–433.
50. Sisto DJ, Warren RF. Complete knee dislocation: a follow-up study of operative treatment. Clin Orthop 1985; 198:94–101.
51. Sedel L, Nizard RS. Nerve grafting for traction injuries of the common peroneal nerve. J Bone Joint Surg Br 1993; 75:772–774.

25. Noyes FR, Dunworth LA, Andriacchi TP, Andrews M, Hewett TE. Knee hyperextension gait abnormalities in unstable knees. Recognition and pre-operative gait retraining. Am J Sports Med 1996; 24:35–45.
26. LaPrade RF, Gilbert TJ, Bollom TS, Wentorf F, Chaljub G. The magnetic resonance imaging appearance of individual structures of the posterolateral knee. A prospective study of normal knees and knees with surgically verified grade III injuries. Am J Sports Med 2000; 28:191–199.
27. Reddy PK, Posteraro R, Schenck RC. The role of magnetic resonance imaging in evaluation of the cruciate ligaments in knee dislocations. Orthopaedics 1996; 19:165–169.
28. Ross G, Chapman AW, Newberg AR, Scheller AD Jr. Magnetic resonance imaging for the evaluation of acute posterolateral complex injuries of the knee. Am J Sports Med 1997; 169:1641–1647.
29. Twaddle BC, Hunter JC, Chapman JR, et al. MRI in acute knee dislocations: a prospective study of clinical, MRI and surgical findings. J Bone Joint Surg Br 1992; 127:1056–1063.
30. Green NE, Allen BL. Vascular injuries associated with dislocation of the knee. J Bone Joint Surg Am 1977; 70:88–97.
31. Hughston JC, Jacobson KE. Chronic posterolateral instability of the knee. J Bone Joint Surg Am 1985; 67:351–359.
32. Baker CL Jr, Norwood LA, Hughston JC. Acute combined posterior cruciate and posterolateral instability of the knee. Am J Sports Med 1984; 12:204–208.
33. DeLee JC, Riley MB, Rockwood CA Jr. Acute posterolateral rotatory instability of the knee. Am J Sports Med 1983; 11:199–207.
34. Waltrip RL, Bennett CH, Irrgang JJ, Harner CD. Surgical management of traumatic knee dislocation: Results of a standardized surgical approach. Poster presentation at: American Association of Orthopaedic Surgeons meeting; March 2001.
35. Fanelli GC, Giannotti BF, Edson CJ. Arthroscopically assisted combined posterior cruciate ligament/posterior lateral complex reconstruction. Arthroscopy 1996; 12:521–530.
36. Noyes FR, Barber-Westin SD. Surgical reconstruction of severe chronic posterolateral complex injuries of the knee using allograft tissues. Am J Sports Med 1995; 23:2–12.
37. Noyes FR, Barber-Westin SD. Surgical restoration to treat chronic deficiency of the posterolateral complex and cruciate ligaments of the knee joint. Am J Sports Med 1996; 24:415–426.
38. Veltri DM, Warren RF. Instructional Course Lecture, American Academy of Orthopaedic Surgeons. Posterolateral instability of the knee. J Bone Joint Surg Am 1994; 76:460–472.
39. Wascher DC, Becker JR, Dexter JG, et al. Reconstruction of the anterior and posterior cruciate ligaments after knee dislocation. Am J Sports Med 1999; 27:189–196.
40. LaPrade RF. Arthroscopic evaluation of the lateral compartment of knees with grade 3 posterolateral knee complex injuries. Am J Sports Med 1997; 25:596–602.
41. Fanelli GC, Giannotti BF, Edson CJ. Arthroscopically assisted combined anterior and posterior cruciate ligament reconstruction. Arthroscopy 1996; 12:5–14.
42. Noyes FR, Barber-Westin SD. Reconstruction of the anterior and posterior cruciate ligaments after knee dislocation. Am J Sports Med 1997; 25:769–778.
43. Shapiro MS, Freedman EL. Allograft reconstruction of the anterior and posterior cruciate ligaments after traumatic knee dislocation. Am J Sports Med 1995; 23:580–587.
44. Terry GC, LaPrade RF. The posterolateral aspect of the knee. Anatomy and surgical approach. Am J Sports Med 1996; 24:732–739.
45. Albright JP, Brown AW. Management of chronic posterolateral rotatory instability of the knee: surgical technique for the posterolateral corner sling procedure. Instr Course Lect 1998; 47:369–378.
46. Clancy WG Jr, Sutherland TB. Combined posterior cruciate ligament injuries. Clin Sports Med 1994; 13:629–647.
47. Latimer HA, Tibone JE, El. Attrache NS, McMahon PJ. Reconstruction of the lateral collateral ligament of the knee with patellar tendon allograft. Report of

2. Seebacher JR, Inglis AE, Marshall JL, Warren RF. The structure of the posterolateral aspect of the knee. J Bone Joint Surg Am 1982; 64:536–541.
3. Meister BR, Michael SP, Moyer RA, Kelly JD, Schneck CD. Anatomy and kinematics of the lateral collateral ligament of the knee. Am J Sports Med 2000; 28:869–878.
4. Maynard MJ, Deng X, Wickiewicz TL, Warren RF. The popliteofibular ligament. Rediscovery of a key element in posterolateral stability. Am J Sports Med 1996; 24:311–316.
5. Terry GC, LaPrade RF. The biceps femoris muscle complex at the knee. Its anatomy and injury patterns associated with acute anterolateral–anteromedial rotatory instability. Am J Sports Med 1996; 24:2–8.
6. Gollehon DL, Torzilli PA, Warren RF. The role of the posterolateral and cruciate ligaments in the stability of the human knee. A biomechanical study. J Bone Joint Surg Am 1987; 69:233–242.
7. Grood ES, Stowers SF, Noyes FR. Limits of movement in the human knee. Effect of sectioning the posterior cruciate ligament and posterolateral structures. J Bone Joint Surg Am 1988; 70:88–97.
8. Veltri DM, Deng XH, Torzilli PA, Warren RF, Maynard MJ. The role of the cruciate and posterolateral ligaments in stability of the knee. A biomechanical study. Am J Sports Med 1995; 23:436–443.
9. Veltri DM, Deng XH, Torzilli PA, Maynard MJ, Warren RF. The role of the popliteofibular ligament in stability of the human knee. A biomechanical study. Am J Sports Med 1996; 24:19–27.
10. Sugita T, Amis AA. Anatomic and biomechanical study of the lateral collateral and popliteofibular ligaments. Am J Sports Med 2001; 29:466–472.
11. Höher J, Harner CD, Vogrin TM, Baek GH, Carlin GJ, Woo SL-Y. *In situ* forces in the posterolateral structures of the knee under posterior tibial loading in the intact and posterior cruciate ligament-deficient knee. J Orthop Res 1998; 16:675–681.
12. Harner CD, Vogrin TM, Hoher J, Ma CB, Woo SL. Biomechanical analysis of a posterior cruciate ligament reconstruction. Deficiency of the posterolateral structures as a cause of graft failure. Am J Sports Med 2000; 28:32–39.
13. LaPrade RF, Resig S, Wentorf F, Lewis JL. The effects of grade III posterolateral knee complex injuries on anterior cruciate ligament graft force. A biomechanical analysis. Am J Sports Med 1999; 27:469–475.
14. Markoff KL, Wascher DC, Finerman GA. Direct in vitro measurement of forces in the cruciate ligaments. II: The effect of section of the posterolateral structures. J Bone Joint Surg Am 1993; 75:387–394.
15. Baker CL Jr, Norwood LA, Hughston JC. Acute posterolateral rotatory instability of the knee. J Bone Joint Surg Am 1983; 65:614–618.
16. Grana WA, Janssen T. Lateral ligament injury of the knee. Orthopedics 1987; 10:1039–1044.
17. LaPrade RF, Terry GC. Injuries to the posterolateral aspect of the knee. Association of anatomic injury patterns with clinical instability. Am J Sports Med 1997; 25:433–438.
18. Wascher DC, Dvirnak PC, DeCoster TA. Knee dislocation: initial assessment and implications for treatment. J Orthop Trauma 1997; 11:525–529.
19. Dennis JW, Jagger C, Butcher JL, et al. Reassessing the role of arteriograms in the management of posterior knee dislocations. J Trauma 1993; 35:692–697.
20. Kendall RW, Taylor DC, Salvia AJR, et al. The role of arteriography in assessing vascular injuries associated with dislocations of the knee. J Trauma 1993; 35:875–879.
21. Treiman GS, Yellin AE, Weaver FA. Examination of the patient with a knee dislocation: the case for selective arteriography. Arch Surg 1992; 127:1056–1063.
22. Veltri DM, Warren RF. Isolated and combined posterior cruciate ligament injuries. J Am Acad Orthop Surg 1993; 1:67–75.
23. Hughston JC, Norwood LA Jr. The posterolateral drawer test and external rotational recurvatum test for posterolateral instability of the knee. Clin Orthop 1980; 147:82–87.
24. Jakob RP, Hassler H, Stoeubli HU. Observations on rotatory instability of the lateral compartment of the knee: experimental studies on the functional anatomy and pathomechanism of the true and reverse pivot shift sign. Acta Orthop Scand 1981; 52(suppl):1–32.

Peroneal Nerve Injuries

The incidence of nerve injury in all knee dislocations is approximately 25% and probably even higher in ACL/PCL/LCL patterns.[18,49,50] The peroneal nerve is more commonly injured than the tibial nerve. Peroneal nerve injuries are usually severe axonotmesis over a long segment of nerve.[18,49] Occasionally, spontaneous nerve recovery will occur; however, more commonly, patients are left with complete or partial nerve palsies. There are reports of nerve recovery following neurolysis,[50] but other authors have had no improvement in peroneal nerve function with neurolysis.[18,49] The lengthy period of nerve injury that occurs with knee dislocations precludes attempts at resection and primary repair. Results of cable grafting of a nerve injury following knee dislocation have not been favorable.[51] Patients with chronic peroneal nerve palsy can have the resultant foot drop managed with an ankle–foot orthosis or with a tendon transfer.

Rehabilitation

Postoperatively, patients are kept non–weight bearing in a postoperative hinged knee brace for 6 weeks. The brace allows motion from 20 to 70°. The patient is allowed to achieve terminal extension out of the brace, but hyperextension is avoided to protect the posterolateral repair/reconstruction. At 6 weeks, full range of motion is allowed in a combined instability functional brace, and progressive weight bearing is begun. If range of motion is not satisfactory at 3 months, a closed manipulation under anesthesia is performed. A closed-chain exercise program is started at 6 weeks. Hip abduction exercises are avoided for 3 to 4 months to prevent a varus load on the posterolateral structures. At 4 to 6 months, open-chain exercises and impact loading are permitted. Agility training begins at 6 to 9 months, but many of these patients are unable to resume sporting activities because of concomitant injuries, peroneal nerve palsy, or residual knee instability.[31,32,36,39,41] A full return to unrestricted activities is discouraged before 1 year.

Conclusions

Combined ACL, PCL, and lateral side injuries of the knee present a difficult challenge for the surgeon. A thorough understanding of the posterolateral anatomy and biomechanics is important for diagnosis and treatment. Treatment should be directed at repairing or reconstructing all injured structures. Cruciate ligament avulsion should be repaired; midsubstance ruptures should be reconstructed with allograft. Primary repair of the lateral structures affords the best chance of a functionally stable knee. A variety of late reconstructive procedures for the posterolateral structures can be performed depending on the severity of the injury. Functional stability can be achieved in the majority of patients, but some patients will be unable to resume sporting activities. With current techniques, a "normal" knee should not be expected after this severe trauma. Injury to the peroneal nerve has a poor prognosis for complete recovery, even with surgical treatment.

References

1. Schenck RC Jr. The dislocated knee. Am Acad Ortho Surg Instr Course Lect 1994; 43:127–136.

Chapter Eight

Combined ACL/PCL/Medial/Lateral Side Injuries of the Knee

Gregory C. Fanelli

The multiple ligament injured knee is a complex problem in orthopaedic surgery. Such injuries may or may not present as acute knee dislocations, and careful assessment of the extremity vascular status is essential because of the possibility of arterial and/or venous compromise. These complex injuries require a systematic approach to evaluation and treatment. Physical examination and imaging studies enable the surgeon to make a correct diagnosis and formulate a treatment plan.

The incidence of injuries to the posterior cruciate ligament (PCL) is reported to be from 1 to 40% of acute knee injuries. This range, which is dependent on the patient population reported, is approximately 3% in the general population and 38% in reports from regional trauma centers.[1-3] Our practice at a regional trauma center has a 38.3% incidence of posterior cruciate ligament tears in acute knee injuries, and 56.5% of these PCL injuries occur in multiple trauma patients. Of these PCL injuries, 45.9% are combined of the anterior cruciate ligament (ACL) and the PCL, while 41.2% are PCL/posterolateral corner tears. Only 3% of acute PCL injuries seen in the trauma center are isolated. This chapter identifies trends that occur with combined ACL/PCL injuries and presents a treatment strategy for these injuries. The reader is referred to other literature that we have published for additional information on this topic.[4-12]

Classification of the Multiple Ligament Injured Knee

Combined ACL/PCL injuries may or may not present as acute knee dislocations. Classification of knee dislocations is based primarily on the direction in which the tibia dislocates relative to the femur.[13,14] This results in five different categories: anterior, posterior, lateral, medial, and rotatory. Other factors to be considered include whether (1) the injury is opened or closed, (2) the injury is due to high energy or low energy trauma, (3) the knee is completely dislocated or subluxed, or (4) there is neurovascular involvement. Furthermore, one should be acutely aware that a complete knee dislocation may spontaneously reduce, and any triple-ligament knee injury is potentially a dislocation.[15-17]

Open knee dislocations are not uncommon. Reported incidence is between 19 and 35% of all dislocations.[18,19] An open knee dislocation carries a worse prognosis secondary to severe injury to the soft tissue envelope. Furthermore, an open injury may require an open ligament reconstruction, or staged reconstruction, since arthroscopically assisted techniques may not be able to be performed in the acute setting with these open injuries.

Distinguishing between low and high energy injuries is important. Low energy or low velocity injuries, usually associated with sports injuries, have a decreased incidence of associated vascular injury. High energy/high velocity injuries secondary to motor vehicle accidents or falls from heights tend to have increased incidence of vascular compromise. Decreased pulse in an injured limb and the history of a high energy injury indicate the need to obtain vascular studies urgently.

Mechanisms of Injury in the Multiple Ligament Injured Knee

The mechanisms of injury for the two most common knee dislocation patterns, anterior and posterior, are well described. Kennedy was able to reproduce anterior dislocation by means of a hyperextension force acting on the knee.[20] At 30° of hyperextension, the posterior capsule failed. When extended further to approximately 50°, the ACL, PCL, and popliteal artery fail. There is some question about whether the ACL or the PCL fails first with hyperextension.[20,21]

The most frequent ACL/PCL/posterolateral corner (PLC) mechanism of injury at our trauma center is forced varus, and knee dislocation. The most frequent ACL/PCL/MCL mechanism of injury at our trauma center is forced valgus, and knee dislocation.[2–4]

Initial Evaluation of the Multiple Ligament Injured Knee

Evaluation of the acute ACL/PCL injured knee includes history of injury mechanism, physical examination with careful neurovascular examination (arteriogram and venogram when indicated), plain radiographs, magnetic resonance imaging (MRI) studies, and examination under anesthesia and diagnostic arthroscopy. For chronic conditions, bone scans may be helpful.[22]

When an acute ACL/PCL injury presents as a dislocated knee, a gentle closed reduction is performed, and the neurovascular status performed is carefully assessed. Acute ACL/PCL injuries that present without documented dislocation must also have careful assessment of the neurovascular status of the extremity, since the knee may have been dislocated "in the field," and spontaneous reduction may have occurred. Wascher has reported a 14% incidence of arterial injury in dislocated knees, while at our center we have reported an 11% incidence of arterial injury in the acute three ligament injured knee.[6,17] Our recommendation is to obtain arteriograms in acute, three ligament injured knees with a clinical examination to rule out vascular damage, especially intimal flap tears that may present several days postinjury. We have also observed deep venous thrombosis associated with acute dislocated/three ligament injured knees and suggest venography in these patients when such a study is clinically indicated.

Physical examination features of the ACL/PCL/PLC injured knee include abnormal anterior and posterior translation at both 25 and 90° of knee flexion. At 90° of knee flexion, the tibial step-off is absent, and the posterior drawer test is 2+ or greater, indicating greater than 10mm of pathologic posterior tibial displacement. The Lachman test and pivot shifting phenomenon are positive, indicating anterior cruciate ligament disruption. We have described three types of posterolateral instability: A, B, and C.[5,6]

Posterolateral instability includes at least 10° of increased tibial external rotation, in comparison to the normal knee at 30 and 90° of knee flexion (positive dial test and external rotation thigh–foot angle test) and variable degrees of varus instability depending on the injured anatomic structures.[23] Posterolateral instability (PLI) type A has increased external rotation only, corresponding to injury to the popliteofibular ligament and popliteus tendon only. PLI type B presents with increased external rotation and mild varus of approximately 5 mm increased lateral joint line opening to varus stress at 30° of knee flexion. This occurs with damage to the popliteofibular ligament and popliteus tendon, and attenuation of the fibular collateral ligament. PLI type C presents with increased tibial external rotation and varus instability of 10 mm greater than the normal knee tested at 30° of knee flexion with varus stress. This occurs with injury to the popliteofibular ligament, popliteus tendon, fibular collateral ligament, and lateral capsular avulsion, in addition to cruciate ligament disruption. The intact medial collateral ligament, tested with valgus stress at 30° of knee flexion, is the stable hinge in the ACL/PCL/PLC injured knee.

The presence of a dimple sign on the anteromedial surface of the knee should be recognized. This indicates a posterolateral dislocation that is associated with a high incidence of irreducibility and potential skin necrosis. Open reduction is indicated.

Combined ACL/PCL/medial side injuries present with the same central pivot physical examination as described earlier plus significant valgus laxity at 0 and 30° of knee flexion. High grade medial side injuries will often present with lateral patellofemoral subluxation or dislocation, with severe tearing of the medial retinaculum and possibly extensor mechanism disruption. These high grade injuries may require immediate surgical repair of the medial side or external fixation to maintain tibiofemoral reduction. Low grade complete medial side injuries have valgus instability at 0 and 30° of knee flexion; however, the tibiofemoral joint stays reduced. Careful assessment of the patellofemoral joint must be undertaken in these injuries, since lateral patellar dislocation can occur.

Diagnostic Imaging Studies in the Multiple Ligament Injured Knee

Plain radiographs include standing anterior–posterior radiographs of both knees if possible, lateral, 30° anterior–posterior axial images of both patellae, and an intercondylar notch view. These radiographic views will help document reduction of the tibiofemoral and patellofemoral joints, assess bony alignment, and evaluate for insertion site bony avulsions of the cruciates, collateral ligament complexes, and extensor mechanisms.

Magnetic resonance imaging has a high diagnostic accuracy in acute posterior cruciate ligament injuries and is helpful both in assessing tear location of the cruciate and collateral ligaments and in formulating a treatment plan.[24,25] Bone scans may be helpful in evaluating subacute and chronic cases. Increased activity in the patellofemoral joint and medial compartment may signify the onset of early degenerative arthrosis, providing an indication for surgical stabilization.[22,26]

In the presence of cyanosis, pallor, weak capillary refill, and decreased peripheral temperature following reduction, arteriography must be considered. Venography is considered when the clinical picture indicates adequate limb perfusion but obstruction of outflow.

Diagnostic Arthroscopy of the Multiple Ligament Injured Knee

The three-zone method of posterior cruciate ligament evaluation enhances the information gained from imaging studies and examination to the injured knee under anesthesia.[4] Zone 1 of the PCL is the femoral insertion to the middle third of the ligament. Zone 2 is the middle third of the PCL, and zone 3 is the tibial insertion site area. A 30° arthroscope, the anterolateral patellar portal, and the posteromedial portal are used in the systematic evaluation of the posterior cruciate ligament and the posterolateral structures. Direct and indirect findings are assessed, and surgical treatment decisions can be made. We have found arthroscopic evaluation of the posterior cruciate ligament most helpful in assessing the interstitial damage of the PCL and ACL in bony insertion site avulsions. Severe interstitial disruption of the posterior cruciate ligament's zone 2 region has indicated reconstruction rather than primary repair as the procedure of choice.

Other Considerations in Evaluation of the Multiple Ligament Injured Knee

An unreduced dislocated knee constitutes an orthopaedic emergency requiring urgent reduction. When there is suspicion of arterial injury, arteriography and vascular surgery consultation are obtained. Popliteal vein injury is also possible, and if the clinical picture warrants, venography is indicated.

A state of irreducibility and/or vascular injury warrants immediate surgical intervention. One should consider four-compartment fasciotomy of the limb when ischemic time is greater than 2.5 h. Inability to maintain reduction mandates early ligamentous reconstruction or external fixation to stabilize the knee, to avoid recurrent vascular compromise. Open dislocations and open fracture dislocations warrant immediate surgical debridement and possible external fixation.

Surgical Indications and Timing

Our goals in the treatment of ACL/PCL injuries are to assess the neurovascular status, restore functional and objective stability to the injured knee, guard against progressive joint degeneration, and provide objective follow-up results regarding the treatment of these patients. The indication for surgery in the ACL/PCL injured knee is severe functional instability. These knees are at high risk for progressive instability and for the development of posttraumatic arthrosis.

Surgery is performed as close to the time of injury as is safely possible. Surgery performed 2 to 3 weeks postinjury allows the acute inflammatory phase to subside and range of motion to be restored. This will lessen the chances of postoperative stiffness, which is a high risk in these multiligament injured knees. The knee is protected in full extension in a long-leg hinged range-of-motion brace. At 2 to 3 weeks postinjury, enough capsular sealing has occurred to allow arthroscopic ACL/PCL reconstruction and

Color Plate I

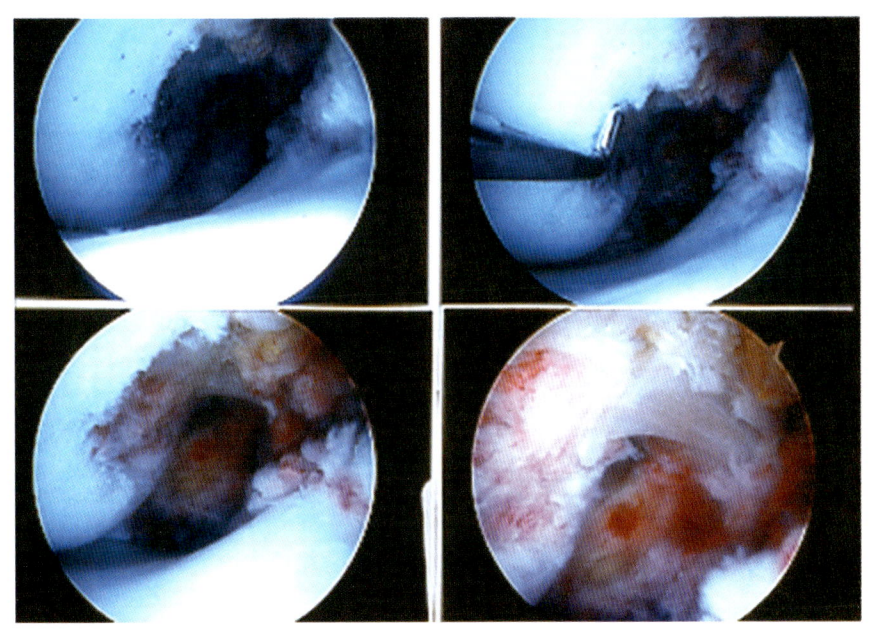

Fig. 3.6C. Arthroscopic preparation of the femoral side of the PCL reconstruction. (From Schenck RC, Injuries of the knee. In: Heckman JD, ed. Rockwood and Green. 5th ed. Philadelphia: Lippincott, Williams & Wilkins. By permission of the publisher.)

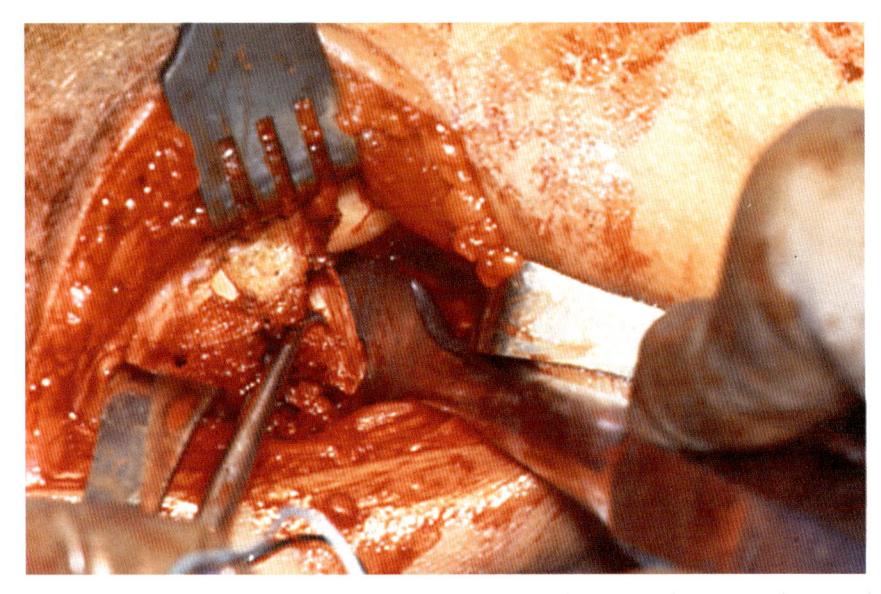

Fig. 3.7C. Open approach to the PCL: avulsion with open reduction and internal fixation using a 4.0 mm cannulated anterior oblique screw through a posteromedial approach. (From Schenck RC, Injuries of the knee. In: Heckman JD ed. Rockwood and Green. 5th ed. Philadelphia: Lippincott, Williams and Wilkins. By permission of the publisher.)

Color Plate II

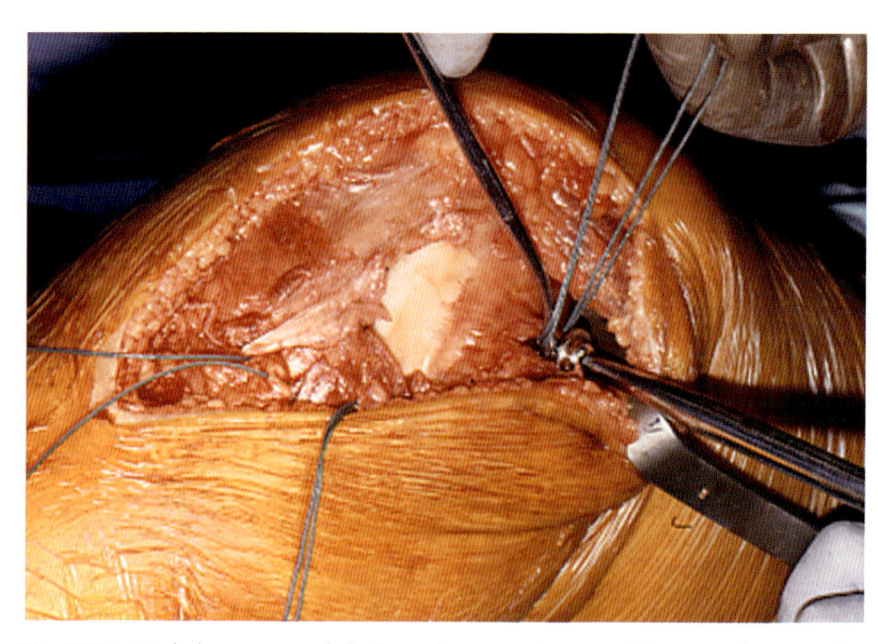

Fig. 3.8B. Medial exposure of the knee for reattachment of the posterior, anterior, and medial collateral ligaments. (From Schenck RC, Injuries of the knee. In: Heckman JD ed. Rockwood and Green. 5th ed. Philadelphia: Lippincott, Williams & Wilkins. By permission of the publisher.)

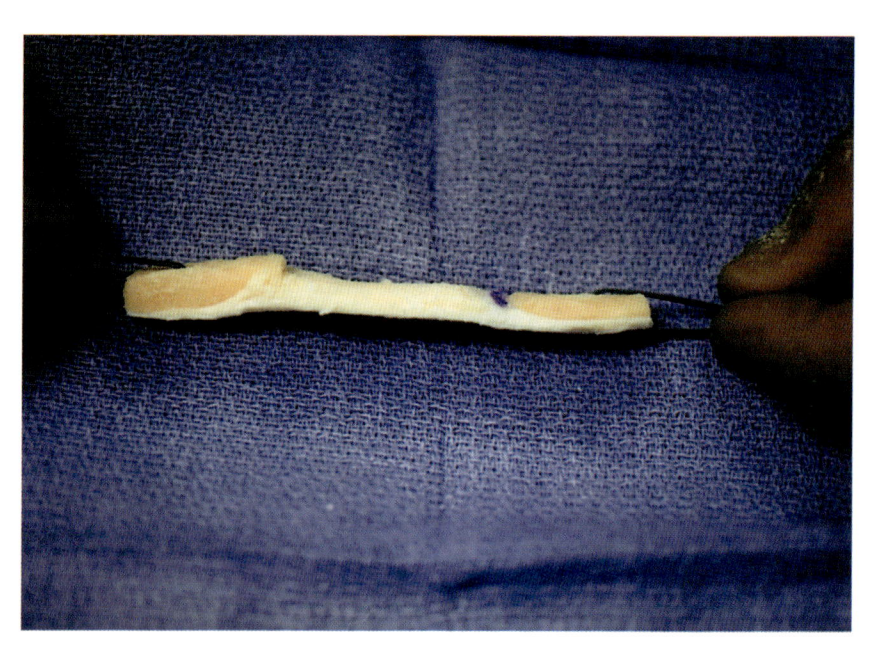

Fig. 5.1. BPTB graft.

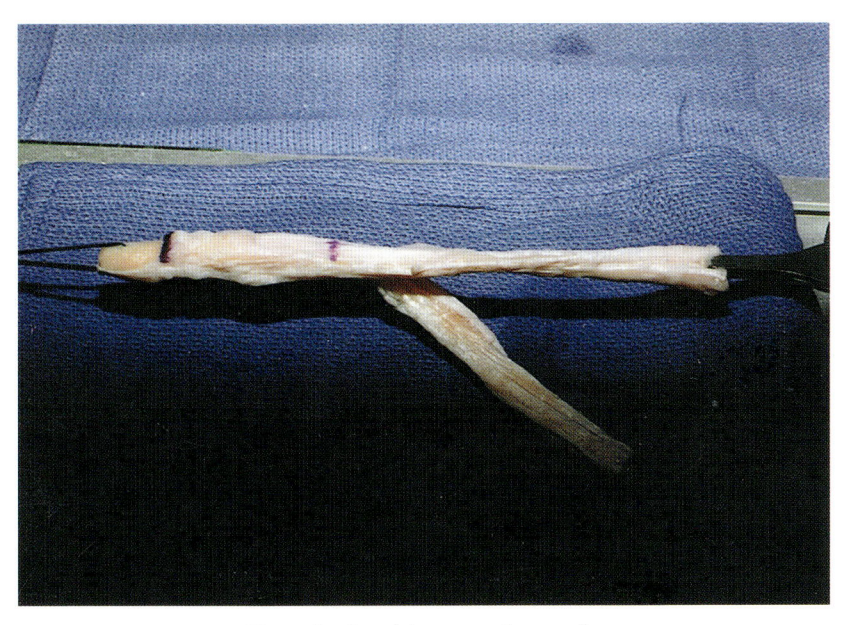

Fig. 5.2. Quadriceps tendon graft.

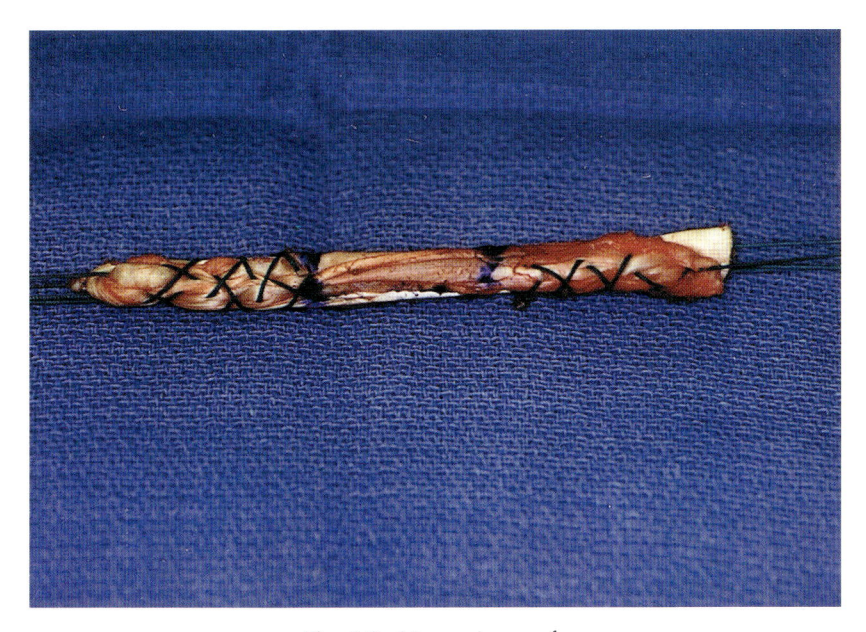

Fig. 5.3. Hamstring graft.

Color Plate IV

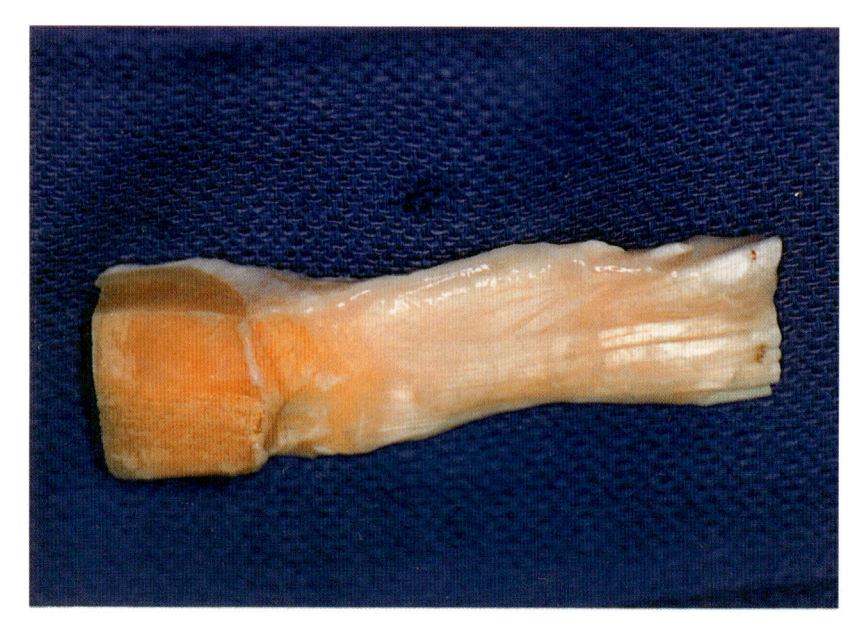

Fig. 5.4. Allograft (Achilles tendon, QT, etc.).

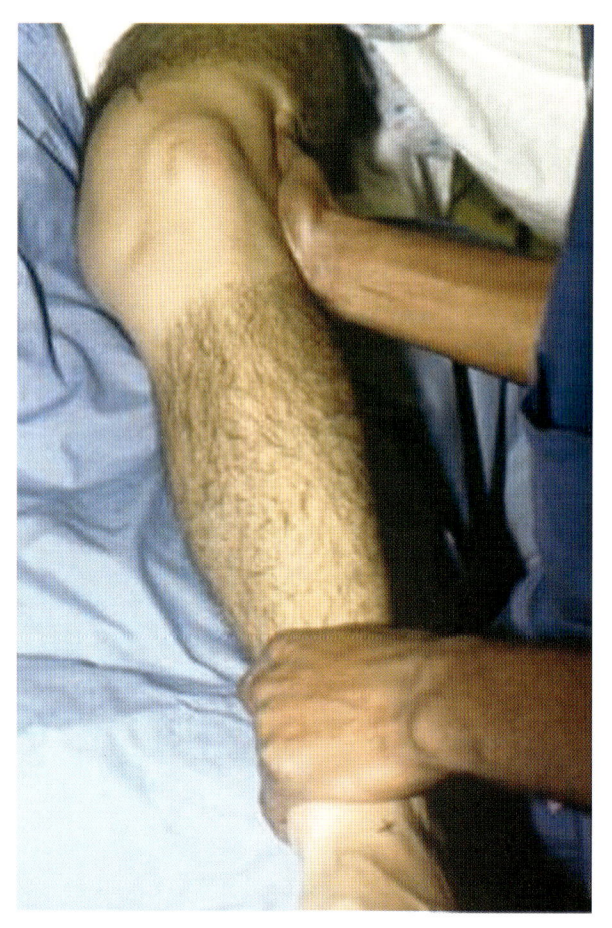

Fig. 6.3. Clinical picture of valgus opening in extension.

Color Plate V

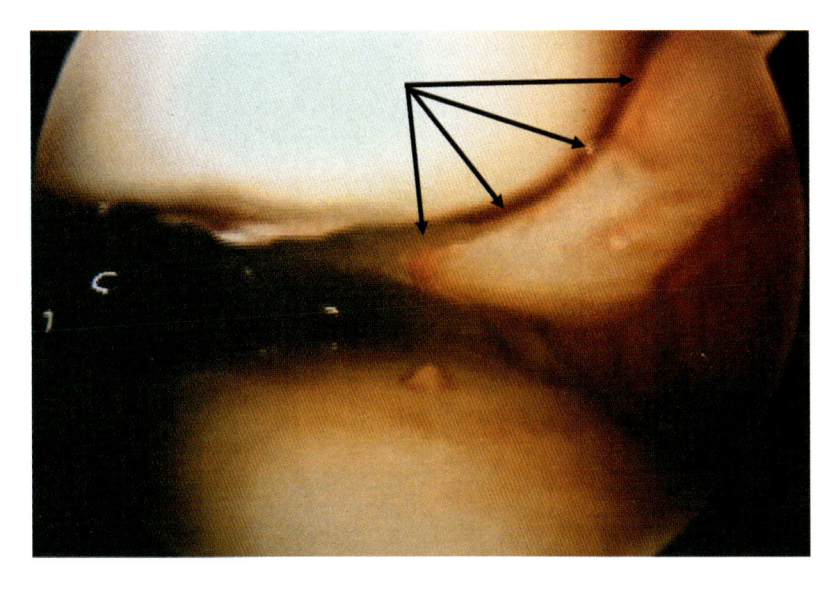

Fig. 6.6B. Arthroscopic image of floating medial meniscus (arrows).

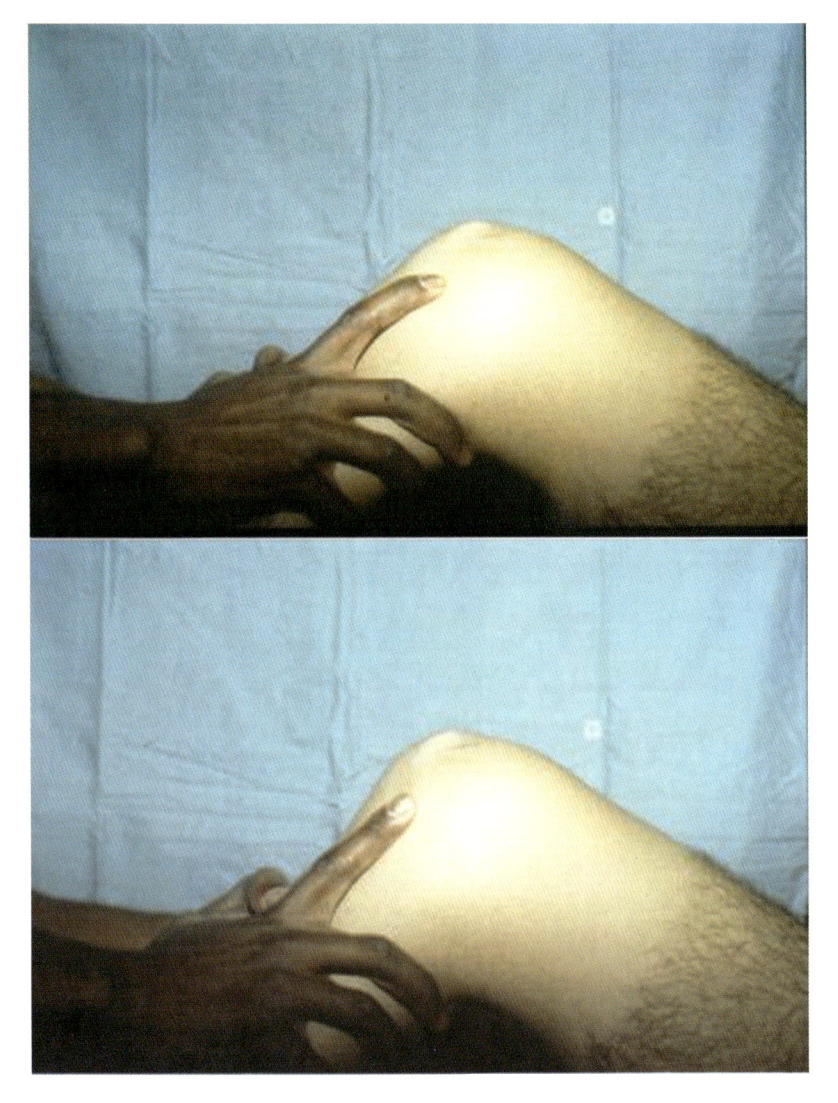

Fig. 6.7. Clinical example of posterior drawer test.

Color Plate VI

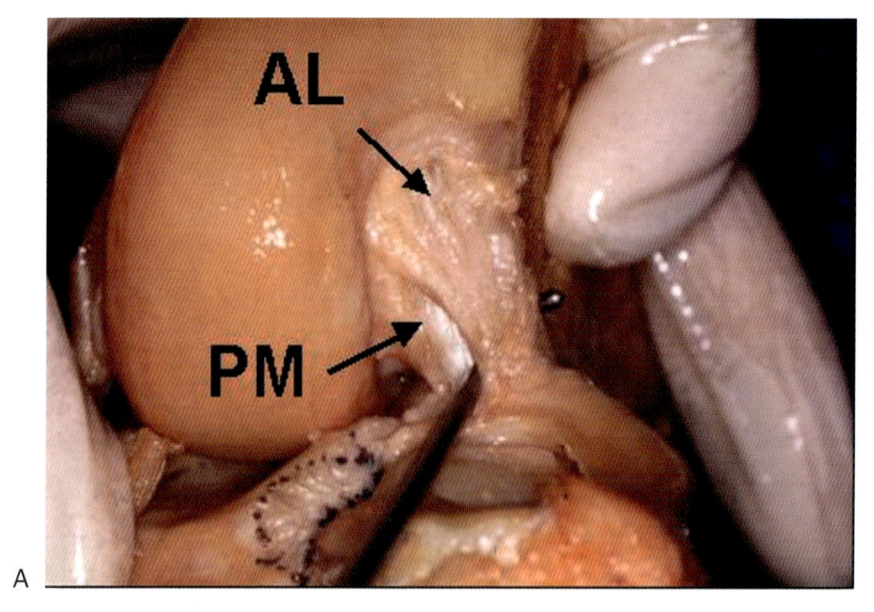

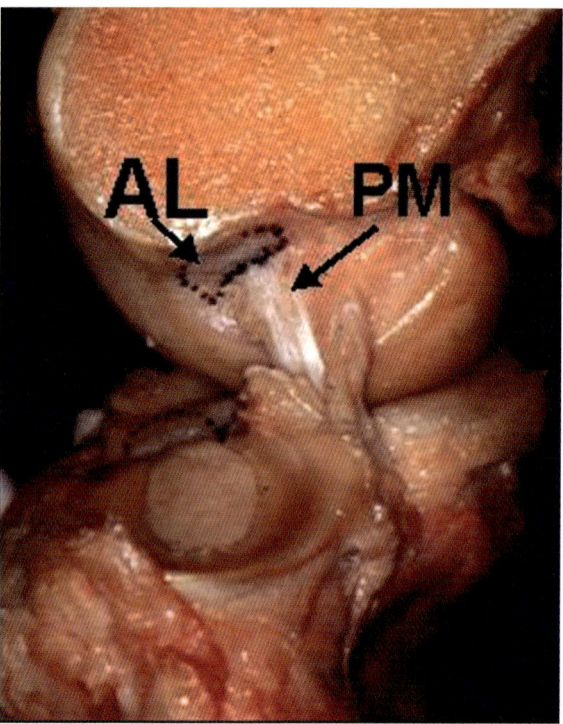

Fig. 6.9. Cadaveric dissection of anterolateral (AL) and posteromedial (PM) components of the PCL in the (A) coronal and (B) sagittal planes.

Color Plate VII

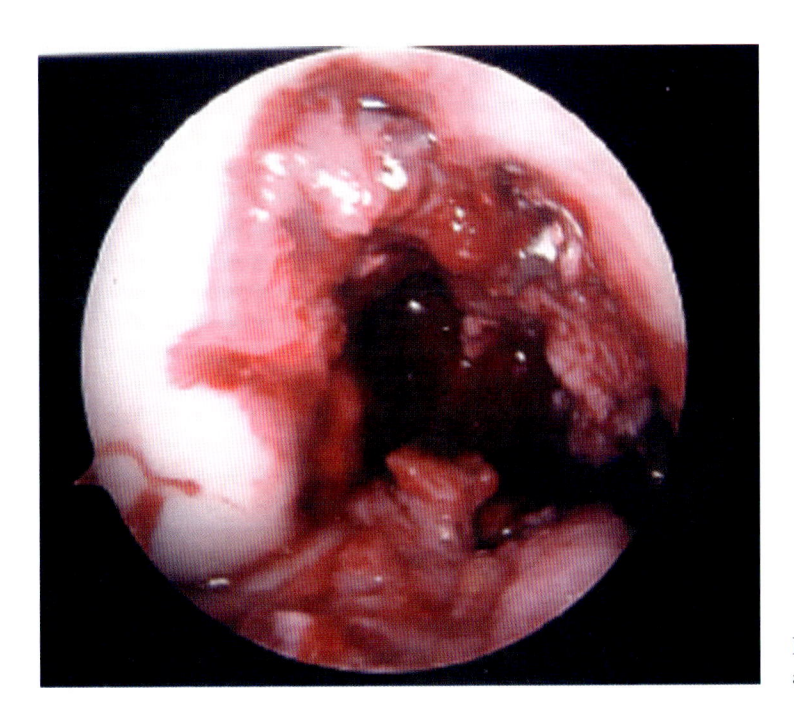

Fig. 6.13. Dry arthroscopic image demonstrating an ACL and PCL tear in the femoral notch.

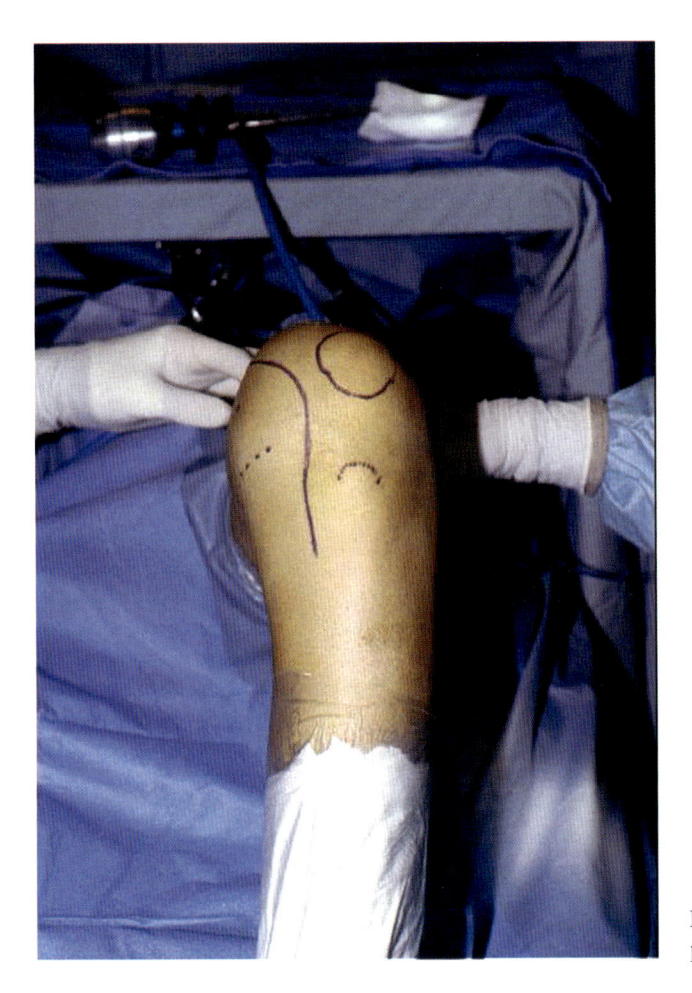

Fig. 6.14. Topographical landmarks (incision, joint line, patella, and tibial tubercle) for the MCL reconstruction.

Color Plate VIII

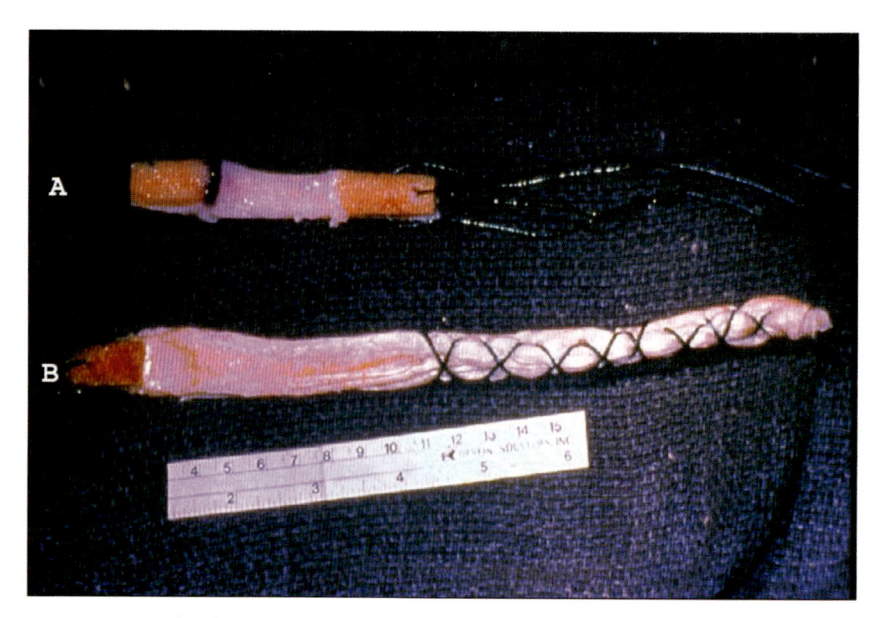

Fig. 6.21. Graft choices: (A) BPTB allograft and (B) Achilles allograft (with whipstitch).

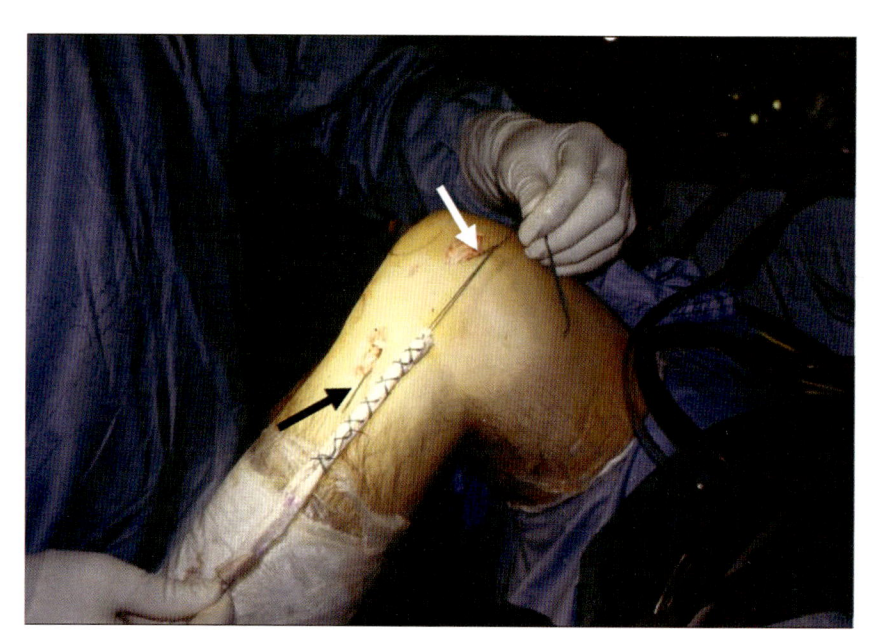

Fig. 6.22. Prepared Achilles graft prior to being passed from the outside in, utilizing an 18-gauge wire. Wire is visualized traversing both tibial and femoral tunnels (arrows).

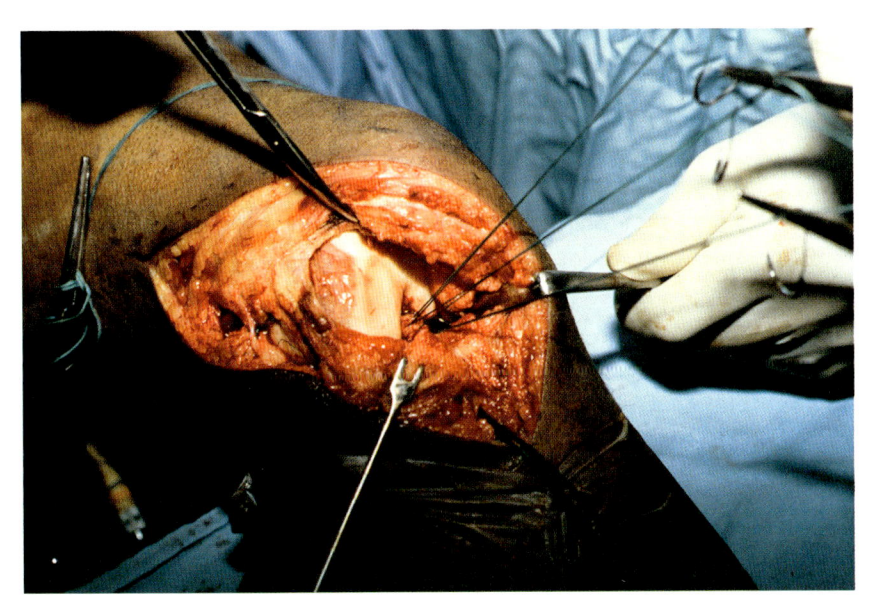

Fig. 6.25C. PCL avulsion repair with associated ACL and medial side injury. Sutures placed in PCL.

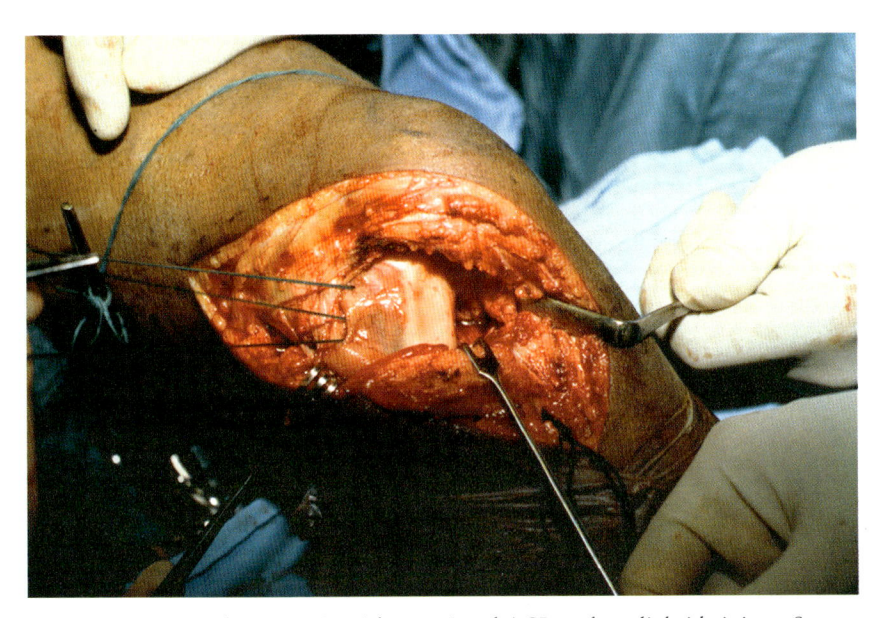

Fig. 6.25F. PCL avulsion repair with associated ACL and medial side injury. Sutures brought through femur.

Color Plate X

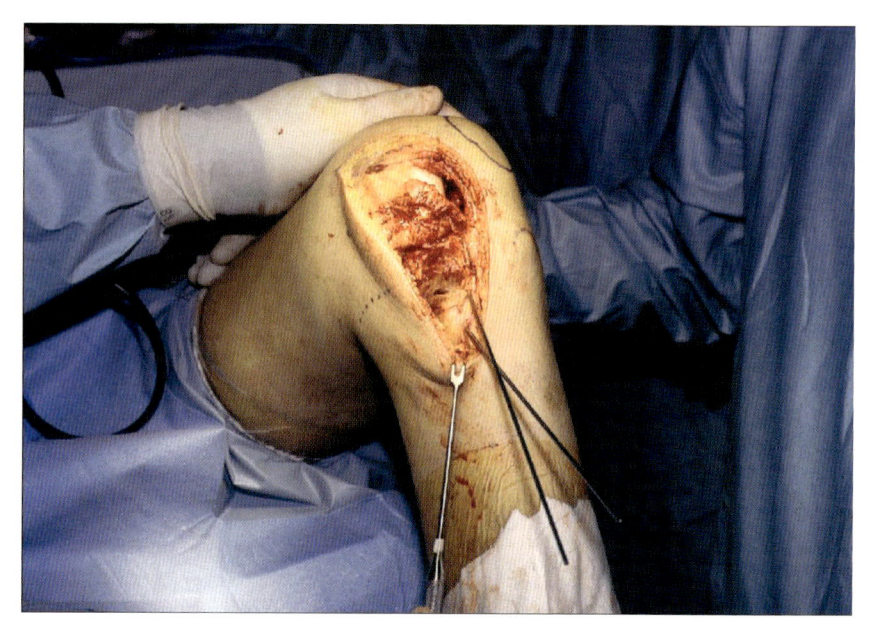

Fig. 6.26. Intraoperative photograph of ACL and PCL guide pin placement.

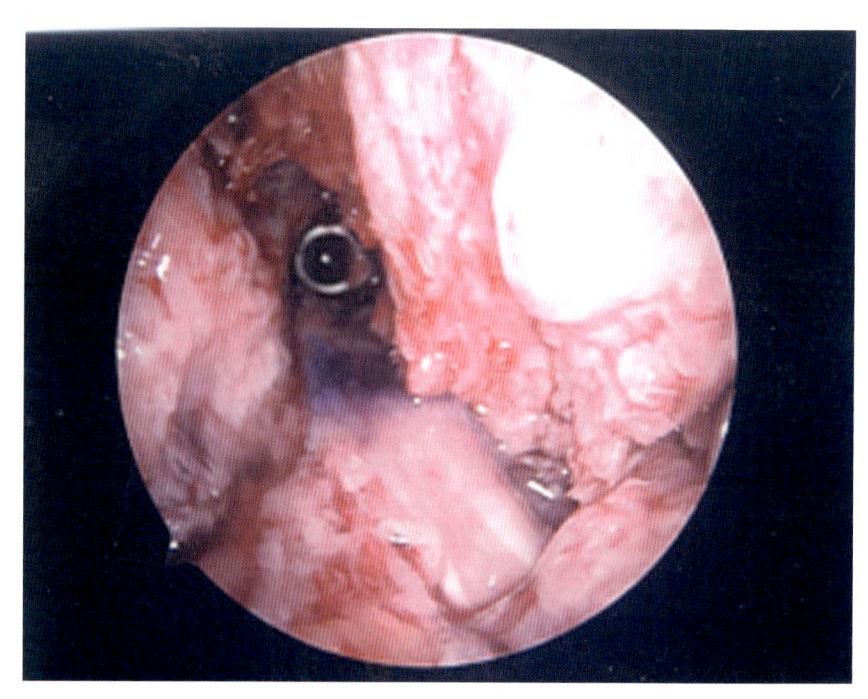

Fig. 6.27. Arthroscopic view of ACL and double-bundle PCL reconstruction.

Color Plate XI

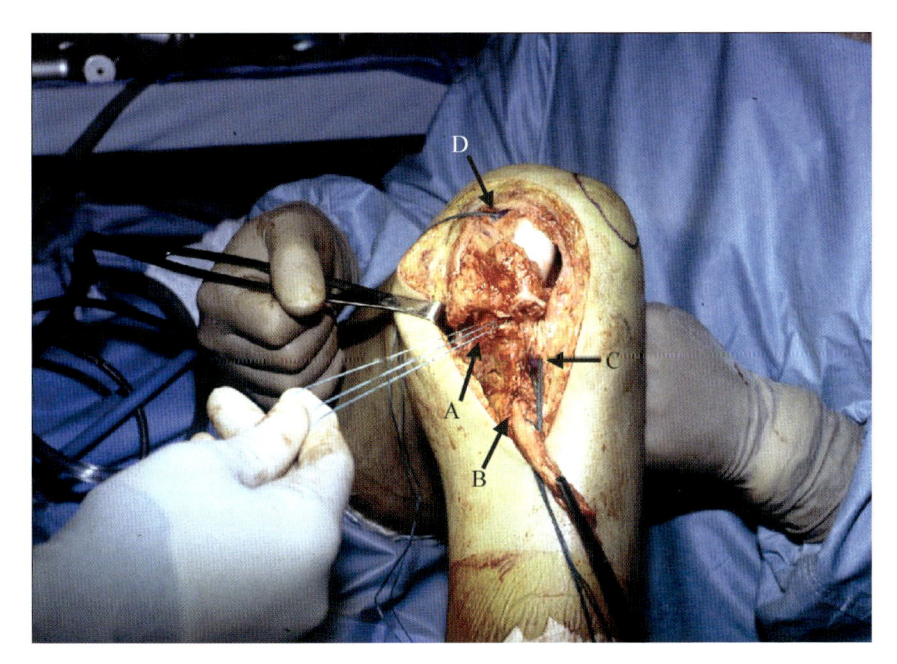

Fig. 6.29A. Repair of medial side injury with associated ACL/PCL injury showing suture anchors in medial tibia to secure medial meniscus and deep medial capsule (A), PCL tibial tunnel and graft (B), ACL tibial tunnel and graft (C), and femoral PCL tunnel and bone plug (D).

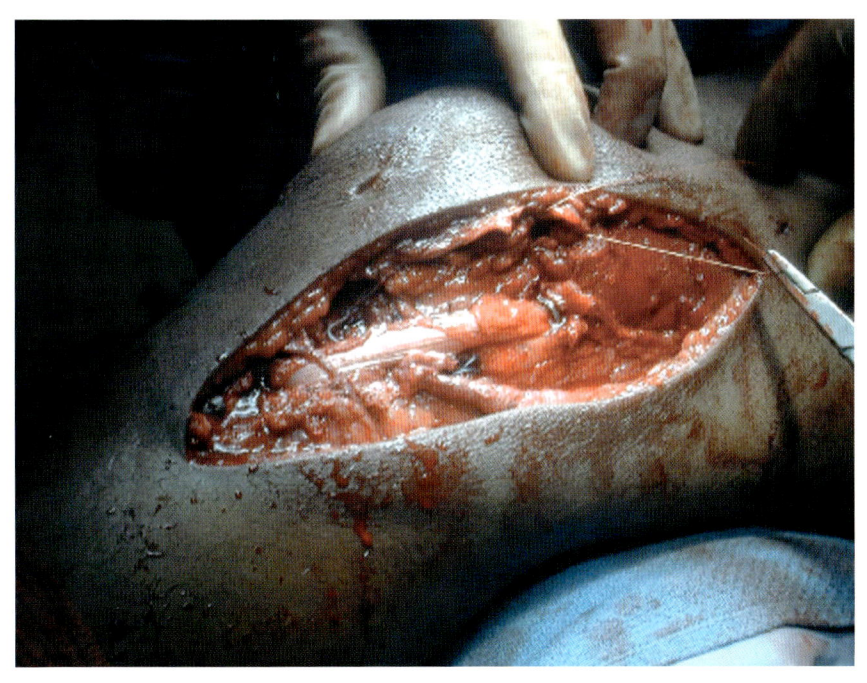

Fig. 6.31. Medial side repair using bone staples for fixation.

Color Plate XII

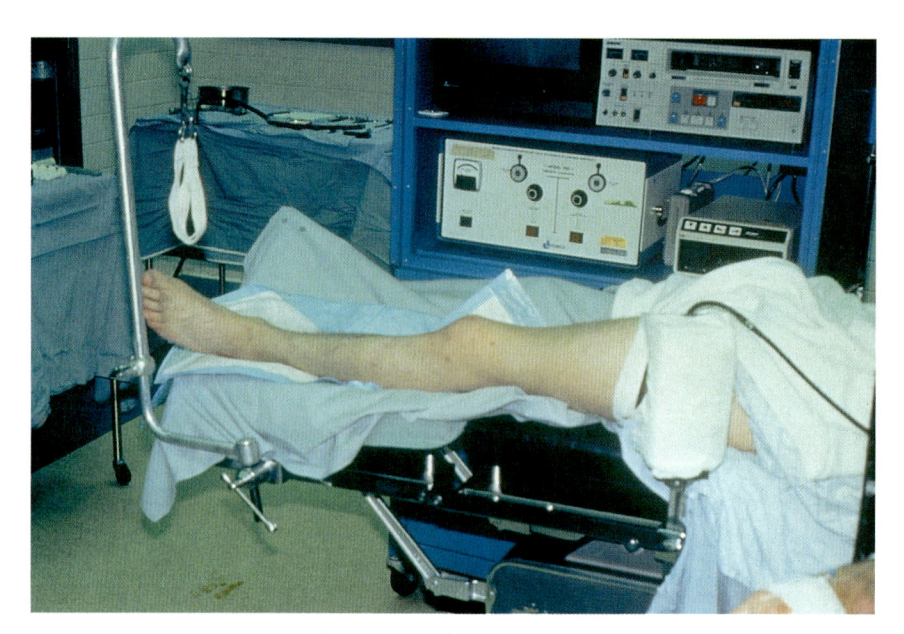

Fig. 8.1. Patient is positioned supine on the operating table with the nonsurgical leg resting on the fully extended operating table. A lateral post is used for control of the surgical lower extremity.

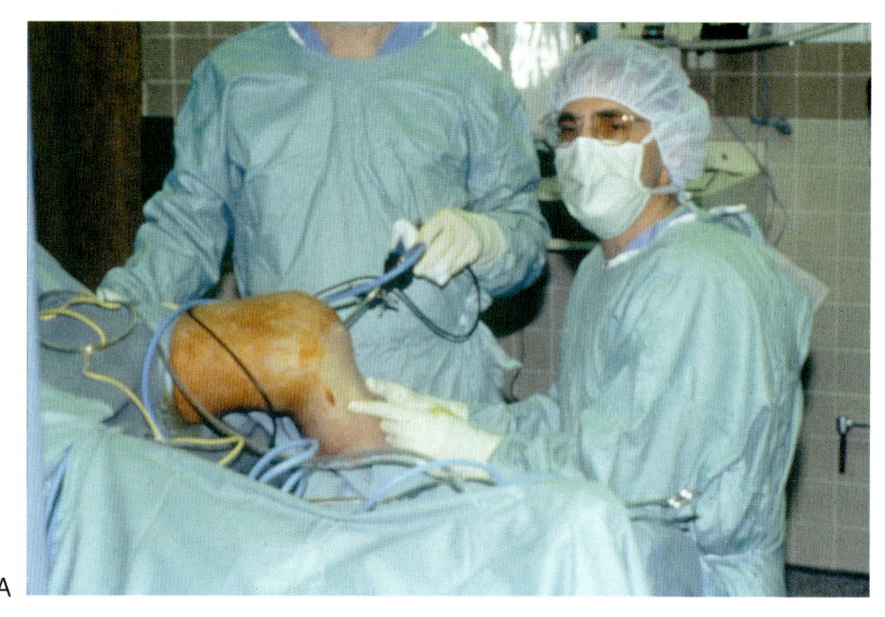

A

Fig. 8.2. A and B. 1 to 2 cm extracapsular posterior medial safety incision allows the surgeon's finger to protect the neurovascular structures and confirm the position of instruments on the posterior aspect of the proximal tibia. (*Continued*)

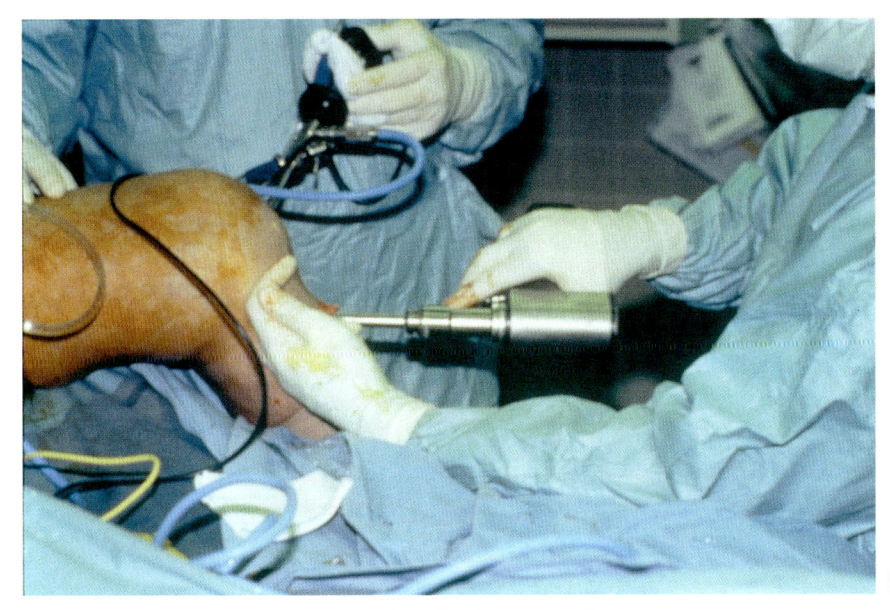

Fig. 8.2. A and B (*Continued*).

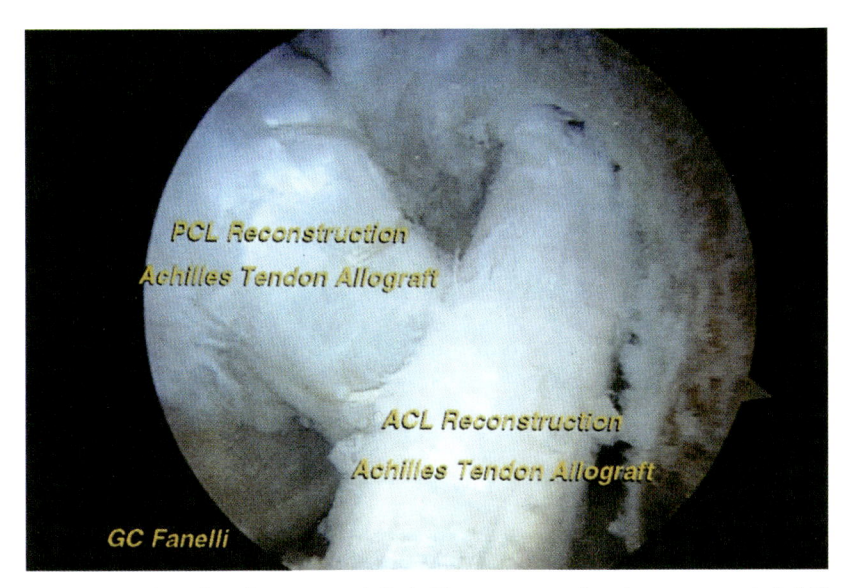

Fig. 8.5. Combined arthroscopic ACL/PCL reconstruction by means of Achilles tendon allograft. The tunnels are precisely created to reproduce the anatomic insertion sites of the anterolateral bundle of the posterior cruciate ligament and the anatomic insertion sites of the anterior cruciate ligament. Correct and accurate tunnel placement is essential for successful combined ACL/PCL reconstructions. The Achilles tendon allograft is preferred because of its large cross-sectional area, strength, and absence of donor site morbidity.

Color Plate XIV

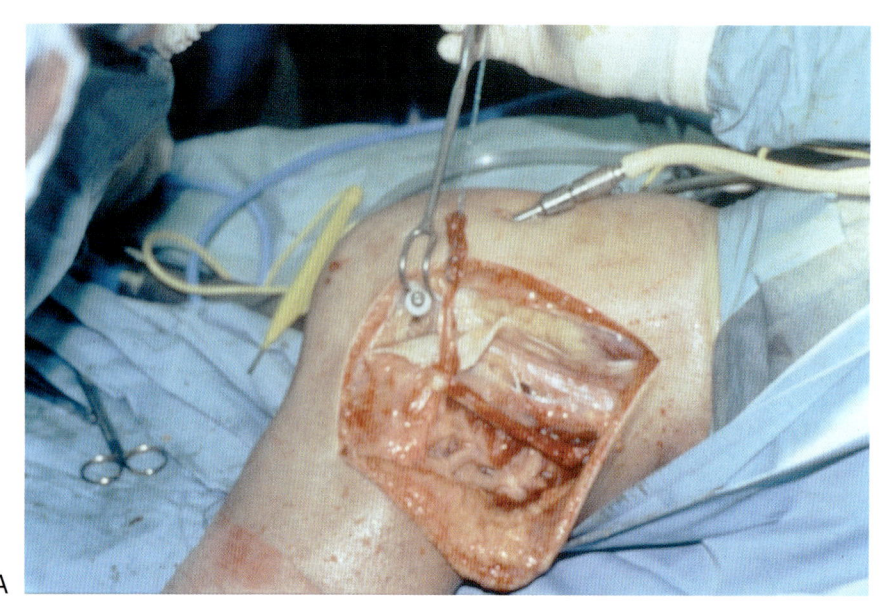

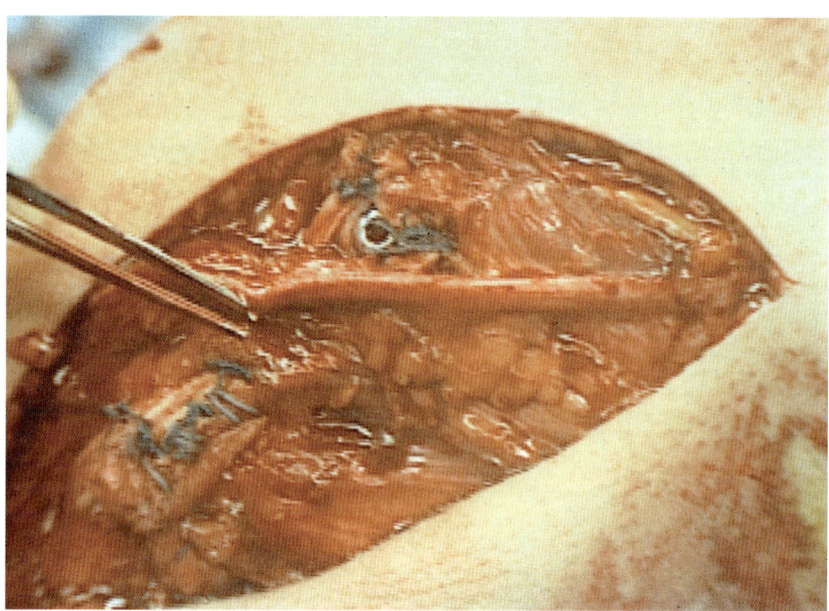

A

B

Fig. 8.6. Our preferred surgical technique for posterolateral and lateral reconstruction is the split biceps tendon transfer (A) or the allograft or autograft figure-of-eight reconstruction (B) combined with posterolateral capsular shift and primary repair of injured structures, as indicated. These complex surgical procedures reproduce the function of the popliteofibular ligament and the lateral collateral ligament and eliminate posterolateral capsular redundancy. The split biceps tendon transfer utilizes anatomic insertion sites and preserves the dynamic function of the long head and common biceps femoris tendon.

Color Plate XV

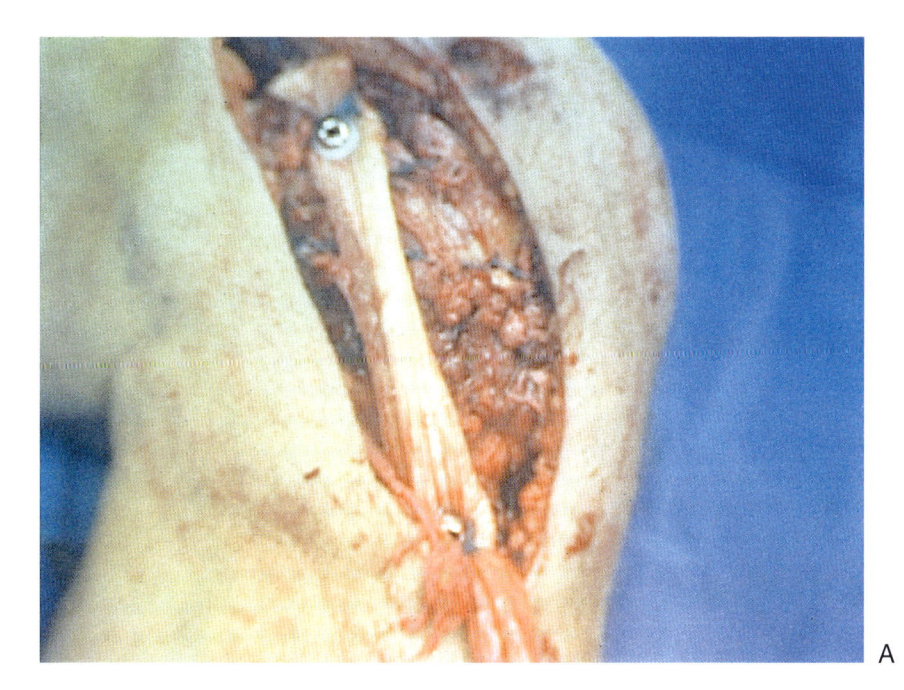

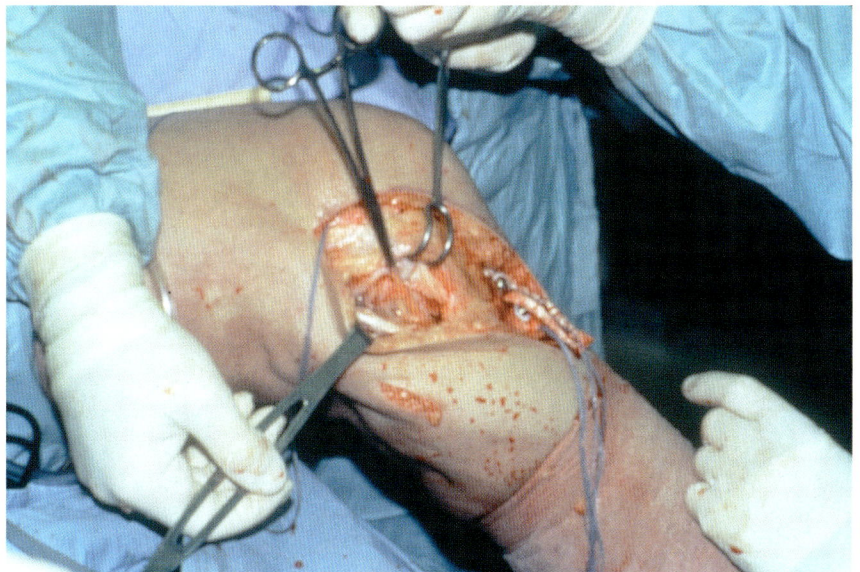

Fig. 8.7. (A) Severe medial side injuries are successfully treated with primary repair by means of the suture anchor technique combined with MCL reconstruction using Achilles tendon allograft. The Achilles tendon allograft's broad anatomy can anatomically reconstruct the superficial medial collateral ligament. The Achilles tendon allograft is secured to the anatomic insertion sites of the superficial MCL by means of screws and spiked ligament washers. The posteromedial capsule can then be secured to the Achilles tendon allograft to eliminate posteromedial capsular laxity. This technique will address all components of the medial side instability. (B) Lesser degrees of medial side instabilities may be treated with posteromedial capsular shift procedures.

Color Plate XVI

Fig. 8.9. Model showing tibial tunnel positions for combined ACL/PCL reconstructions. It is essential to have an adequate bone bridge between the two tunnels. (From Fanelli GC, Giannotti BF, Edson CJ. Current concepts review. The posterior cruciate ligament arthroscopic evaluation and treatment. Arthroscopy 1994; 10(6):673–688. Used with permission.)

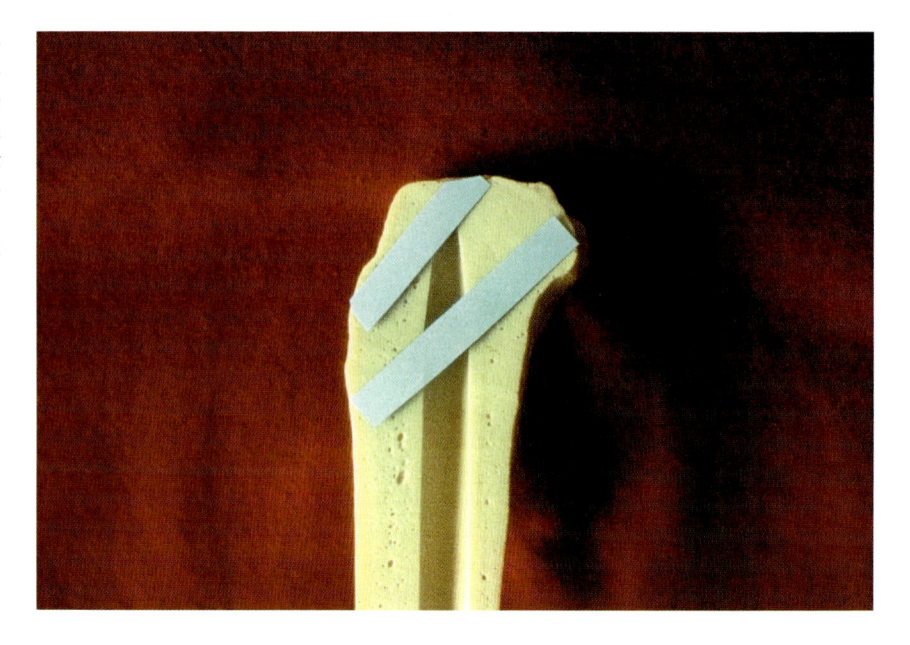

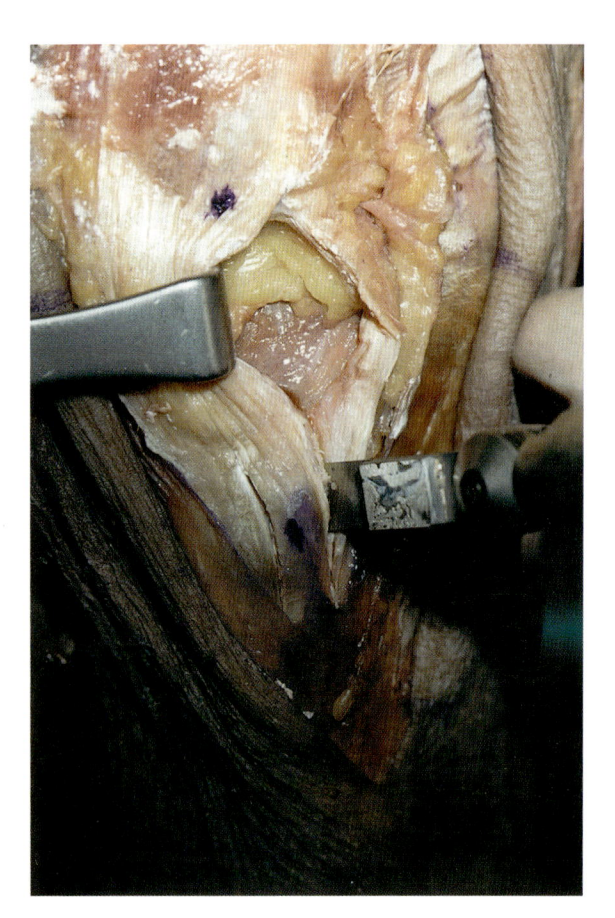

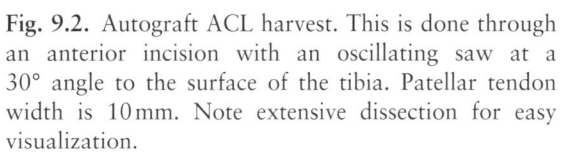

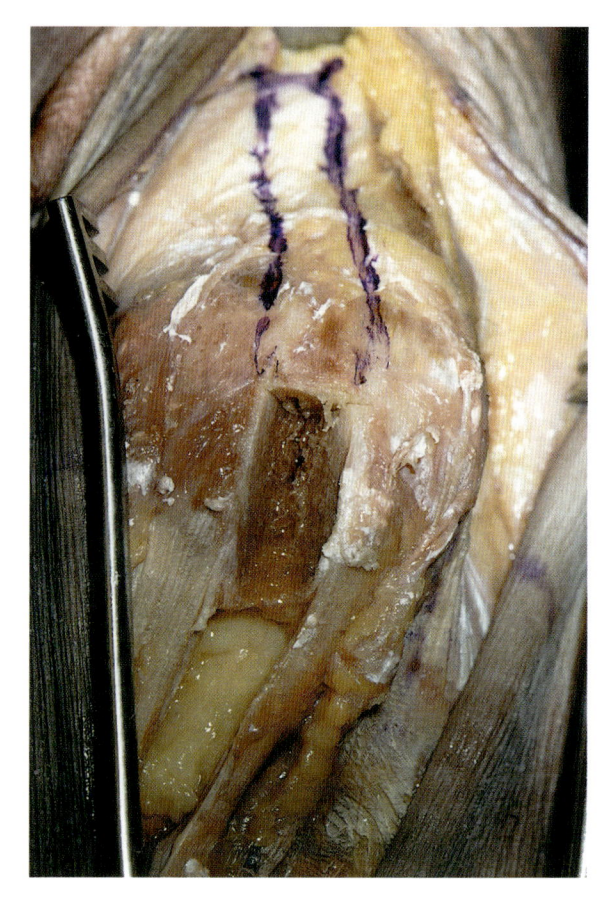

Fig. 9.2. Autograft ACL harvest. This is done through an anterior incision with an oscillating saw at a 30° angle to the surface of the tibia. Patellar tendon width is 10 mm. Note extensive dissection for easy visualization.

Fig. 9.3. Autograft quadriceps tendon harvest. A marker is used to show the dimensions of the patellar bone plug and appropriate length of quadriceps tendon.

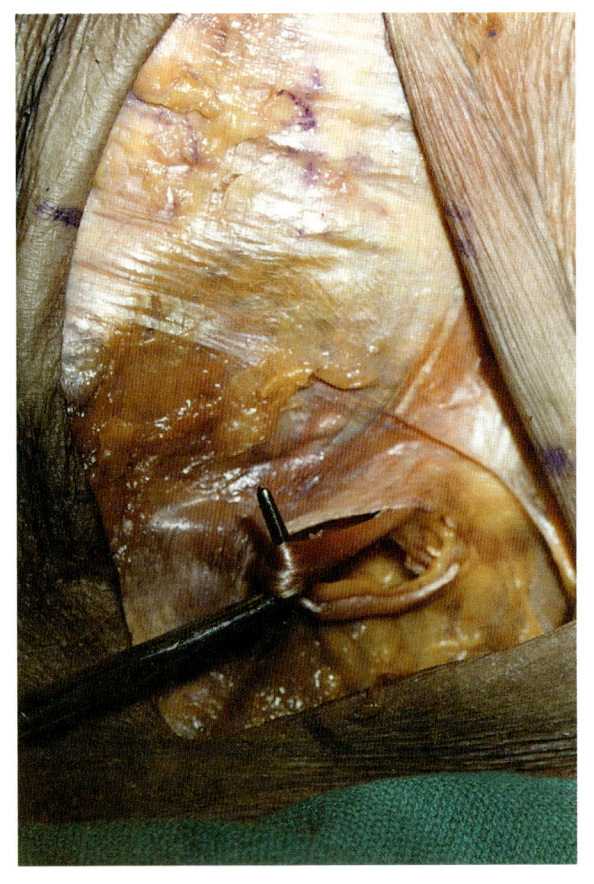

Fig. 9.4. Autograft hamstring harvest with use of right angle forceps to identify the two hamstrings. This is done through an incision in line with the fibers of the sartorius fascia.

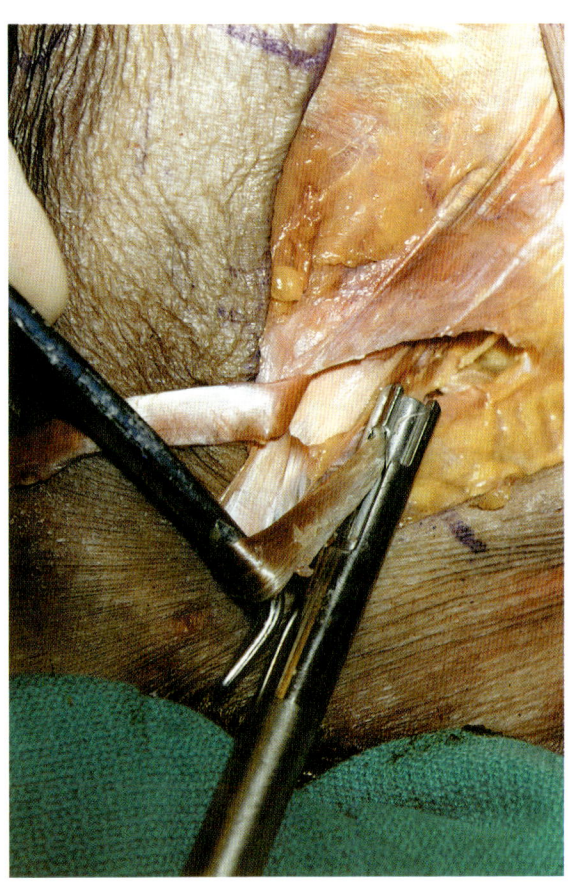

Fig. 9.5. Autograft hamstring harvest with tendon stripper. Care is taken to remove all fascial bands and vinculae to prevent a premature harvest of the hamstrings.

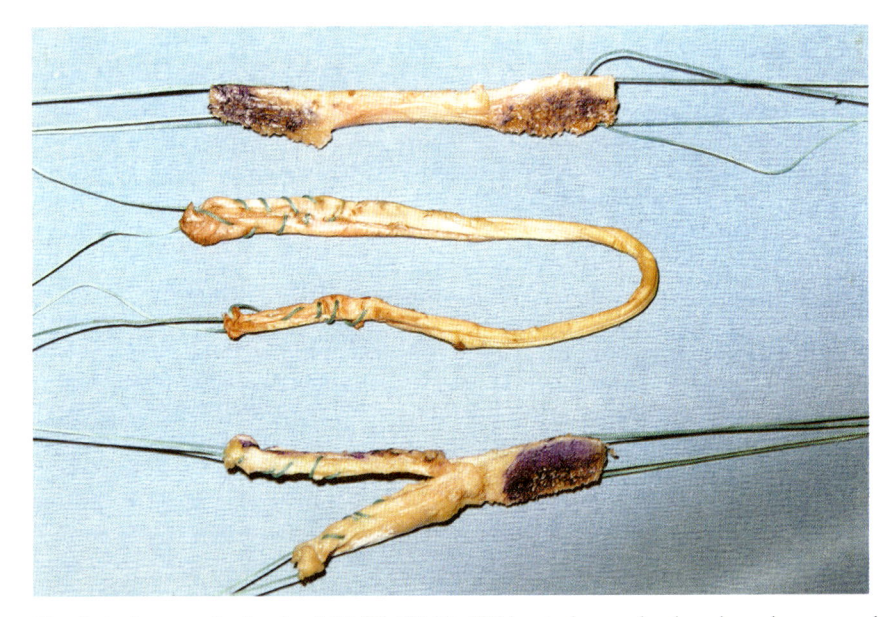

Fig. 9.6. Autografts for the ACL/PLC/PCL. Whipstitches and colored marks are used to facilitate graft passage and fixation.

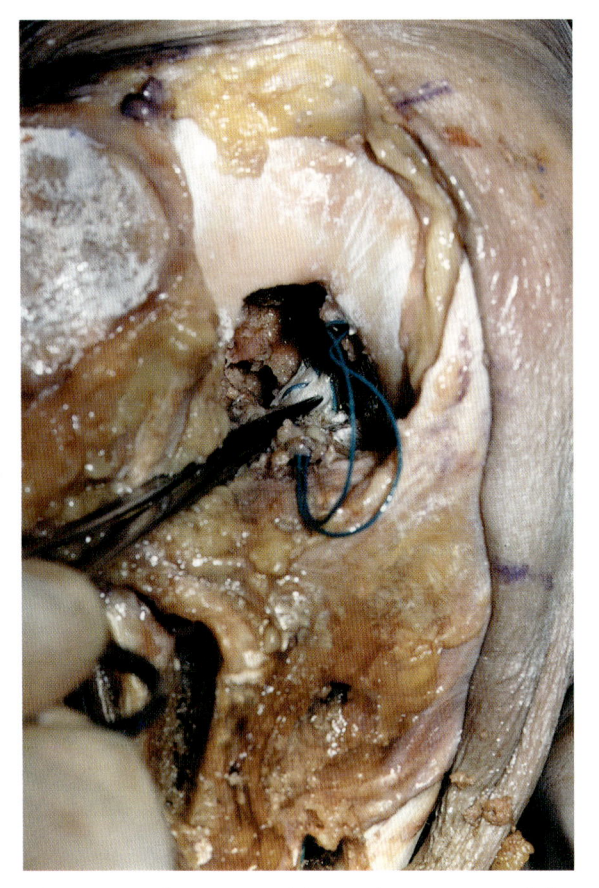

Fig. 9.11. (Left) Passage of the quadriceps autograft for reconstruction of the PCL. The tibial plug has already been passed anterograde through the tibial tunnel. Note the two limbs of the autograft: the posteromedial is already through the femoral tunnel, and the anterolateral limb is anterior as identified by the Ethibond whipstitches.

Fig. 9.13. (Right) Fixation of the anterolateral limb of the PCL reconstruction with a cannulated soft tissue screw in a retrograde fashion through the notch.

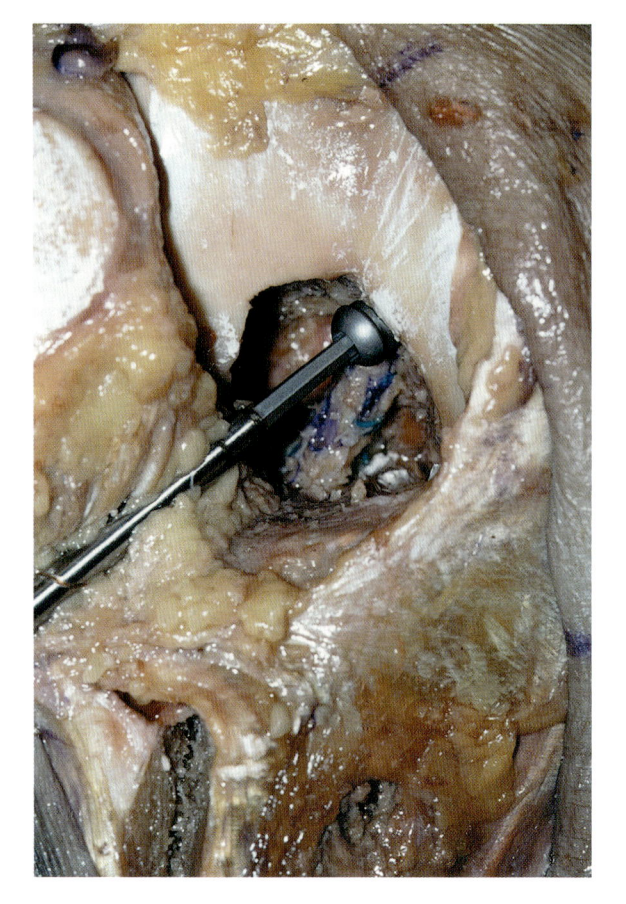

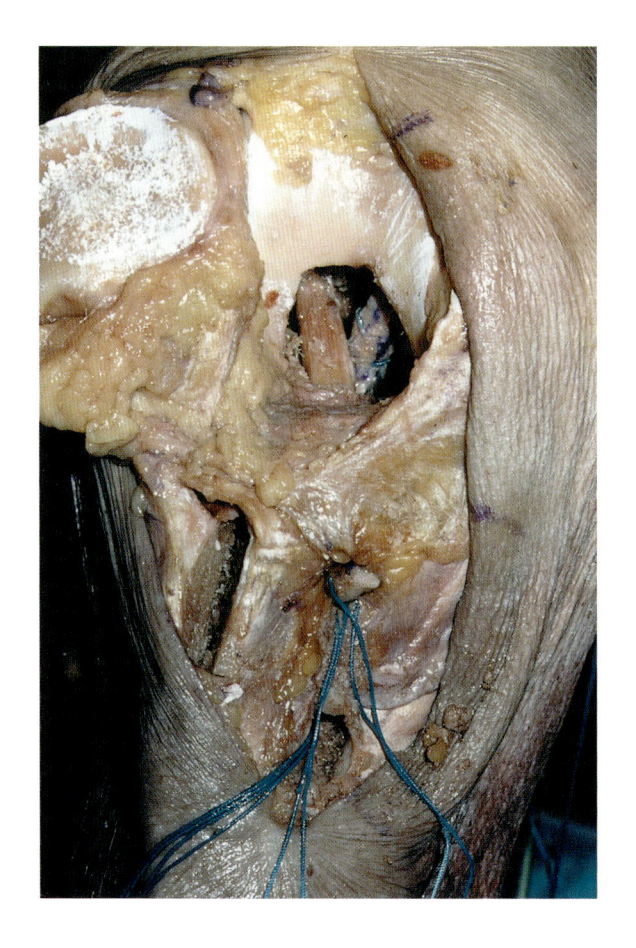

Fig. 9.14. Passage of the PCL and ACL autografts as seen from the anteromedial aspect of the knee. Note position of the femoral grafts and the relationships of the tibial ACL autograft harvest site and the tibial tunnels of the PCL (inferior) and ACL (superior).

Color Plate XIX

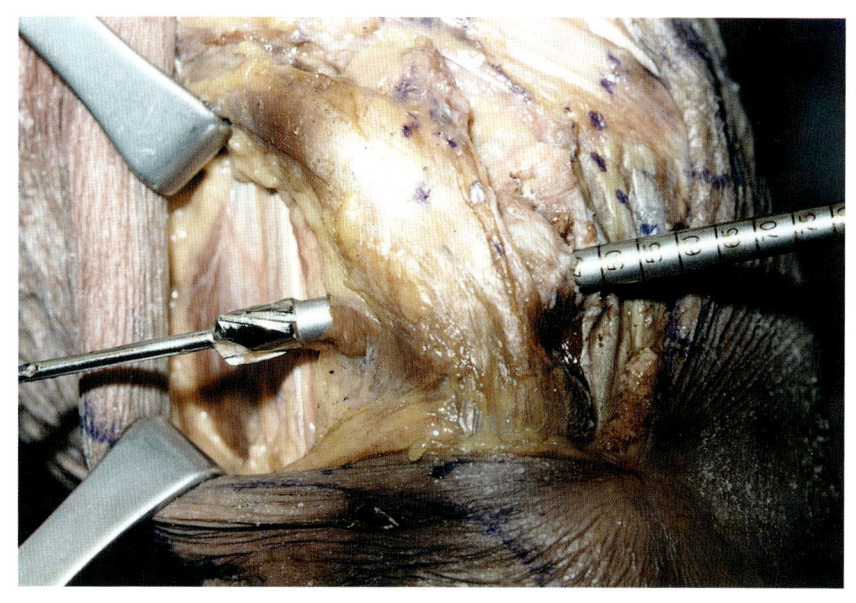

Fig. 9.21. Preparation of the fibular head for passage of double-hamstring autograft. A 7 mm reamer is used in an anterior-to-posterior direction over a guide wire.

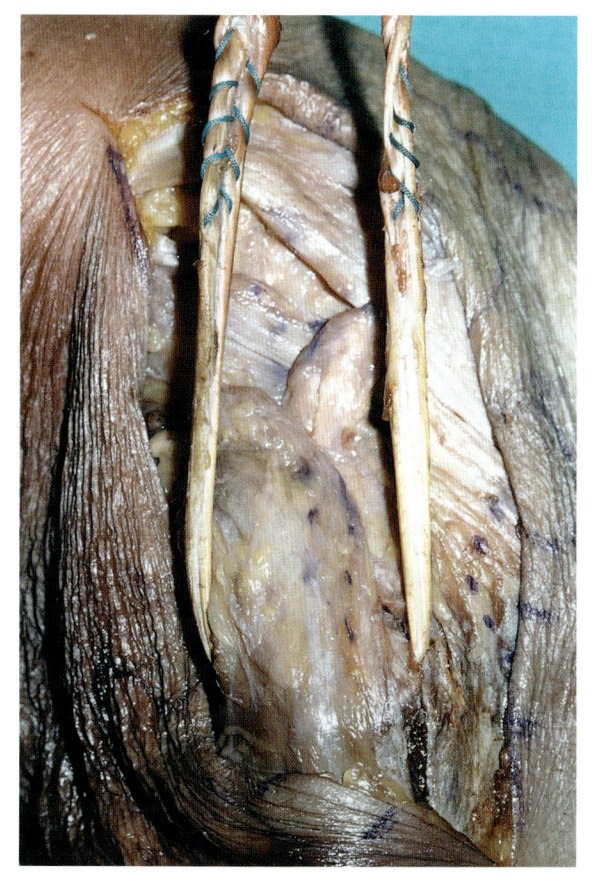

Fig. 9.22. Passage of the double-hamstring autograft through the fibular head.

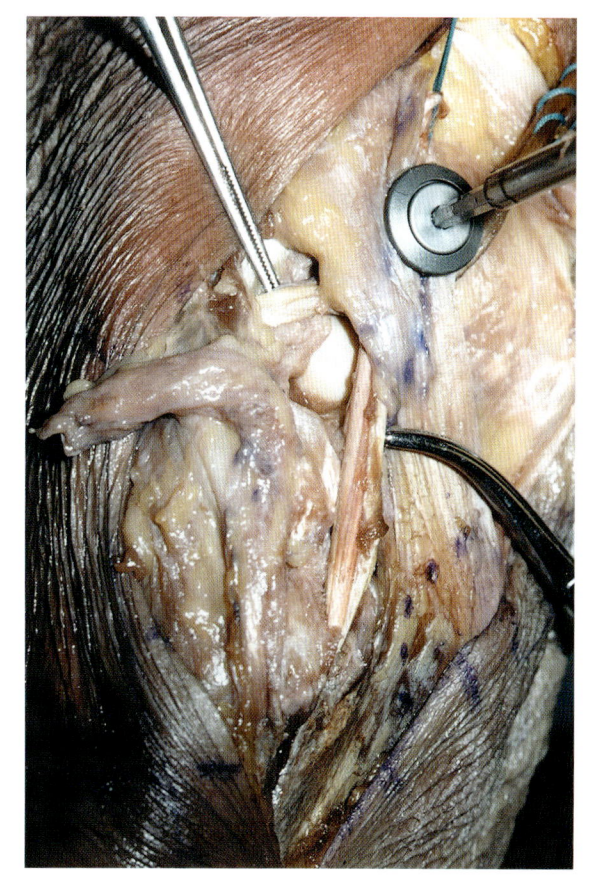

Fig. 9.23. Fixation of the PLC fibular "O" autograft. The graft is passed in a figure-of-eight fashion such that the posterior limb (left) serves as the popliteofibular complex and the anterior limb (right) serves as the reconstructed LCL.

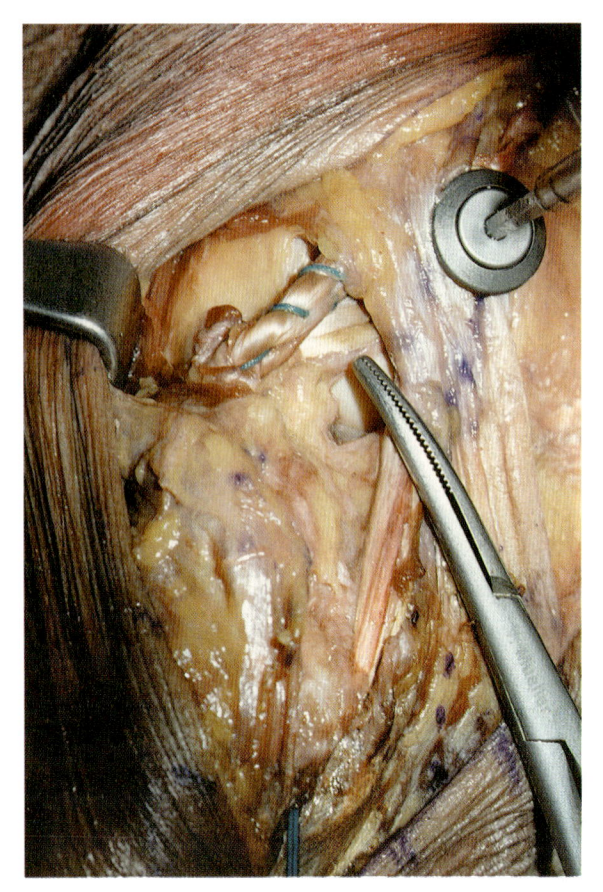

Fig. 9.24. Fixation of the PLC graft often allows for overlapping of the anterior and posterior limbs with extra tendon. Care is taken to ensure that the tendon is captured by the soft tissue washer.

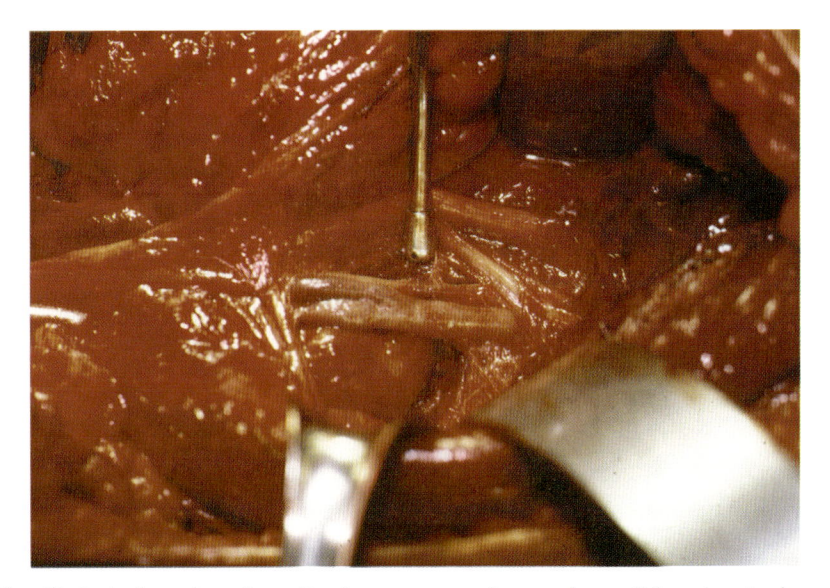

Fig. 10.6. A thrombosed popliteal artery secondary to knee dislocation is shown from a posterior approach. The contused popliteal artery is inferior to the suction tip; the popliteal vein and tibial nerve are also well visualized.

Color Plate XXI

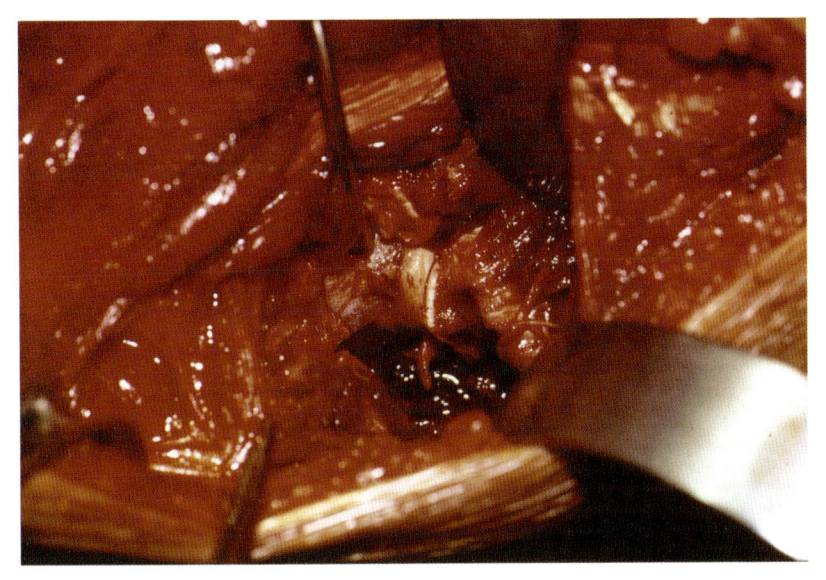

Fig. 10.9. Open joint secondary to a knee dislocation shown from the posterior approach during surgery for a popliteal artery occlusion. The extensive amount of tissue injury is evident, as is the large hematoma that was evacuated from the lateral aspect of the wound.

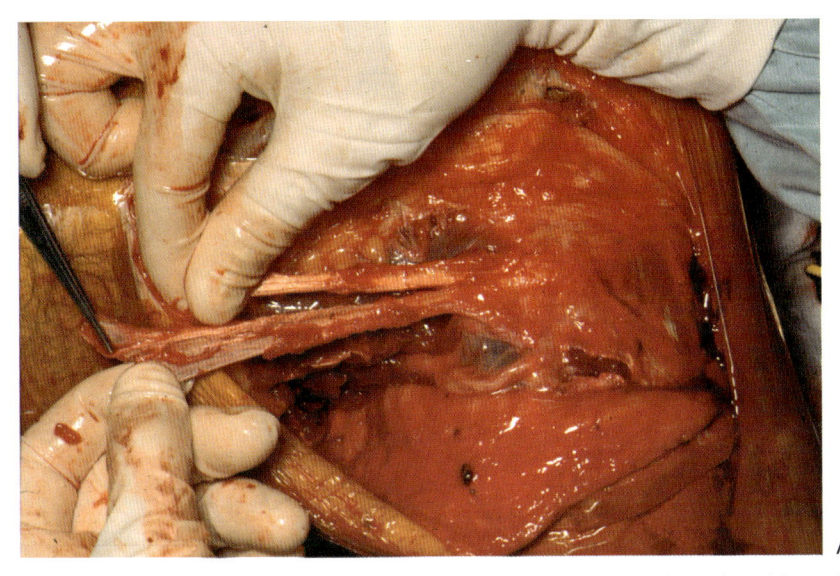

Fig. 16.10A and B. Our preferred surgical technique for posterolateral and lateral reconstruction is the split biceps tendon transfer (A) or the allograft or autograft figure-of-eight reconstruction (B) combined with posterolateral capsular shift and primary repair of injured structures as indicated. *(Continued)*

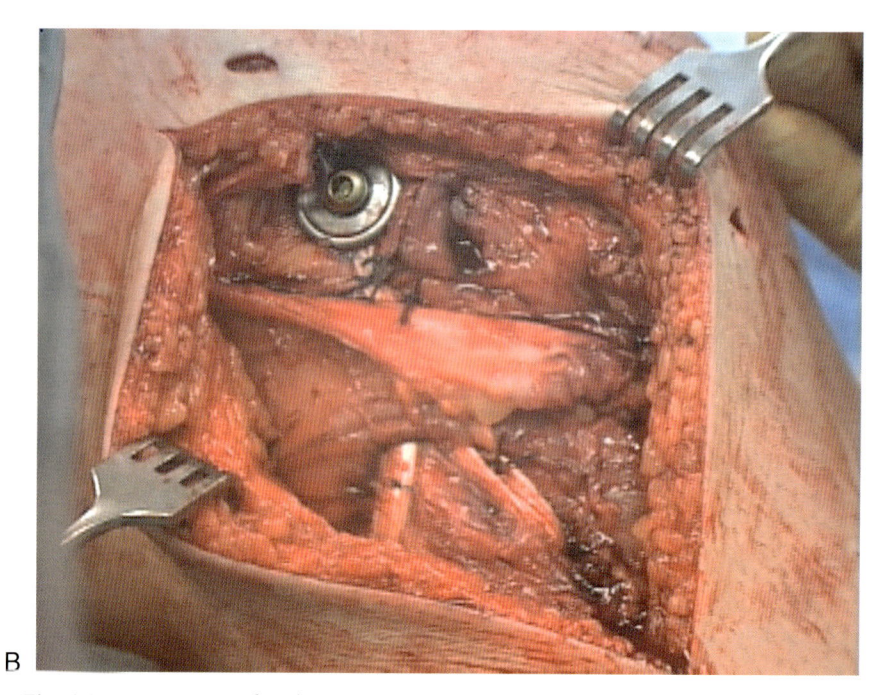

Fig. 16.10. (*Continued*). These complex surgical procedures reproduce the function of the popliteofibular ligament and the lateral collateral ligament and eliminate posterolateral capsular redundancy. The split biceps tendon transfer utilizes anatomic insertion sites and preserves the dynamic function of the long head and common biceps femoris tendon.

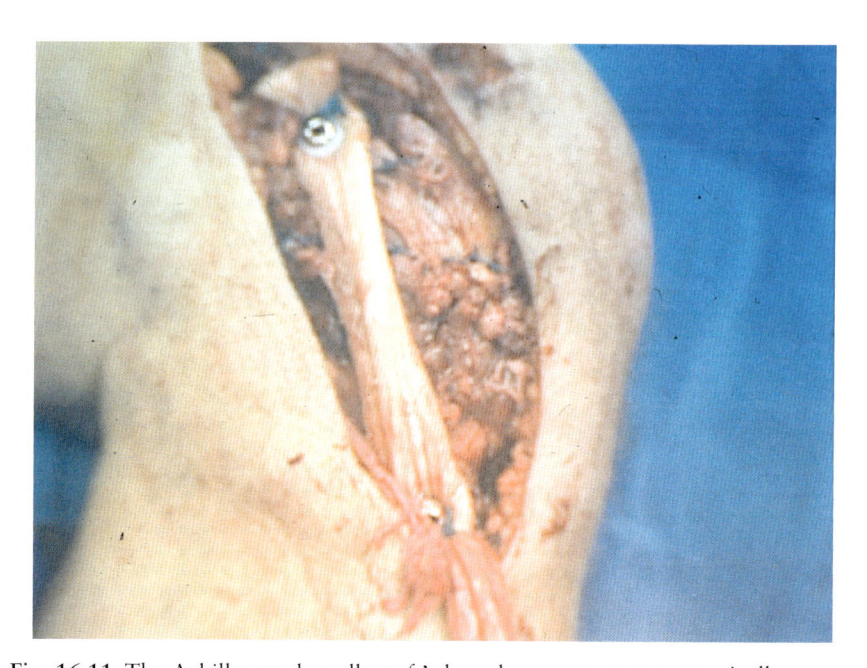

Fig. 16.11 The Achilles tendon allograft's broad anatomy can anatomically reconstruct the superficial medial collateral ligament. Screws and spiked ligament washers are used to secure the Achilles tendon allograft to the anatomic insertion sites of the superficial MCL. The posteromedial capsule can then be secured to the Achilles tendon allograft to eliminate posteromedial capsular laxity. This technique will address all components of the medial side instability.

Color Plate XXIII

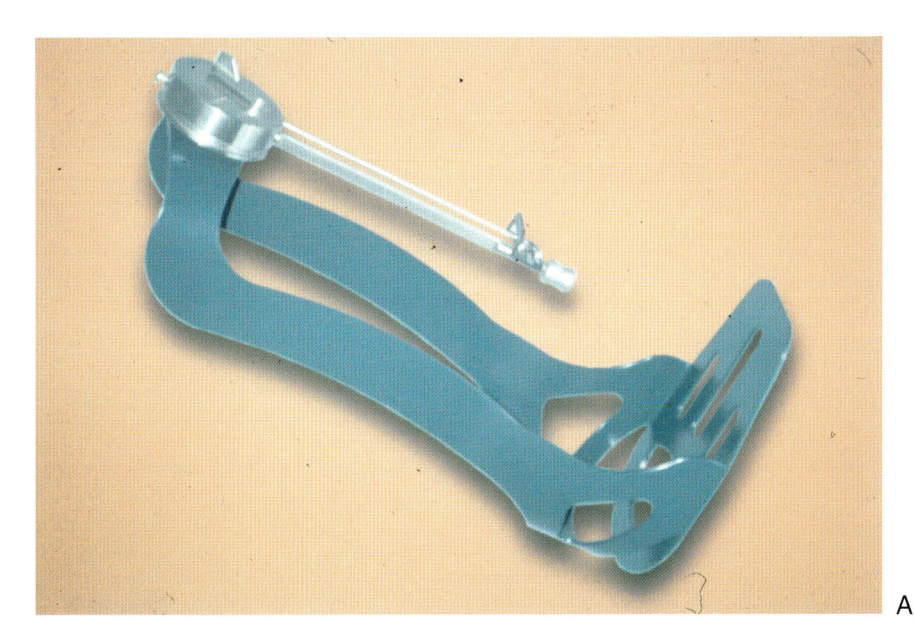

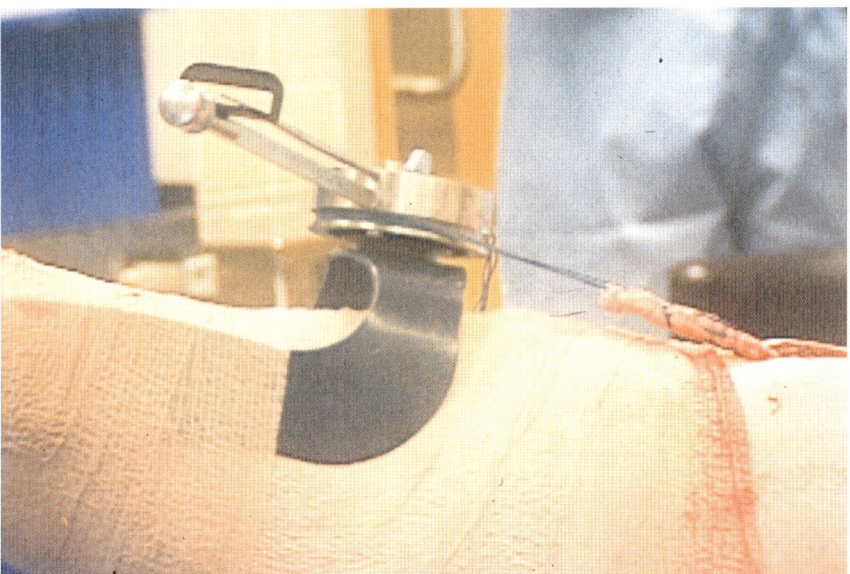

Fig. 16.12 The mechanical graft knee ligament tensioning device (A) is used as in (B) to precisely tension PCL and ACL grafts. During PCL reconstruction, the tensioning device is attached to the tibial end of the graft and the torque wrench ratchet is set to 20 lb to restore the anatomic tibial step-off. The knee is cycled through 25 full flexion–extension cycles, and with the knee at 70° of flexion, final PCL tibial fixation is achieved with a Lactosorb resorbable interference screw; backup fixation is provided by screw and spiked ligament washer. The tensioning device is applied to the ACL graft, and set to 20 lb, whereupon the graft is tensioned with the knee in 70° of flexion. Final ACL fixation is achieved with Lactosorb bioabsorbable interference screws and spiked ligament washer backup fixation. The mechanical tensioning device ensures consistent graft tensioning and eliminates graft advancement during interference screw insertion. It also restores the anatomic tibial step-off during PCL graft tensioning and applies a posterior drawer force during ACL graft tensioning. (Photograph 16.12A courtesy of Arthrotek, Inc., Warsaw, IN, used with permission.)

also to allow primary repair and/or reconstruction of the injured collateral ligament structures. Specific cases of ACL/PCL/MCL injuries are amenable to brace treatment of the medial collateral ligament for 4 to 6 weeks, followed by combined ACL/PCL reconstruction.[4,6,7,9–12,27,28]

Special considerations that affect the timing of surgery include vascular status of the extremity, reduction stability in dislocated knees, skin condition, multiple system injuries, open injuries, and other orthopaedic injuries. These overriding conditions may necessitate performing the surgery earlier or later than ideally planned. We have reported excellent results with delayed reconstruction of the multiligament injured knee.[4,15,27,28]

Graft Selection

The ideal graft material is strong, provides secure fixation, is easy to pass and readily available, and has low donor site morbidity. The available options in the United States are autograft and allograft sources. Our preferred graft for the posterior cruciate ligament is the Achilles tendon allograft because of its large cross-sectional area and strength, absence of donor site morbidity, and easy passage with secure fixation. We currently prefer Achilles tendon allograft for the ACL reconstruction.[29] The preferred graft material for the posterolateral corner is a split biceps tendon transfer, free autograft or allograft semitendinosus, or allograft Achilles tendon tissue when the biceps tendon is not available. Medial side reconstruction is performed with Achilles tendon or other allograft tissue, capsular shift procedures, or a combination of both procedures.

Surgical Technique

This section describes our surgical technique for reconstruction of the multiple ligament injured knee.[4,15,27,28,30–32] The patient is positioned supine on the operating room table. The surgical leg hangs over the side of the operating table, and the well leg is supported by the fully extended operating table. A lateral post is used for control of the surgical leg (Figure 8.1; see

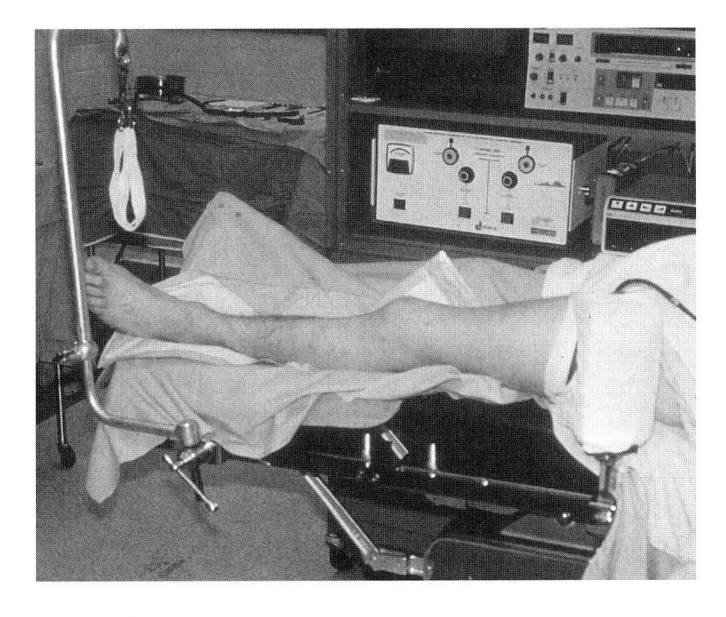

Fig. 8.1. Patient is positioned supine on the operating table with the nonsurgical leg resting on the fully extended operating table. A lateral post is used for control of the surgical lower extremity. (See color plate.)

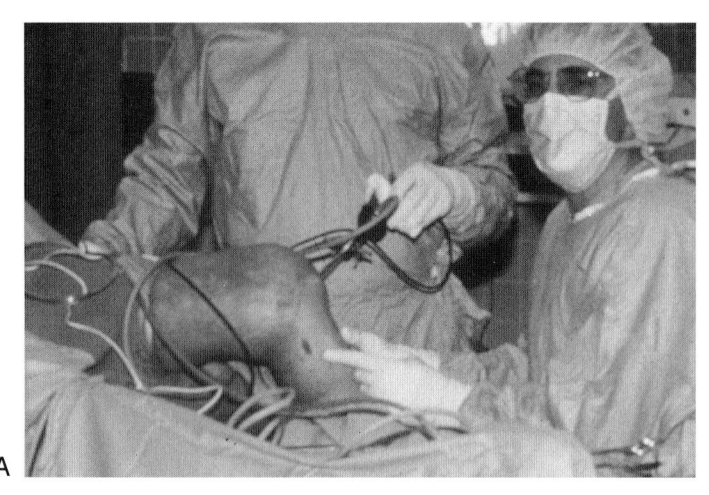

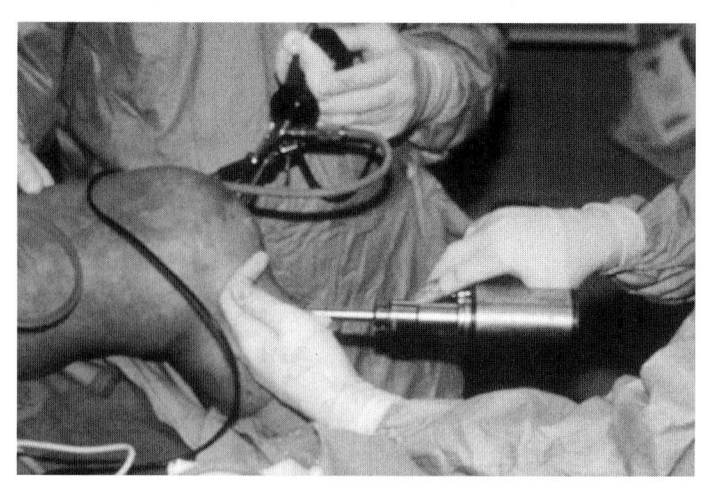

Fig. 8.2A and B. 1 to 2 cm extracapsular posterior medial safety incision allows the surgeon's finger to protect the neurovascular structures and confirm the position of instruments on the posterior aspect of the proximal tibia. (See color plate.)

color plate). The surgery is done under tourniquet control. Fluid inflow is by gravity. We do not routinely use an arthroscopic fluid pump.

Arthroscopic instruments are placed with the inflow in the superior lateral patellar portal, arthroscope in the inferior lateral patellar portal, and instruments in the inferior medial patellar portal. These portals are interchanged as necessary. An accessory extracapsular, extra-articular posteromedial safety incision is used to protect the neurovascular structures and to confirm the accuracy of tibial tunnel placement (Figure 8.2; see color plate).

The notchplasty is performed first and consists of ACL and PCL stump debridement, bone removal, and contouring of the medial wall of the lateral femoral condyle and the intercondylar roof. This allows visualization of the over-the-top position, and prevents ACL graft impingement throughout the full range of motion. Specially curved PCL instruments (Arthrotek, Warren, IN) are used to elevate the capsule from the posterior aspect of the tibia (Figure 8.3).

ACL/PCL Reconstruction

The PCL tibial and femoral tunnels are created with the help of the Fanelli PCL/ACL drill guide (Arthrotek: Figure 8.4). The transtibial PCL tunnel is

Fig. 8.3. Specially curved instruments used to elevate the capsule from the posterior aspect of the tibial ridge during PCL reconstruction. Posterior capsular elevation is critical in transtibial PCL reconstruction because it facilitates accurate PCL tibial tunnel placement and subsequent graft passage.

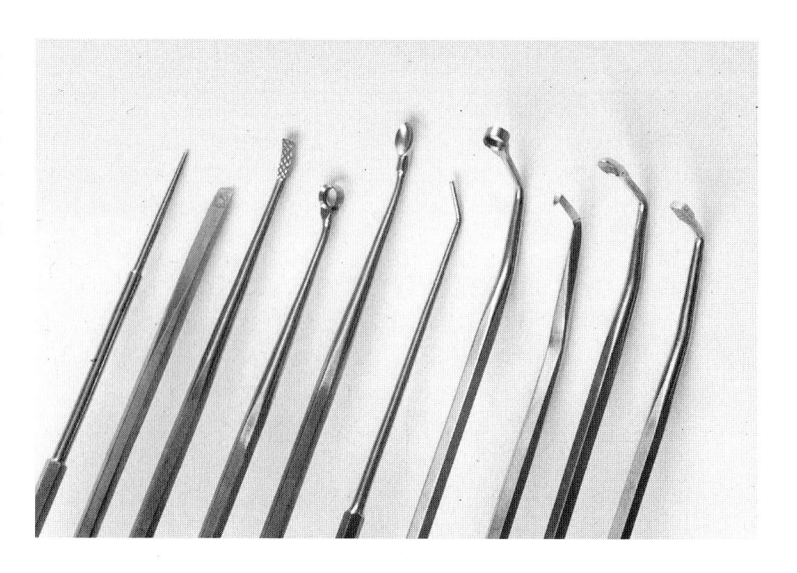

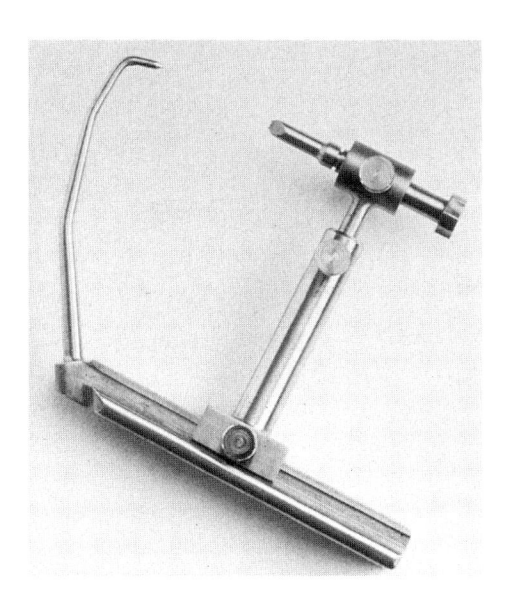

Fig. 8.4. The PCL/ACL drill guide system is used to precisely create both the PCL femoral and tibial tunnels and the ACL single-incision technique and double-incision technique tunnels. The drill guide is positioned for the PCL tibial tunnel so that a guide wire enters the anteromedial aspect of the proximal tibia approximately 1 cm below the tibial tubercle, at a point midway between the posteromedial border of the tibia and the tibial crest anteriorly. The guide wire exits in the inferior lateral aspect of the PCL tibial anatomic insertion site. The guide is positioned for the PCL femoral tunnel so that the guide wire enters the medial aspect of the medial femoral condyle midway between the medial femoral condyle articular margin and the medial epicondyle 2 cm proximal to the medial femoral condyle distal articular surface (joint line). The guide wire exits through the center of the stump of the anterolateral bundle of the posterior cruciate ligament. The drill guide is positioned for the single-incision endoscopic ACL technique so that the guide wire enters the anteromedial surface of the proximal tibia approximately 1 cm proximal to the tibial tubercle at a point midway between the posteromedial border of the tibia and the tibial crest anteriorly. The guide wire exits through the center of the stump of the tibial ACL insertion. (Photograph courtesy of Arthrotek, Inc., Warsaw, Indiana. Used with permission.)

drilled from the anteromedial aspect of the proximal tibial 1 cm below the tibial tubercle to exit in the inferior lateral aspect of the PCL anatomic insertion site. The PCL femoral tunnel originates externally between the medial femoral epicondyle and the medial femoral condylar articular surface approximately 2 cm proximal to the distal medial femoral condyle articular surface, emerging through the center of the stump of the anterolateral bundle of the posterior cruciate ligament. This external position of the femoral tunnel, in our experience, decreases the chance of avascular necrosis or subchondral fracture of the medial femoral condyle. The PCL graft is positioned and anchored on the femoral side and left free on the tibial side.

The ACL tunnels are created using the single-incision technique.[30–32] The tibial tunnel begins externally at a point 1 cm proximal to the tibial tubercle on the anteromedial surface of the proximal tibia to emerge through the center of the stump of the ACL tibial footprint. The femoral tunnel is positioned next to the over-the-top position on the medial wall of the lateral femoral condyle near the ACL anatomic insertion site. The tunnel is created to leave a 1 to 2 mm posterior cortical wall so that interference fixation can be used. The ACL graft is positioned and anchored on the femoral side, with the tibial side left free (Figure 8.5; see color plate).

Posterolateral Reconstruction Surgical Technique

Surgical techniques we use for posterolateral reconstruction are the split and full biceps tendon transfer to the lateral femoral epicondyle and the allograft or autograft figure-of-eight technique combined with posterolateral capsular shift as indicated.[6,22,23,34] The requirements for the biceps tendon procedures include an intact proximal tibiofibular joint, intact posterolateral capsular attachments to the common biceps tendon, and an intact biceps femoris tendon insertion into the fibular head. These techniques reproduce the function of the popliteofibular ligament and lateral collateral ligament, tighten the posterolateral capsule, and provide a post of strong autogenous tissue to reinforce the posterolateral corner.

A lateral hockey stick incision is made.[5,6,33] The peroneal nerve is dissected free and protected throughout the procedure. The long head and common biceps femoris tendon are isolated, and the anterior two thirds is separated

Fig. 8.5. Combined arthroscopic ACL/PCL reconstruction by means of Achilles tendon allograft. The tunnels are precisely created to reproduce the anatomic insertion sites of the anterolateral bundle of the posterior cruciate ligament and the anatomic insertion sites of the anterior cruciate ligament. Correct and accurate tunnel placement is essential for successful combined ACL/PCL reconstructions. The Achilles tendon allograft is preferred because of its large cross-sectional area, strength, and absence of donor site morbidity. (See color plate.)

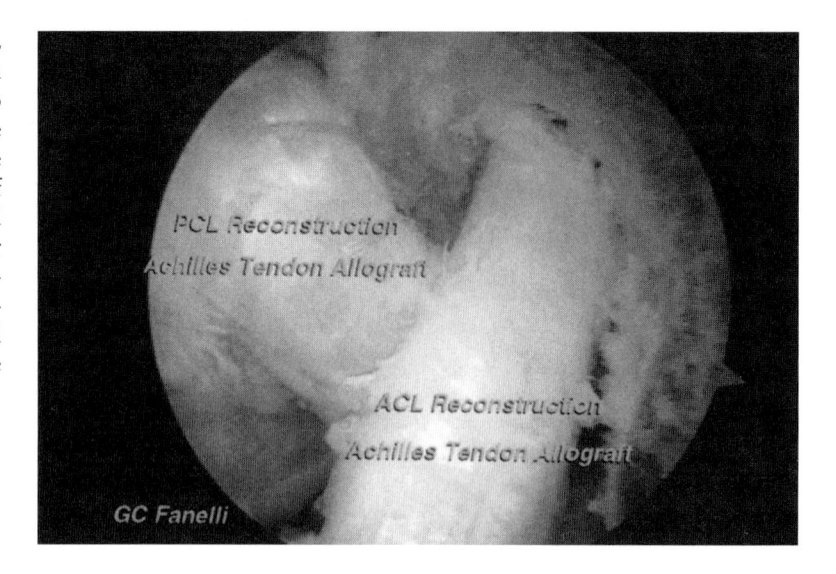

from the short head muscle. The tendon is detached proximally and left attached distally to its anatomic insertion site on the fibular head. The strip of biceps tendon is approximately 12 to 14 cm long. The iliotibial band is incised in line with its fibers, and the fibular collateral ligament and popliteus tendon are exposed. A drill hole is made 1 cm anterior to the fibular collateral ligament femoral insertion. A longitudinal incision is made in the lateral capsule just posterior to the fibular collateral ligament. The split biceps tendon is passed medial to the iliotibial band and secured to the lateral femoral epicondylar region with a screw and spiked ligament washer. The residual tail of the transferred split biceps tendon is passed medial to the iliotibial band and secured to the fibular head. The posterolateral capsule that had been incised is then shifted and sewn into the strut of transferred biceps tendon to eliminate posterolateral capsular redundancy (Figure 8.6A; see color plate). In cases of a proximal tibiofibular joint that has been disrupted, a two-tailed allograft reconstruction is used to control the tibia and fibula independently.[35]

Posterolateral reconstruction with the free graft figure-of-eight technique uses semitendinosus autograft or allograft, Achilles tendon allograft, or other soft tissue allograft material. A curvilinear incision is made in the lateral aspect of the knee extending from the lateral femoral epicondyle to the interval between Gerdy's tubercle and the fibular head. The fibular head is exposed, and a tunnel is created in an anterior-to-posterior direction at the area of maximal fibular diameter. The tunnel is created by passing a guide pin followed by a cannulated drill, usually 7 mm in diameter. The peroneal nerve is protected during tunnel creation and throughout the procedure. The free tendon graft is then passed through the fibular head drill hole. An incision is then made in the iliotibial band in line with the fibers directly overlying the lateral femoral epicondyle. The graft material is passed medial to the iliotibial band, and the limbs of the graft are crossed to form a figure-of-eight. A drill hole is made 1 cm anterior to the fibular collateral ligament femoral insertion. A longitudinal incision is made in the lateral capsule just posterior to the fibular collateral ligament. The graft material is passed medial to the iliotibial band and secured to the lateral femoral epicondylar region with a screw and spiked ligament washer. The posterolateral capsule that had been incised is then shifted and sewn into the strut of figure-of-eight graft tissue material to eliminate posterolateral capsular redundancy.

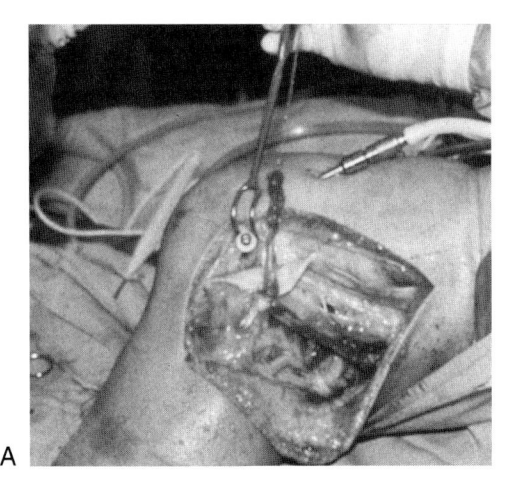

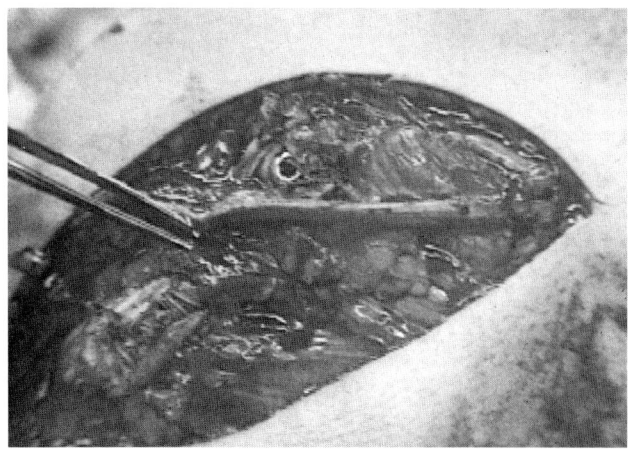

8. Combined ACL/PCL/Medial/Lateral Side Injuries

The anterior and posterior limbs of the figure-of-eight graft material are sewn to each other to reinforce and tighten the construct (Figure 8.6B; see color plate). The iliotibial band incision is closed. The procedures described are intended to eliminate posterolateral and varus rotational instability.

Medial Reconstruction Surgical Technique

Posteromedial and medial reconstructions are performed through a medial hockey stick incision. Care is taken to maintain adequate skin bridges between incisions. The superficial medial collateral ligament (MCL) is exposed, and a longitudinal incision is made just posterior to the posterior border of the MCL. Care is taken not to damage the medial meniscus during the capsular incision. The interval between the posteromedial capsule and the medial meniscus is developed. The posteromedial capsule is shifted anterosuperiorly. The medial meniscus is repaired to the new capsular position, and the shifted capsule is sewn into the medial collateral ligament. When superficial MCL reconstruction is indicated, it is performed with allograft or autograft tissue. This graft material is attached at the anatomic insertion sites of the superficial medial collateral ligament on the femur and tibia. The posteromedial capsular advancement is performed and sewn into the newly reconstructed MCL (Figure 8.7A; see color plate). Lower degree medial side instabilities may be treated with posteromedial capsular shift procedures (Figure 8.7B; see color plate).

Graft Tensioning and Fixation

The PCL is reconstructed first, followed by the ACL, followed by the posterolateral complex and the medial ligament complex. Tension is placed on the PCL graft distally by using the Arthrotek knee ligament tensioning device, and the tension is set for 20 lb (Figure 8.8). This restores the anatomic tibial step-off. The knee is cycled through a full range of motion 25 times to allow pretensioning and settling of the graft. After the knee has been placed in 0 or 70° of flexion, fixation is achieved on the tibial side of the PCL graft with a bioabsorbable interference screw, and backup fixation with a screw and spiked ligament washer. Next the Arthrotek knee ligament tensioning device is applied to the ACL graft and set to 20 lb. The knee is placed in 0 or 70° of flexion, and final fixation is achieved of the ACL graft

Fig. 8.6. Our preferred surgical technique for posterolateral and lateral reconstruction is the split biceps tendon transfer (A) or the allograft or autograft figure-of-eight reconstruction (B) combined with posterolateral capsular shift and primary repair of injured structures, as indicated. These complex surgical procedures reproduce the function of the popliteofibular ligament and the lateral collateral ligament and eliminate posterolateral capsular redundancy. The split biceps tendon transfer utilizes anatomic insertion sites and preserves the dynamic function of the long head and common biceps femoris tendon. (See color plate.)

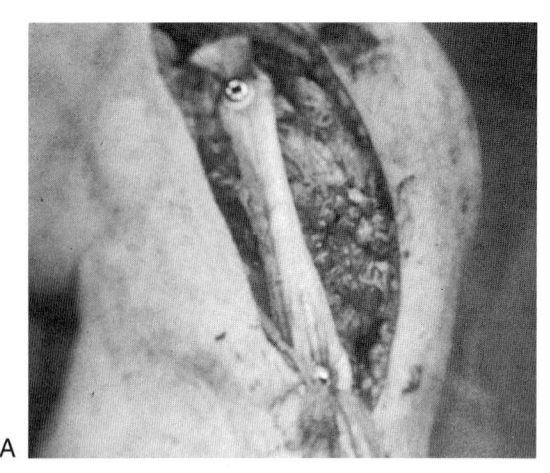

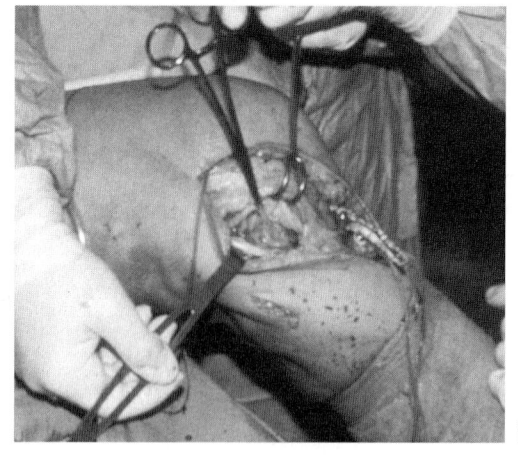

Fig. 8.7. (A) Severe medial side injuries are successfully treated with primary repair by means of the suture anchor technique combined with MCL reconstruction using Achilles tendon allograft. The Achilles tendon allograft's broad anatomy can anatomically reconstruct the superficial medial collateral ligament. The Achilles tendon allograft is secured to the anatomic insertion sites of the superficial MCL by means of screws and spiked ligament washers. The posteromedial capsule can then be secured to the Achilles tendon allograft to eliminate posteromedial capsular laxity. This technique will address all components of the medial side instability. (B) Lesser degrees of medial side instabilities may be treated with posteromedial capsular shift procedures. (See color plate.)

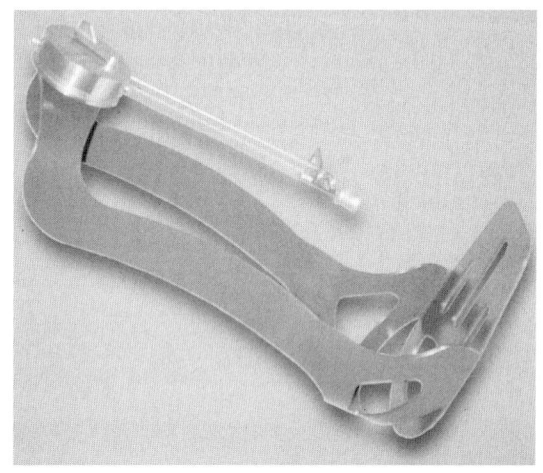

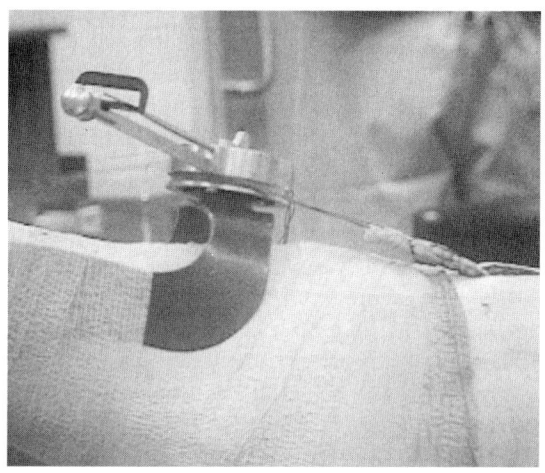

Fig. 8.8. (A) The mechanical graft knee ligament tensioning device is used to precisely tension PCL and ACL grafts. (Photograph courtesy of Arthrotek, Inc., Warsaw, Indiana. Used with permission.) (B) During PCL reconstruction, the tensioning device is attached to the tibial end of the graft and the torque wrench ratchet set to 20 lb. This restores the anatomic tibial step-off. The knee is cycled through 25 full flexion–extension cycles, and with the knee at 70° of flexion, final PCL tibial fixation is achieved with a Lactosorb resorbable interference screw and screw and spiked ligament washer for backup fixation. The tensioning device is applied to the ACL graft and set to 20 lb, and the graft is tensioned with the knee in 70° of flexion. Final ACL fixation is achieved with Lactosorb bioabsorbable interference screws and spiked ligament washer backup fixation. The mechanical tensioning device assures consistent graft tensioning and eliminates graft advancement during interference screw insertion. It also restores the anatomic tibial step-off during PCL graft tensioning and applies a posterior drawer force during ACL graft tensioning.

8. Combined ACL/PCL/Medial/Lateral Side Injuries

with a bioabsorbable interference screw and spiked ligament washer backup fixation. The knee is then placed in 30° of flexion, the tibial internally rotated, and slight valgus force applied to the knee, resulting in final tensioning and fixation of the posterolateral corner is achieved. The MCL reconstruction is tensioned with the knee in 30° of flexion with the leg in a figure-of-four position. Full range of motion is confirmed on the operating table to ensure that the knee is not "captured" by the reconstruction.

Surgical Technique Technical Hints

The posteromedial safety incision protects the neurovascular structures, confirms accurate tibial tunnel placement and allows the pace of the surgical procedure to be accelerated. The single-incision ACL reconstruction technique prevents lateral cortex crowding and eliminates multiple through-and-through drill holes in the distal femur, reducing stress riser effect. It is important to be aware of the two tibial tunnel directions and to have a bone bridge of 1 cm or greater between the PCL and ACL tibial tunnels. This will reduce the possibility of fracture (Figure 8.9; see color plate). We have found it useful to use primary and backup fixation. Primary fixation is done with bioabsorbable interference screws, and backup fixation is performed with a screw and spiked ligament washer. Secure fixation is critical to the success of this surgical procedure (Figure 8.10).

Patients with chronic multiple ligament injured knee may present with varus deformity combined with a lateral thrust. This may result from the ligament injury alone or a combination of the ligament injury and a malunited tibial plateau fracture. These conditions require a high tibial osteotomy to correct bony malalignment prior to ligament reconstruction. The correction of the bony malalignment will eliminate the varus thrust and

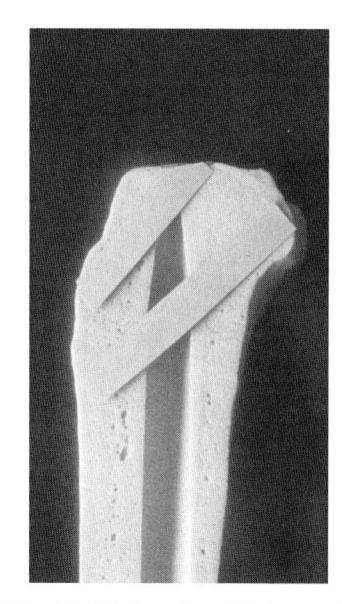

Fig. 8.9. Model showing tibial tunnel positions for combined ACL/PCL reconstructions. It is essential to have an adequate bone bridge between the two tunnels. (From Fanelli GC, Giannotti BF, Edson CJ. Current concepts review. The posterior cruciate ligament arthroscopic evaluation and treatment. Arthroscopy 1994; 10(6):673–688. Used with permission.) (See color plate.)

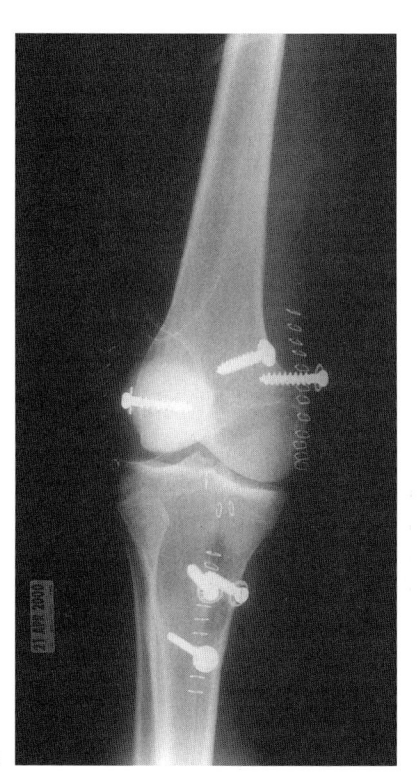

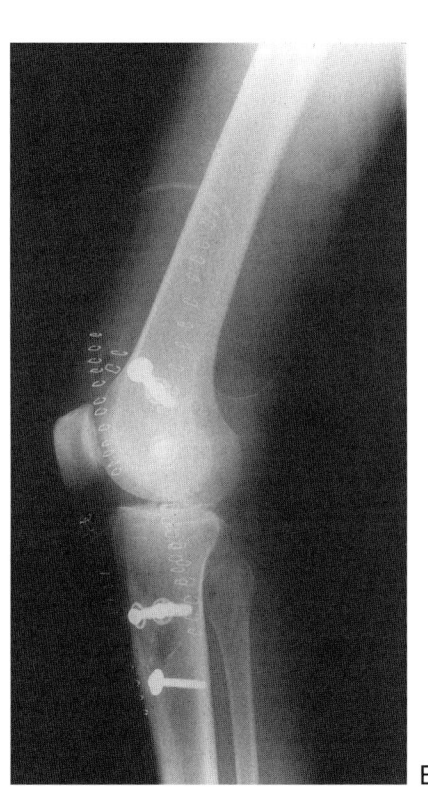

Fig. 8.10. (A) Anteroposterior and (B) lateral radiographs after combined ACL/PCL reconstruction. Note position of tibial tunnel on lateral x-ray. The tibial tunnel guide wire exits at the apex of the tibial ridge posteriorly, which places the graft at the anatomic tibial insertion site after the tibial tunnel has been drilled. We have found it useful to use primary and backup fixation. Primary fixation is with bioabsorbable interference screws, and backup fixation is performed with a screw and spiked ligament washer. Secure fixation is critical to the success of this surgical procedure.

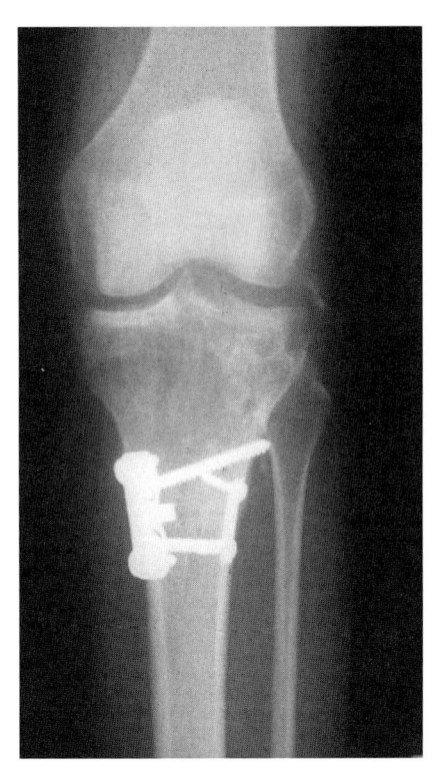

Fig. 8.11. Opening wedge high tibial osteotomy in a patient with a multiple ligament injured knee. This patient had a malunited tibial plateau fracture in addition to cruciate ligament and lateral side injuries, which had resulted in a lateral thrusting gait during ambulation. Opening wedge high tibial osteotomy was performed below the level of the tibial tubercle to avoid interference with cruciate ligament reconstruction tunnels. The realignment of the lower extremity after the osteotomy eliminated the varus thrusting gait even before ligament reconstruction was performed.

improve the chance of successful ligament surgical reconstruction (Figure 8.11).

Postoperative Rehabilitation

Rehabilitation following multiple ligament reconstruction is an ever evolving process. Rehabilitation guidelines consider surgical technique and the natural alignment of the lower extremity. Postoperative weeks 1 to 6 comprise the maximum protection phase. During this period, the patient is non–weight bearing, and the surgical extremity is braced in full extension. During postoperative weeks 4 through 6, range of motion is progressed. In postoperative weeks 7 to 10, the rehabilitation brace is unlocked and weight bearing is progressed at 25% of body weight per week over the next 4 weeks. The patient is fully weight bearing, using crutches, at the end of postoperative week 10. Varus and/or valgus forces are avoided during range-of-motion exercises to protect the collateral ligaments that have been reconstructed. The long-leg rehabilitation brace is discontinued at the end of postoperative week 10, and an ACL-PCL functional brace is used for activities of daily living for continued protection. Range-of-motion exercises on a stationary bicycle are progressed, and closed-chain exercises are performed with stair-stepping machines, rowing machines, and elliptical trainers; leg presses are performed, as well. Proprioceptive skill training is advanced. Straight-line jogging is initiated between postoperative months 4 and 5, depending on the patient's strength and proprioceptive skill level.

Sport-specific exercises and training begin between postoperative months 4 and 5, with a return to sports at the end of postoperative month 6 to 9 if the following criteria are met: quadriceps and hamstring strength is 90% or greater than the uninvolved extremity; patient can perform all necessary skills without pain or restriction; and a functional brace (combined instability brace) has been obtained. It should be noted that a loss of 10 to 15° of terminal flexion can be expected in these complex knee ligament reconstructions. This does not cause a functional problem for these patients and is not a cause for alarm.

Results of Surgical Reconstruction in the Multiple Ligament Injured Knee

We have published elsewhere the results of our arthroscopically assisted combined ACL/PCL and PCL/posterolateral complex reconstructions in which we used the reconstructive technique described in this chapter.[4,15,27] More recently, Ibrahim reported on the results of 41 traumatic knee dislocations treated with ACL and PCL reconstructions. In these young patients (mean age 26.3 years), early mobilization with continuous passive motion and active range-of-motion exercises were started on postoperative day 2. Based on these results, at a mean follow-up of 39 months, Ibrahim recommended early reconstruction of the cruciate ligaments, early repair of the collateral ligaments, and aggressive rehabilitation in these young, active patients.[36]

Other recent reports that evaluate results based on arthrometric data support early reconstruction of the cruciate ligaments and early repair of the collateral ligaments. Although results vary, they all demonstrate that residual laxity is present in a certain portion of reconstructed knees.[37–39]

Yeh et al. reported on the results of PCL reconstruction with ACL debridement. This study did not report mean side-to-side difference in anterior–posterior laxity, but the authors reported good range of motion and a mean Lysholm score of 84 at a follow-up period of 27 months.[40]

Fanelli Sports Injury Clinic Results: Combined ACL/PCL Reconstruction

Thirty-five patients treated surgically for combined ACL/PCL instability of the knee are presented.[10,28] These patients were evaluated preoperatively, and postoperatively on an annual basis by means of the Lysholm, Tegner, and Hospital for Special Surgery (HSS) knee ligament rating scales, the KT1000 knee ligament arthrometer, and stress radiography.[41,42] All evaluations were performed by an independent examiner, thus eliminating surgeon bias. Statistical analysis was performed by an independent statistician who was not a member of the surgical team.

Thirty-five arthroscopically assisted combined ACL/PCL reconstructions were performed by a single surgeon (G.C.F.). The minimum follow-up is 24 months, with a follow-up range of 24 to 120 months. There were 26 men and 9 women, and 19 acute and 16 chronic combined ACL/PCL injuries. Acute injuries were defined as those the operating surgeon had control of since the time of injury and had performed the surgery less than 8 weeks postinjury (this allowed for bracing of acute MCL tears). Chronic injuries were defined as those of patients who had had surgery more than 8 weeks postinjury. Chronic injuries presented with functional instability of the knee as the chief complaint. These chronic patients had been initially treated with immobilization and were later referred for definitive treatment. The time of reconstruction in these chronic knee injuries was 3 to 26 months postinjury. No reconstructions were performed in patients with arthrosis.

The ligaments injured in the study group included 1 ACL/PCL tear, 19 ACL/PCL/posterior lateral corner tears, 9 ACL/PCL/MCL tears, and 6 ACL/PCL/MCL/posterior lateral corner tears. Mechanisms of injury were as follows: 20 motorcycle/motor vehicle accidents, 9 sports-related accidents, 4 falls, 1 industrial accident, and 1 pedestrian/automobile accident. Six of the acute knee injuries presented as tibiofemoral dislocations, and 4 of the chronic knee injuries had been documented earlier as tibiofemoral dislocations. Twenty-six fresh-frozen irradiated Achilles tendon allografts, 7 bone–patellar tendon–bone (BPTB) autografts, and 2 semitendinosus–gracilis autografts were used for the posterior cruciate ligament reconstructions. Sixteen autograft BPTB units, 12 fresh-frozen irradiated BPTB allografts, 6 fresh-frozen irradiated Achilles tendon allografts, and 1 semitendinosus–gracilis autograft were used for the ACL reconstruction.

Statistical Analysis

The statistical analysis was performed by an independent statistician who was not associated with the surgical team. The statistical tests used to analyze the data were the Wilcoxon signed rank test and the paired *t* test. When no statistically significant difference was found between groups of paired numbers, power analysis was performed to assess the sample size. Statistical analysis was performed using the SigmaStat computer program (version 2.0; SPSS, Chicago).

Knee Ligament Rating Scales

Patients were evaluated using Tegner, Lysholm, and HSS knee ligament rating scales.[41,42] The mean preoperative Lysholm score for 30 knees was 32.1 (range 0–75). The mean postoperative Lysholm score for 35 knees was 91.2 (range 70–100). This is a statistically significant improvement ($p = 0.001$).

The mean preoperative Tegner score for 30 knees was 1.4 (range 0–7). The mean postoperative Tegner score for 35 knees was 5.3 (range 3–7). This is a statistically significant improvement from preoperative to postoperative values ($p = 0.001$). Mean preoperative HSS score for 30 knees was 19.9 (range 0–51), and mean postoperative HSS score for 35 knees was 86.8 (range 71–96). This is a statistically significant improvement ($p = 0.001$).

When the groups were divided into acute and chronic and evaluated with all three knee ligament rating scales, all patients showed a statistically significant improvement from preoperative to postoperative ($p = 0.001$). There was, however, no statistically significant difference between acute and chronic knees evaluated postoperatively with Tegner ($p = 0.907$), Lysholm ($p = 0.083$), and HSS ($p = 0.422$) knee scales.

When the knees were divided into autograft PCL and allograft PCL groups and evaluated with all three knee ligament rating scales, all patients showed a statistically significant improvement from preoperative to postoperative status ($p = 0.001$). There was, however, no statistically significant difference between autograft PCL and allograft PCL groups evaluated postoperatively with Tegner ($p = 0.640$), Lysholm ($p = 0.533$), and HSS ($p = 0.558$) knee ligament rating scales.

KT1000 Arthrometer Measurements

Knees in the series were evaluated with the KT1000 knee ligament arthrometer (MEDmetric, San Diego, CA) to attempt to quantitate pre- and postoperative anterior and posterior tibial translation in millimeters. Corrected anterior, corrected posterior, and PCL screen measurements were used, and the results were recorded as a side-to-side difference between the involved and the normal knee according to the methods of Daniel.[1] The mean preoperative corrected anterior side-to-side difference value in 21 knees was 3.4 mm (range 0.0–6.5 mm), and the mean postoperative corrected anterior side-to-side difference in 35 knees was 1.0 mm (range 0.0–3.5 mm). The mean preoperative corrected posterior side-to-side difference value in 21 knees was 6.1 mm (range 2.0–12.5 mm), and the mean postoperative corrected posterior side-to-side difference value in 35 knees was 2.6 mm (range 0–9.0 mm). The mean preoperative PCL screen side-to-side difference value in 24 knees was 5.2 mm (range 0.5–11.0 mm), and the mean postoperative PCL screen side-to-side difference value in 35 knees was 2.7 mm (range 0–7.0 mm).

All three KT1000 scores (corrected anterior, corrected posterior, and PCL screen) demonstrated a statistically significant improvement from preoperative to postoperative values ($p = 0.001$).

An attempt was made to determine the significance of KT1000 data between acute and chronic knees, and between allograft PCL and autograft PCL knees. The Mann-Whitney rank sum test, and the paired t test with power analysis were used to calculate p values. The KT1000 arthrometer data did not demonstrate any significant differences between acute and chronic conditions, and there were no significant differences between allograft PCL knees and autograft PCL knees.

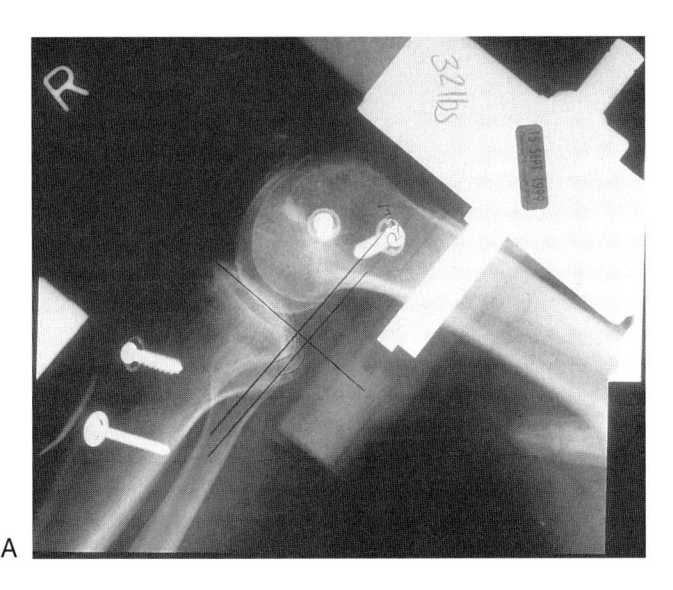

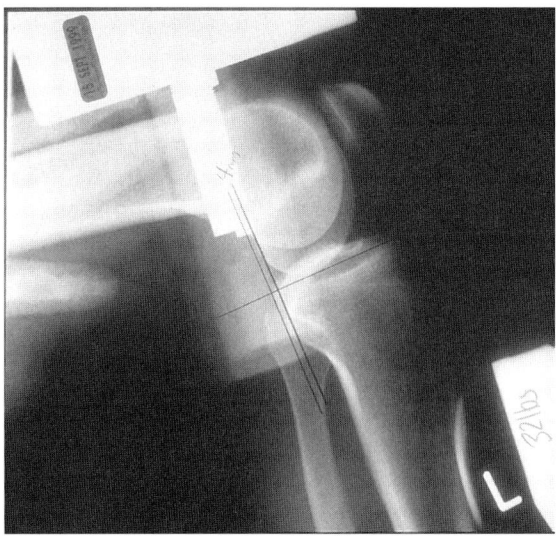

Fig. 8.12. Telos stress radiographs demonstrating a 1mm side-to-side difference in the PCL reconstruction component of an ACL-PCL-PLC-MCL reconstructed knee.

Stress Radiography

Stress radiographic measurements obtained with the Telos stress radiographic device (Telos Corporation, Germany) were used to assess the static stability of the PCL reconstruction. The knee to be tested is placed in the Telos frame in 90° of flexion. A 32 lb posterior displacement force is applied to the tibial tubercle area, and a lateral x-ray is performed. The study is performed on the surgical and nonsurgical knees, and the difference in posterior displacement measured in millimeters between the normal and the surgical knee is recorded (Figure 8.12).

The postoperative side-to-side differences comparing the surgical and nonsurgical knees were obtained in 21 patient knees. Eleven of 21 knees (52.3%) had a side-to-side difference of 0 to 3 mm. Five of 21 (23.8%) knees had a side-to-side difference of 4 to 5 mm. Four of 21 knees (19.0%) had a side-to-side difference of 6 to 10 mm.

Since there were only 4 preoperative Telos stress radiographic measurements and 21 postoperative measurements, the sample size was not large enough to permit the calculation of an accurate p value. The mean postoperative side-to-side Telos difference in the allograft PCL reconstructed knees was 2.8 mm (range 0.0–9.0 mm), while the mean side-to-side difference in the autograft PCL reconstructed knees was 3.0 mm (range 2.0–4.0 mm). Statistical analysis using the paired t test with power analysis demonstrated no statistical difference between the allograft and autograft PCL groups ($p = 0.901$). The mean postoperative side-to-side Telos difference in the acute ACL/PCL reconstructed knees was 3.2 mm (range 0.0–9.0 mm), while the mean side-to-side difference in the chronic ACL/PCL reconstructed knees was 3.2 mm (range 0.0–8.0 mm). Statistical analysis using the paired t test with power analysis demonstrated no statistical difference between the acute and chronic groups ($p = 1.000$).

Physical Examination

The posterior cruciate ligament was assessed on physical examination by the proximal tibial step-off and the posterior drawer test.[14,35] Preoperatively, 32 knees had a decreased tibial step-off of 15 mm or greater, corresponding to a grade III+ posterior drawer, and 3 knees had a decreased tibial step-off of 10 to 15 mm, corresponding to a grade II+ posterior drawer. Postoperatively, 16 of 35 (46%) knees had a normal tibial step-off and normal posterior drawer, and 19 of 35 (54%) knees had a tibial step-off decreased 5 mm, corresponding to a grade I posterior drawer.

The anterior cruciate ligament was evaluated by using the Lachman test and the pivot shifting phenomenon.[43,44] Preoperatively, 35 knees had a grade III Lachman test and a grade III pivot shifting phenomenon. Postoperatively, 33 of 35 (94%) knees had normal Lachman and pivot shift tests.

Medial collateral ligaments were evaluated by using valgus stress with the knee in 30° of flexion. Seven medial collateral ligament tears were treated surgically, while 8 were treated with bracing. Seven of 7 (100%) of the surgically treated MCL tears were equal to the normal knee when evaluated postoperatively with the 30° valgus stress test. Seven of 8 (87.5%) of the brace-treated MCL tears were equal to the normal knee when evaluated postoperatively with the 30° valgus stress test.

Posterior lateral instability was evaluated on physical examination by using the reverse pivot shift test, the external rotation thigh–foot angle test (dial test), and the varus stress test at 30° of knee flexion.[45,46] There were 25 patients in this group with posterior lateral instability combined with ACL/PCL injuries. All 25 patients had a positive reverse pivot shift test and an external rotation thigh–foot angle test (ERTFAT) that was increased 20° over the uninvolved extremity preoperatively, and tested with the knee in 30 and 90° of knee flexion. Postoperatively, the ERTFAT done at 30 and 90° of knee flexion revealed equal external rotation to the uninvolved lower extremity in 6 of 25 (24%) knees, and less external rotation in 19 of 25 (76%) knees, indicating overcorrection of the posterior lateral instability. Postoperatively, all 25 knees had elimination of the reverse pivot shift. Varus stress testing performed in 30° of knee flexion demonstrated the surgical knee equal to the normal knee in 22 of 25 (88%) and grade 1 varus laxity in 3 of 25 (12%).

Fanelli Sports Injury Clinic Results: Combined PCL–Posterolateral Reconstruction

Another group of patients to be included in the results of multiple ligament injured knee treatment is the combined posterior cruciate ligament–posterolateral complex instability knee injury group. While not dislocated knees, these are severe multiple ligament injured knees that typically present to our institution as a result of high energy trauma.[2,3]

Materials and Methods

This case series type of study presents the 2- to 10-year (24–120 month) follow-up results of 41 chronic posterior cruciate ligament–posterolateral complex reconstructions performed by a single surgeon (G.C.F.). All patients were evaluated by an independent examiner who was not a member of the surgical team. This was done to eliminate operating surgeon bias. An independent statistician, not associated with the surgical team, performed the statistical analysis.

The study group of patients consisted of 31 males and 10 females. There were 17 right and 24 left knees, and all 41 patients had chronic PCL/posterior lateral corner knee injuries with functional instability that interfered with the desired activities of daily living.

The surgical technique chosen for the 41 posterior cruciate ligament reconstruction procedures was a single femoral tunnel, single-bundle, transtibial tunnel, arthroscopically assisted reconstruction using fresh-frozen Achilles tendon allograft. The surgical technique for the 41 postero-lateral reconstructions was a biceps tendon tenodesis combined with a posterolateral capsular shift procedure.

Physical examination tests that were used to evaluate the posterior cruciate ligament included the proximal tibial step-off and the posterior drawer test. Physical examination tests used to evaluate the posterior lateral corner were the external rotation thigh–foot angle test, the posterior lateral drawer test, and the reverse pivot shift test. KT1000 arthrometer measurements as described by Daniel were used to enhance the physical examination for posterior cruciate ligament evaluation.[1]

Statistical Analysis

Statistical analysis was performed by an independent statistician using SigmaStat, version 2.0. Knee ligament rating scales, arthrometer measurements, and stress radiographic measurement results were analyzed. The paired *t* test and the power analysis were the statistical tests used. Throughout the analysis, 95% confidence intervals were used.

Results

The follow-up range for these patients was 24 to 120 months (2–10 years), with a minimum follow-up of 24 months. The patients were evaluated pre-operatively and postoperatively by means of the Tegner, Lysholm, and Hospital for Special Surgery knee ligament rating scales.[20,21] The patients were also evaluated with the KT1000 knee ligament arthrometer using the PCL screen, corrected anterior, and corrected posterior measurements. These measurements and the KT1000 techniques we used to obtain them are described in detail by Daniel and Stone.

Physical Examination Results

Physical examination criteria used to evaluate these patients included tibial step-off, posterior drawer, varus stress test, external rotation thigh–foot angle test at 30 and 90° of flexion, posterior lateral drawer, and range of knee motion in comparison to the uninvolved knee.

The tibial step-off and posterior drawer examinations were performed with the knee at 90° of flexion comparing the involved and the uninvolved knee. Both the posterior drawer and tibial step-off were considered to be normal when there was no difference between the involved and uninvolved knees. Grades 1, 2, and 3 posterior drawer and decreased tibial step-offs are described as having a proximal tibial posterior displacement, in comparison to the normal knee, of 5, 10, and 15 mm, respectively.

Preoperatively, 33 knees had a grade 3 posterior drawer and decreased tibial step-off of 15 mm or greater. Eight patients had a grade 2 posterior drawer and a decreased tibial step-off of 10 to 15 mm. Postoperatively, 29 of 41 (70%) patients had a normal posterior drawer and normal tibial step-off. Eleven of 41 (27%) patients had a grade 1 posterior drawer with a decreased tibial step-off of approximately 5 mm. One of 41 (3%) patients had a grade II posterior drawer with a tibial step-off decreased approximately 10 mm.

The varus stress test, posterior lateral drawer, and external rotation thigh–foot angle at 30 and 90° of flexion were used to document posterior lateral instability on physical examination. Preoperatively, all 41 knees had a positive posterior lateral drawer test. Preoperatively, all 41 knees had an external rotation thigh–foot angle (tested at 30 and 90° of knee flexion) that was 20° greater than the uninvolved normal knee. Postoperatively, 40 posterior lateral drawer tests and varus stress tests were restored to normal (98%). Postoperatively, the external rotation thigh–foot angle, tested at 30 and 90° of flexion, was tighter (less external rotation) than the normal knee in 29 of 41 (71%) patients, equal to the normal knee in 11 of 41 (27%) patients, and greater than the normal knee in 1 of 41 (2%) patients. This indicates that the posterior lateral instability was corrected in 40 of 41 (98%) of the cases.

Postoperative range of motion demonstrated a mean range of motion loss of 10° of terminal flexion in comparison to the uninvolved knee. There were no flexion contractures in this series.

Knee Ligament Rating Scale Results

All 41 patients were evaluated preoperatively and postoperatively using the Lysholm, Tegner, and Hospital for Special Surgery knee ligament rating scales. The paired t test was used to determine the level of statistical significance between the pre- and postoperative knee ligament rating scale values.

Pre- and postoperative Lysholm mean values were 65.48 (range 31–94) and 91.67 (range 73–100), respectively. Pre- and postoperative Tegner mean values were 2.71 (range 0–5) and 4.92 (range 3–7), respectively. Pre- and postoperative HSS mean values were 50.84 (range 13–78) and 88.69 (range 65–98), respectively. There was a statistically significant improvement from preoperative to postoperative values for all three knee ligament rating scales ($p = 0.001$).

KT1000 Knee Ligament Arthrometer Results

The KT1000 knee ligament arthrometer was used to evaluate all 41 knees in this series both pre- and postoperatively. The PCL screen, corrected anterior, and corrected posterior measurements were used to compare the involved and uninvolved knees according to the methods of Daniel.[1] The paired t test was used to determine the level of statistical significance between the pre- and postoperative KT1000 arthrometer values.

Preoperative mean PCL screen side-to-side difference measurement was 4.64 mm (range 0–10.0 mm), and postoperative mean PCL screen side-to-side difference measurement was 1.80 mm (range −2.5 to 6.5 mm). This is a statistically significant improvement from pre- to postoperative ($p = 0.001$).

Preoperative mean corrected posterior side-to-side difference measurement was 5.44 mm (range 0.0–14.0 mm), and postoperative mean corrected posterior side-to-side difference measurements was 2.11 mm (range −2.5 to 7.0 mm). This was a statistically significant improvement from pre- to postoperative status ($p = 0.001$).

Preoperative mean corrected anterior side-to-side difference measurement was 1.24 mm (range −3.0 to 7.0 mm), and postoperative mean corrected anterior side-to-side difference measurement was 0.63 mm (range −3.0 to 6.0 mm). There is no statistically significant difference between KT1000 corrected anterior preoperative and postoperative scores ($p = 0.175$). Power analysis was performed. The power of the paired t test was 0.144, which is below the desired power of 0.8000, suggesting that lack of significance must be cautiously interpreted. The lack of significance between pre- and postoperative corrected anterior scores does not necessarily indicate that this treatment was not successful. This result was expected, since the corrected anterior measurement evaluates the anterior cruciate ligament, and all anterior cruciate ligaments were intact in this series.

Stress Radiography Results

Stress radiography was performed pre- and postoperatively by means of the Telos stress radiography device (Austin and Associates, Maryland). Lateral radiographs of the surgical and normal knees were taken with the knees secured in the Telos device at 90° of knee flexion, with a 32 lb force applied at the tibial tubercle directed in a posterior direction. The preoperative mean side-to-side difference was 10.40 mm (range 7–14 mm), and the postoperative mean side-to-side difference was 2.26 mm (range −1 to 7 mm). The statistical test used was the paired t test, and the statistical analysis demonstrated a statistically significant improvement from pre- to postoperative measurements ($p = 0.001$).

Complications

Potential complications in the treatment of combined ACL/PCL/posterolateral corner injuries include failure to recognize and treat vascular injuries (both arterial and venous), iatrogenic neurovascular injury at the time of reconstruction, iatrogenic tibial plateau fractures at the time of reconstruction, failure to recognize all components of the instability, medial femoral condyle osteonecrosis, loss of knee motion, and postoperative anterior knee pain.[47-51] Our complications included postoperative adhesions requiring arthroscopic lysis and manipulation in 3 patients, and removal of painful hardware in 5 patients.

Conclusions

ACL/PCL injuries are most frequently seen in multiple trauma patients but do occur in the athletic injury population. Acute three ligament injured knees may have been tibiofemoral dislocations with spontaneous reduction in the field. Careful documentation of the neurovascular status is essential in these cases to avoid the complications associated with limb ischemia. Systematic evaluation of these patients with history, physical examination, imaging studies, examination under anesthesia, and diagnostic arthroscopy will aid in arriving at the correct diagnosis and treatment plan formulation.

Combined ACL/PCL instabilities can be successfully treated with arthroscopic reconstruction and the appropriate collateral ligament surgery. Statistically significant improvement is noted from the preoperative condition at 2- to 10-year follow-up when the evaluators used objective parameters of knee ligament rating scales, arthrometer testing, stress radiography, and physical examination. Postoperatively, these knees are not normal, but they are functionally stable. Continuing technical improvements will most likely produce better results in the future.

References

1. Daniel DM, Akeson W, O'Conner J, eds. Knee Ligaments—Structure, Function, Injury, and Repair. New York: Raven Press; 1990.
2. Fanelli GC. PCL injuries in trauma patients. Arthroscopy 1993; 9(3):291–294.
3. Fanelli GC, Edson CJ. Posterior cruciate ligament injuries in trauma patients. Part II. Arthroscopy 1995; 11(5):526–529.

4. Fanelli GC, Giannotti BF, Edson CJ. Current concepts review. The posterior cruciate ligament arthroscopic evaluation and treatment. Arthroscopy 1994; 10(6):673–688.
5. Fanelli GC, Feldmann DD. Management of combined ACL/PCL/posterolateral complex injuries of the knee. Oper Techniques Sports Med 1999; 7(3):143–149.
6. Fanelli GC, Feldmann DD. The dislocated/multiple ligament injured knee. Oper Techniques Orthop 1999; 9(4):298–308.
7. Fanelli GC. Combined anterior and posterior cruciate ligament injuries: the multiple ligament injured knee. Sports Med Arthrosc Rev 1999; 7(4):289–295.
8. Fanelli GC. Treatment of combined anterior cruciate ligament–posterior cruciate ligament–lateral side injuries of the knee. Clin Sports Med 2000; 19(3): 493–502.
9. Fanelli GC, Edson CJ, Maish DR. Management of combined ACL/PCL injuries. Techniques Orthop 2001; 16(2):157–166.
10. Fanelli GC. Surgical treatment of the acute and chronic ACL/PCL/medial side/lateral side injuries of the knee. Sports Med Arthrosc Rev 2001; 9(3).
11. Fanelli GC. Arthroscopic combined ACL/PCL reconstruction. In: Fanelli GC, ed. Posterior Cruciate Ligament Injuries. A Practical Guide to Management. New York: Springer-Verlag; 2001.
12. Fanelli GC, Feldmann, Edson CJ, Maish DR. The multiple ligament injured knee. In: DeLee JC, Drez D, Miller M, eds. DeLee and Drez's Orthopaedic Sports Medicine. 2nd ed. In press.
13. Ghalambor N, Vangsness CT. Traumatic dislocation of the knee: a review of the literature. Bull Hosp Joint Dis 1995; 54(1):19–24.
14. Good L, Johnson RJ. The dislocated knee. J Am Assoc Orthop Surg 1995; 3(5):284–292.
15. Fanelli GC, Giannotti BF, Edson CJ. Arthroscopically assisted combined posterior cruciate ligament/posterior lateral complex reconstruction. Arthroscopy 1996; 12(5):521–530.
16. Shelbourne KD, Porter DA, Clingman JA, et al. Low velocity knee dislocation. Orthop Rev 1991; 20:995–1004.
17. Wascher DC, Dvirnak PC, DeCoster TA. Knee dislocation: initial assessment and implications for treatment. J Orthop Trauma 1997; 11(7):525–529.
18. Shields L, Mital M, Cave EF. Complete dislocation of the knee: experience at the Massachusetts General Hospital. J Trauma 1969; 9:192–215.
19. Meyers MH, Harvey JP. Traumatic dislocation of the knee joint: a study of eighteen cases. J Bone Joint Surg Am 1971; 53:16–29.
20. Kennedy JC. Complete dislocation of the knee joint. J Bone Joint Surg Am 1963; 45:889–904.
21. Girgis FG, Marshall JL, Al Monajem ARS. The cruciate ligaments of the knee joint: anatomic, functional, and experimental analysis. Clin Orthop 1975; 106:216–231.
22. Clancy WG. Repair and reconstruction of the posterior cruciate ligament. In: Chapman M, ed. Operative Orthopaedics. Philadelphia: JB Lippincott; 1988:1651–1665.
23. Bleday RM, Fanelli GC, Giannotti BF, Edson CJ, Barrett TA. Instrumented measurement of the posterolateral corner. Arthroscopy 1998; 14(5):489–494.
24. Fowler PJ. Imaging of the posterior cruciate ligament. In: Fanelli GC, ed. Posterior Cruciate Ligament Injuries. A Practical Guide to Management. New York: Springer-Verlag; 2001, pp. 77–86.
25. Harner CD, Hoher J. Current concepts. Evaluation and treatment of posterior cruciate ligament injuries. Am J Sports Med 1998; 26(3):471–482.
26. Skyhar MJ, Warren RF, Oritz GJ, et al. The effects of sectioning the posterior cruciate ligament and the posterolateral complex on the articular contact pressure within the knee. J Bone Joint Surg Am 1993; 75:694–699.
27. Fanelli GC, Giannotti BF, Edson CJ. Arthroscopically assisted combined anterior and posterior cruciate ligament reconstruction. Arthroscopy 1996; 12(1):5–14.
28. Fanelli GC, Edson CJ. Arthroscopically assisted combined ACL/PCL reconstruction. 2–10 year follow-up. Arthroscopy 2002; 18(7):703–714.
29. Fanelli GC, Feldman DM. The use of allograft tissue in knee ligament reconstruction. In: Parisien JS, ed. Current Techniques in Arthroscopy. Philadelphia: Current Medicine; 1998, pp. 47–55.

30. Malek MM, Fanelli GC, DeLuca JV. Intraarticular and extraarticular anterior cruciate ligament reconstruction. In: Scott WN, ed. The Knee. St Louis, MO: CV Mosby; 1994:791–812.
31. Malek MM, Fanelli GC, Golden MD. Combined intraarticular and extraarticular anterior cruciate ligament reconstruction. In: Scott WN, ed. Ligament and Extensor Mechanism Injuries of the Knee. St Louis, MO: CV Mosby; 1991:267–284.
32. Fanelli GC, Desai BM, Cummings PD, Hanks GA, Kalenak A. Divergent alignment of the femoral interference screw in single incision endoscopic reconstruction of the anterior cruciate ligament. Contemp Orthop 1994; 28(1):21–25.
33. Fanelli GC, Larson RV. Practical management of posterolateral instability of the knee. Arthroscopy 2002; 18(2, suppl 1):1–8.
34. Wascher DC, Grauer JD, Markoff KL. Biceps tendon tenodesis for posterolateral instability of the knee. An in vitro study. Am J Sports Med 1993; 21(3):400–406.
35. Muller W. The Knee: Form, Function, and Ligamentous Reconstruction. New York: Springer-Verlag; 1983.
36. Ibrahim SA. Primary repair of the cruciate and collateral ligaments after traumatic dislocation of the knee. J Bone Joint Surg Br 1999; 81(6):987–990.
37. Martinek V, Imhoff AB. Combined anterior cruciate ligament and posterior cruciate ligament injury—technique and results of simultaneous arthroscopic reconstruction. Zentralbl Chir 1998; 123(9):1027–1032.
38. Noyes FR, Barber-Westin SD. Reconstruction of the anterior and posterior cruciate ligaments after knee dislocation. Use of early protected motion to decrease arthrofibrosis. Am J Sports Med 1997; 25(6):769–778.
39. Wascher DC, Becker JR, Dexter JG, Blevins FT. Reconstruction of the anterior and posterior cruciate ligaments after knee dislocation. Results using fresh frozen nonirradiated allografts. Am J Sports Med 1999; 27(2):189–196.
40. Yeh WL, Tu YK, Su JY, Hsu RW. Knee dislocation: treatment of high velocity knee dislocation. J Trauma Inj Infect Crit Care 1999; 46(4):693–701.
41. Tegner Y, Lysholm J. Rating system in the evaluation of knee ligament injuries. Clin Orthop 1985; 198:43–49.
42. Windsor RE, Insall JN, Warren RF, Wickiewicz TL. The Hospital for Special Surgery knee ligament rating form. Am J Knee Surg 1988; 1:140–145.
43. Torg JS, Conrad W, Kalen V. Clinical diagnosis of anterior cruciate ligament instability in the athlete. Am J Sports Med 1976; 4:84.
44. Galway HR, MacIntosh DL. The lateral pivot shift: a symptom and sign of anterior cruciate ligament insufficiency. Clin Orthop 1980; 147:45–50.
45. Veltri DM, Warren RF. AAOS Instructional Course Lecture. Posterolateral instability of the knee. J Bone Joint Surg Am 76; 3:460–472.
46. Jakob RP, Hassler H, Staubli HU. Experimental studies on the functional anatomy and the pathomechanism of the true and reversed pivot shift sign. Acta Orthop Scand 1981; 5(suppl):18–32.
47. Fanelli GC, Monahan TJ. Complications and pitfalls in posterior cruciate ligament reconstruction. In: Malek MM, Fanelli GC, Johnson Darren, Johnson Don, section eds. Knee Surgery: Complications, Pitfalls, and Salvage. New York: Springer-Verlag; 2001, pp. 121–128.
48. Fanelli GC, Monahan TJ. Complications of posterior cruciate ligament reconstruction. Sports Med Arthrosc Rev 1999; 7(4):296–302.
49. Fanelli GC, Monahan TJ. Complications in posterior cruciate ligament and posterolateral complex surgery. Oper Techniques Sports Med 2001; 9(2):96–99.
50. Fanelli GC. Complications in PCL surgery. In: Fanelli GC, ed. Posterior Cruciate Ligament Injuries. A Practical Guide to Management. New York: Springer-Verlag; 2001, pp. 291–302.
51. Fanelli GC. Complications in the multiple ligament injured knee. In: Schenck RC Jr, ed. Monograph on Multiple Ligamentous Injuries of the Knee in the Athlete. Rosemont, IL: American Association of Orthopaedic Surgeons; 2002: 101–107.

Chapter Nine

Open Surgical Treatment

Richard S. Richards II and Claude T. Moorman III

The multiple ligament injured knee remains a complex problem for the orthopaedic surgeon. Controversy surrounds the myriad vascular, neurologic, and ligament injuries that often accompany this trauma. Though most often seen in motor vehicle accidents (MVA) and industrial accidents, this injury pattern has been occurring with increasing frequency in athletes participating in sporting events.[1] The difficulty in management of the multiple ligament injured knee is compounded by the relative infrequency of occurrence and the paucity of literature on the subject. The rate of dislocation as a percentage of all injuries seen in the emergency department has been reported to be 0.001 to 0.013% per year.[2-6] Because of the likelihood of a spontaneous reduction in the field, there needs to be a high index of suspicion for this diagnosis when there is biplanar laxity in any knee, even with a radiographically reduced joint.[7] Until proven otherwise, evaluation of the neurovascular status of the limb and subsequent management should be carried out under the assumption that a dislocation has occurred.[5]

Initial management focuses on the ABCs of trauma.[7] A dislocated joint is reduced, and vascular status is assessed. Vascular, neurologic, and skeletal injuries take precedence over ligament trauma. The timing and extent of surgical intervention for ligament injuries are driven by the vascular stability and comorbidities.[5] The approach of the senior author is to proceed with ligament reconstruction as soon as the vascular status has been stabilized and the comorbidities have been successfully treated. Reconstructive options include arthroscopic, hybrid, and open approaches. This chapter describes our preferred open approach.

Classification

Knee dislocation is the most common trauma resulting in multiple ligament injury.[8-10] This trauma can result from high energy trauma, such as MVA or industrial accidents, or low energy trauma, such as can be incurred in sporting events.[1] High energy trauma results in a higher incidence of vascular injury and comorbidity and requires a careful query to illuminate additional ipsilateral injury.[7] Knee dislocation has traditionally been classified in the reference to where the tibia ends up relative to the femur.[11] The causes of dislocations are attributed as follows: anterior to a hyperextension force, posterior to a posteriorly directed force applied to the anterior tibia with the knee flexed, lateral to a valgus force, medial to a varus force, and rotational dislocation to a combination of the foregoing. Anterior and posterior dislocations make up the majority, and they have the highest incidence of vascular injury.[11]

At our institution we have attempted to determine the energy level involved and to classify the energy level of the injury as high or low to reflect the magnitude of trauma. We then use the injury pattern discerned from the history, examination, and imaging findings to classify the patient into a category based on the pattern of injury. The most common injury patterns are ACL/PCL/medial side injury and ACL/PCL/posterolateral corner (PLC) injury patterns. These two injury patterns are managed quite differently. Strategic planning is then based on this determination.

Mechanisms of Injury

Injuries to the anterior cruciate ligament (ACL) usually result from non-contact sports involving plant-and-pivot or stop-and-jump mechanisms. Injuries to the posterior cruciate ligament (PCL) occur with abrupt posterior translation of a flexed knee or secondary to excessive tension overload in the PCL. Injuries to the medial collateral ligament (MCL) are caused by contact or noncontact valgus stresses to a flexed knee. PLC injuries occur from a blow to the anteromedial aspect of the knee, contact and noncontact hyperextension injuries, and varus contact forces to a flexed knee. Reports in the literature demonstrate that the most frequent mechanism for a combined ACL/PCL/PLC injury is forced varus and knee dislocation.[9,10,12] A combination injury to the ACL/PCL/MCL complex results from a high-energy mechanism of combined valgus and external axial moment.[13]

Initial Evaluation

Most knee dislocations are obvious on initial presentation, whereas patients with multiple ligament knee injuries require a high index of suspicion to rule out the possibility of knee dislocation with spontaneous reduction.[12] The evaluation of ACL/PCL/PLC/MCL injuries must include a history of the mechanism of injury, and a physical examination with careful serial neurovascular examination and plain radiographs.[13] Magnetic resonance imaging (MRI), evaluation under anesthesia and diagnostic arthroscopy may also be necessary to complete the workup.[14]

There is controversy regarding the use of angiography in acute multiple ligament knee injuries. Wascher reported a 14% incidence of vascular injury in dislocated knees, and Fanelli reported an 11% incidence of arterial injury in the acute three ligament injured knee.[14–16] This information suggests the value of angiography in the majority of cases. There is emerging information suggesting the value of a more selective approach.[17] The approach of the senior author is to use the ankle–brachial index (ABI) as an initial screening measure. Pulses are considered to be "normal" when the ABI is greater than or equal to 0.80. Patients in this category do not undergo routine angiography but are followed with careful serial neurovascular examinations. We have not had any negative sequelae of this approach in this category.[17] Patients with adequate perfusion whose ABI is less than 0.80 are referred to vascular radiology for arteriography. Patients with absent pulses and/or obviously impaired perfusion are referred directly to the vascular surgery service for immediate intervention in the radiology suite. These patients often undergo single-pass angiography in the operating room to confirm the site of vascular injury.

Ligament examination is initiated with a Lachman test at 25° of flexion to assess the integrity of the ACL. End point determination is critical as well as zero-point determination due to the likelihood of a concomitant PCL injury. Pivot shift may be helpful but may be false negative in the face of concomitant medial side injury.[7] The PCL is evaluated with a posterior drawer test at 90° of flexion in addition to a side-to-side measure of posterior sag or step-off. The MCL is evaluated with valgus stress at both 30° of flexion and full extension. Varus stability is tested in 30° of flexion and with the knee in full extension. Posterolateral integrity is tested in 30° of knee flexion with external rotation torque applied to the tibia with the knees held together. A positive test is 10° of increased external rotation versus the opposite side.

Plain radiography includes lateral, Merchant, and bilateral standing posteroanterior views, when possible, to confirm reduction and to evaluate osseous injury. Attention should be focused on documenting joint reduction and avulsion injuries of the capsule, cruciates, collaterals, and the extensor mechanism. MRI should be performed after acute stabilization/reduction has been achieved. MRI has demonstrated its usefulness in visualizing and characterizing both osseous and soft tissue injury patterns.[18-20] We have found it to be of particular value in evaluating the posterolateral corner in subtle cases.

Surgical Indications

Immediate operative intervention is necessary for irreducible dislocations.[21,22] This rare injury results from a rotatory injury pattern in which the medial femoral condyle buttonholes through the medial capsule with the MCL invaginated into the joint, thus preventing reduction. Prompt surgical action is needed to prevent skin necrosis secondary to contact pressure.

For stable reduced knees, we prefer to perform elective reconstruction in the first 3 weeks after injury. Obviously, this choice is predicated on the vascular stability of the knee. When repair/grafting of the artery is required, we prefer to wait 6 weeks following the vascular reconstruction to ensure safety of tourniquet use. There has been no published information on tourniquet use following vascular reconstruction/repair. We have not had any vascular sequelae with tourniquet use 6 weeks after injury.

We prefer to stratify treatment into the following two major injury patterns: ACL/PCL/medial side and ACL/PCL/PLC injuries. Additional differentiation is made for acute (≤6 weeks) versus chronic (>6 weeks) management of ligament injury. Consideration is given in the acute situation for repair of the collateral and capsular structures, whereas in patients presenting for surgery after 6 weeks, reconstruction is more often necessary. Reconstruction is generally required for definitive management of ACL/PCL/PLC regardless of tissue condition.

The literature supports the operative reconstruction of the cruciate and posterolateral corner with variability in the approach toward the medial complex.[3,12,23-28] The MCL, as an extra-articular structure, has the potential to heal without reconstruction. Both clinical and basic science studies support a conservative approach in dealing with isolated MCL injuries.[29-34] Although this approach is accepted for grades I and II MCL injuries combined with ACL/PCL/PLC injuries, a more aggressive approach is used for grade III injuries.[34,35] In patients with low grade MCL injury combined with ACL/PCL injuries, it is recommended that surgical reconstruction of the cruciates be delayed to allow the MCL to heal before definitive reconstruction.[34–36] Patients with multiple ligament injuries that involve high grade MCL injuries and gross instability should acutely undergo reconstruction and repair of all injured structures. In fact, the literature supports the notion of multiple ligament reconstruction and repair as close to the time of injury as is clinically feasible.[14] General guidelines that have been reported include operative intervention within the 2- to 3-week window after the injury. This allows both restoration of adequate range of motion and resolution of the acute inflammatory phase. This delay will decrease the chances of arthrofibrosis, a significant risk in the multiple ligament injured knee.[12] Other conditions that can affect the timing of surgery include vascular status of the extremity, reduction stability, condition of the soft tissue envelope, multiple system injuries, and other orthopaedic injuries.[12] These special considerations may require the operative intervention to be performed earlier or later than expected. The literature does support the delayed reconstruction of the multiple ligament injured knee.[12,27,28]

The operative indication for surgery in the multiple ligament injured knee is severe functional instability. Such knees are at increased risk for progressive instability and development of posttraumatic arthrosis. Thus, the goal of surgical intervention of the multiple ligament injured knee is to ensure a stable neurovascular extremity, to reestablish functional and objective stability, and to attempt to retard the development of degenerative joint disease.

Surgical Technique

The senior author prefers to reconstruct the ACL/PCL/PLC injured knee by using the following open surgical technique. After the foregoing benefits and risks of the procedure have been discussed with the patient, both verbal and written consents are obtained. The patient is placed supine on the operating room table, and the uninjured leg and body are supported in the extended position. A lateral valgus bar is placed next to the injured thigh with a bump made of towels and coband placed under the working knee. After Esmark exsanguination, the tourniquet is inflated to 300 to 350 mm Hg.

An anterior incision is made biased slightly medial to allow for hamstring harvest and tunnel placement for the ACL and PCL reconstruction. Next, the lateral incision for the posterolateral corner reconstruction is marked, keeping a 6 to 8 cm skin bridge between the incisions depending on previous incisions or scars (Figure 9.1). The quadriceps tendon, the patella, the MCL complex, and the hamstring insertions can be reached through the midline incision.

The anterior incision is made and developed to the patellar paratenon, making sure that the fibers of the patellar tendon are not violated. The paratenon is dissected off the patellar tendon both superiorly and inferiorly. The entire distal quadriceps tendon to just distal to the tibial tubercle should be exposed. A marker is used to point the center of the inferior pole of the patella, as well as the center of the tibial tubercle. A no. 10 blade is used to develop a 10 mm wide one-third patellar tendon autograft. An oscillating saw is used to create patellar and tibial tubercle bone plugs that are approximately 25 mm long (Figure 9.2; see color plate). The saw cuts for the tibial tubercle plug are made at a 30° angle from the axis, while the patellar cuts are created from a 45° angle. Curved osteotomes (half and quarter-inch) are used to complete the harvest. Metzenbaum scissors are used to remove the tendon from the underlying fat pad and periosteum.

9. Open Surgical Treatment

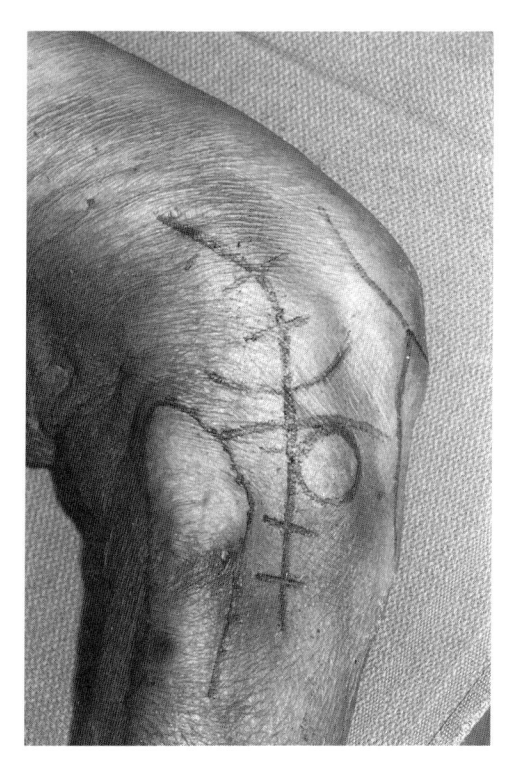

Fig. 9.1. Marking of lateral skin incision. Note position of fibular head and Gerdy's tubercle.

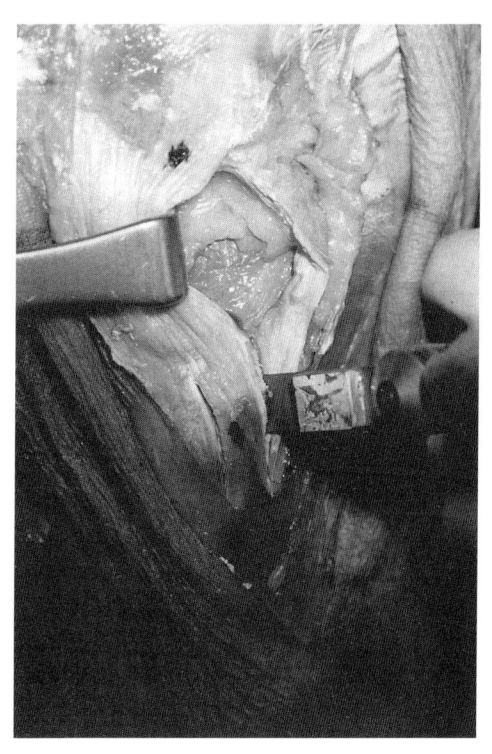

Fig. 9.2. Autograft ACL harvest. This is done through an anterior incision with an oscillating saw at a 30° angle to the surface of the tibia. Patellar tendon width is 10 mm. Note extensive dissection for easy visualization. (See color plate.)

A 10 mm × 70 mm quadriceps tendon graft is harvested for a double-bundle PCL autograft. A similar 25 mm patellar bone plug is created with an oscillating saw. The center of the quadriceps tendon, which should be 10 mm wide, is harvested full thickness (Figure 9.3; see color plate). The quadriceps tendon has a natural cleavage in the coronal plane, which allows for creation of two equal soft tissue limbs. The gracilis and semitendinosus are harvested for a double-bundle hamstring autograft. The sartorius fascia is incised along its fibers with a no. 15 blade. Right angle forceps are used to locate and isolate the gracilis and the semitendinosus (Figure 9.4; see color plate). Careful attention is paid to make sure that the crossing fascia slings and vinculae are released around the distal tendon insertion. A tendon harvester, such as Lineate, is then used to harvest each respective tendon (Figure 9.5; see color plate). The distal insertion site is removed with sharp dissection to create a doubled free-tendon graft.

The three autografts are prepared on the back table (Figure 9.6; see color plate). A colored marker is used on the flat bone side where the interference screw will be placed. Then whipstitching is used to place no. 2 Ethibond sutures on the free tendon ends. Bone plug sizes and free-tendon edge sizes are assessed with cylindrical sizers. The ACL and PCL stumps are debrided with rongeurs, and the notchplasty is done with curved osteotomes and a medium-sized curette (Figure 9.7). This allows clear visualization of the over-the-top position for the ACL and for the proper PCL position placement, along with prevention of ACL graft impingement.

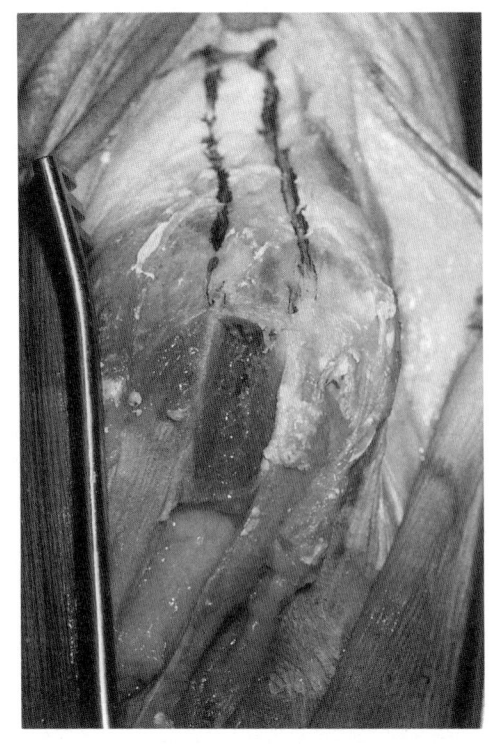

Fig. 9.3. Autograft quadriceps tendon harvest. A marker is used to show the dimensions of the patellar bone plug and appropriate length of quadriceps tendon. (See color plate.)

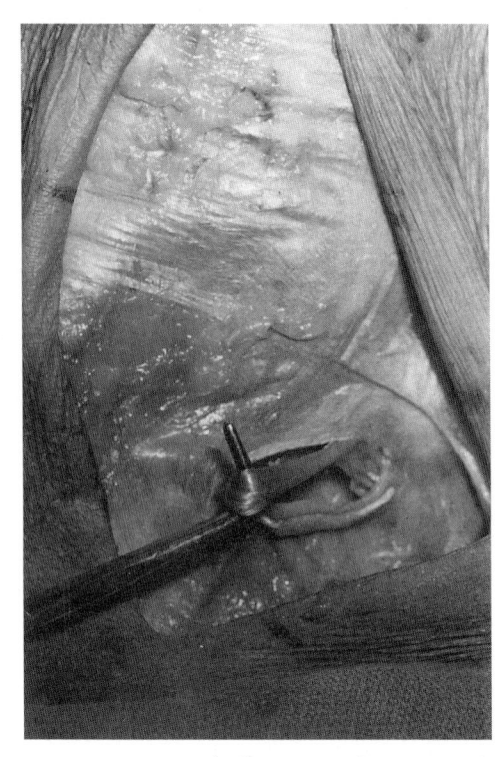

Fig. 9.4. Autograft hamstring harvest with use of right angle forceps to identify the two hamstrings. This is done through an incision in line with the fibers of the sartorius fascia. (See color plate.)

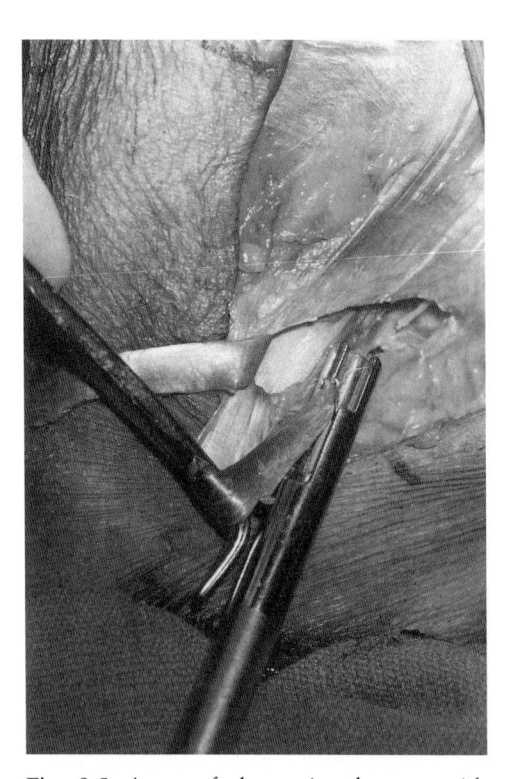

Fig. 9.5. Autograft hamstring harvest with tendon stripper. Care is taken to remove all fascial bands and vinculae to prevent a premature harvest of the hamstrings. (See color plate.)

9. Open Surgical Treatment

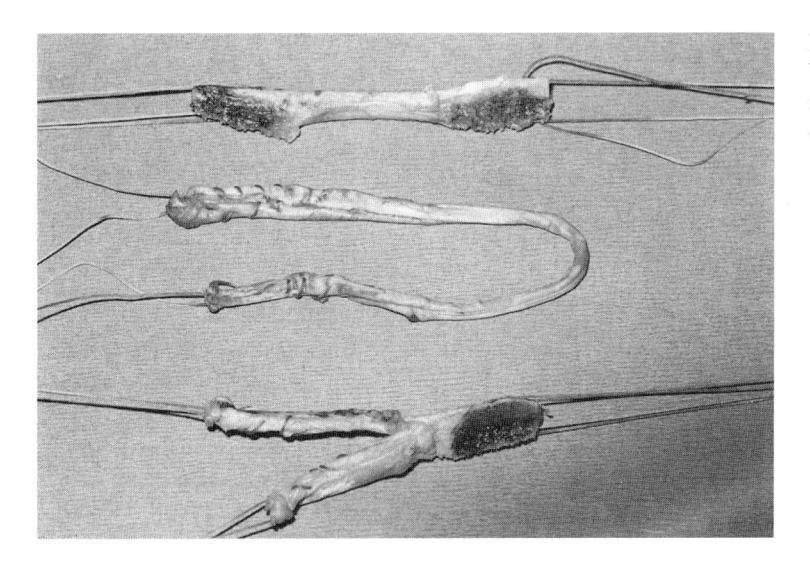

Fig. 9.6. Autografts for the ACL/PLC/PCL. Whipstitches and colored marks are used to facilitate graft passage and fixation. (See color plate.)

The PCL tunnels are created with the tunnel diameter based on the bone and tendon plug sizes. The PCL Arthrex guide is used at approximately 50 to 60°, with the guide pin being drilled under fluoroscopic guidance. The starting point for the tibial tunnel is on the anteromedial aspect of the tibia, below the level of the tibial tubercle (Figure 9.8). This inferior position allows for tunnel stacking with later ACL tunnel placement. The guide pin should exit the posterior proximal tibia in the distal lateral third of the PCL insertion site. On the lateral radiograph, this position is located on the posteriorly sloping "PCL facet" approximately 1 cm from the posterior cortex. Next, the medial tibial periosteum around the guide pin is incised down to bone with electrocautery and elevated with a periosteal elevator. An appropriately sized reamer is chosen, and the tunnel is drilled; great care is necessary upon exiting the posterior tibial cortex.

The PCL femoral tunnels are created in an inside-out manner. After the notchplasty is performed, the anterolateral tunnel on the medial femoral condyle is created. This site is located at the junction of the roof and notch, 10 mm posterior to the articular margin within the footprint of the PCL. The appropriately sized reamer is then used to drill the tunnel. A second guide pin is then directed 5 mm posterior from the edge of the first tunnel.[36]

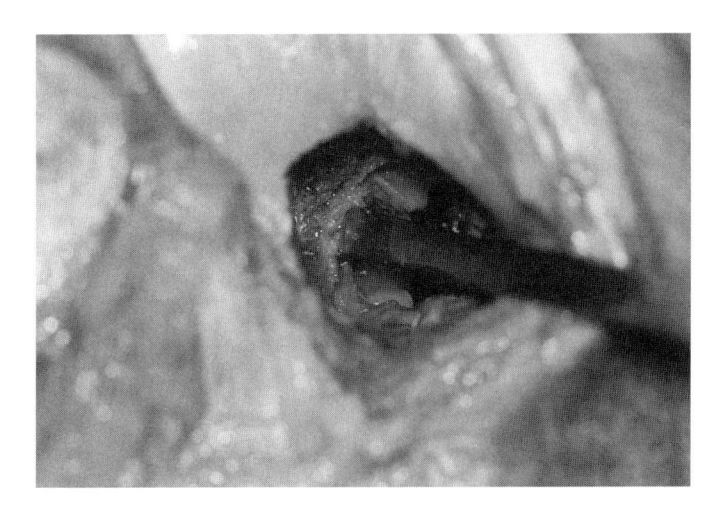

Fig. 9.7. Notchplasty is performed with straight osteotomes and curved curettes. Open approach allows excellent visualization of the over-the-top position.

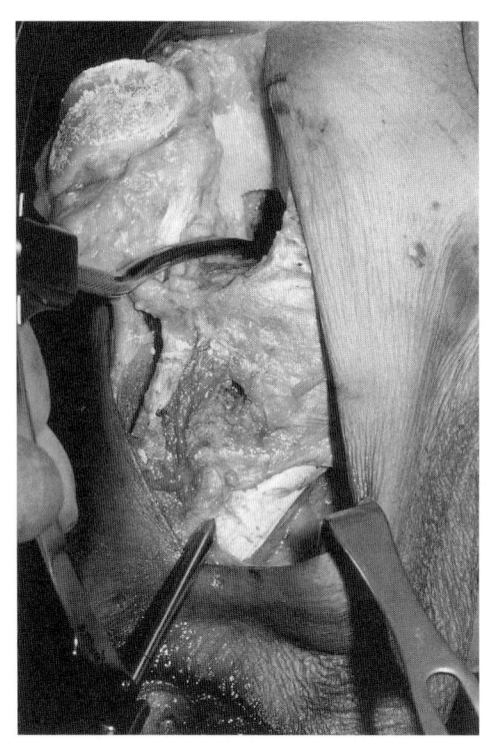

Fig. 9.8. PCL guide used make tibial tunnel. Image intensification is used to achieve proper position on the "PCL facet." Note inferior start position of the PCL tunnel in reference to the tibial tubercle.

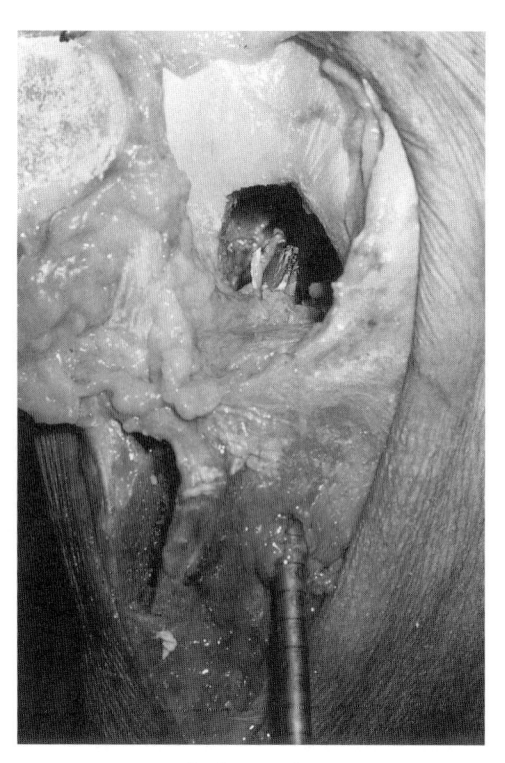

Fig. 9.9. ACL tibial tunnel preparation with cannulated reamer over a guide wire. Note location of tunnel in reference to the tibial tubercle.

This tunnel is then drilled, ensuring that the bone bridge between the tunnels is not violated.

The ACL tunnels are created by starting the tibial tunnel 1 cm proximal to the tibial tubercle on the anteromedial surface of the proximal tibia, using a 55° ACL guide (i.e., Arthrex), allowing the guide pin to emerge through the center of the stump of the ACL footprint (Figure 9.9). Care is taken to have at least a 1 cm bone bridge between the ACL and PCL tunnels. The placement of the femoral tunnel is determined using the over-the-top position on the medial wall of the lateral femoral condyle as a reference. The bone plug size is taken into account (Figure 9.10), and then a 5 to 7 mm offset guide is used to create a posterior wall 1 to 2 mm thick.

Passage and fixation of the PCL graft occur next. The quadriceps double-bundle graft with bone plug is used to reconstruct the PCL. This graft type has been chosen to avoid the risks of allograft disease transmission and long-term loosening, and to obtain more accurate physiologic posterior translation throughout the range of motion.[37–40] A suture passer or a long Kelly clamp is placed retrograde through the tibial PCL tunnel to appear in the posterior medial aspect of the notch. The Ethibond sutures from the bone plug end of the graft are fed into the open Kelly arms and pulled antero-grade through the tibial tunnel. Care is taken to keep the bone plug oriented properly. Next, a Beath needle is used to place the free tendon ends into the anterolateral and posteromedial femoral positions. The postero-medial free tendon end is secured with soft tissue screw over a guide pin through the femoral notch in retrograde fashion. Tensioning of the

9. Open Surgical Treatment

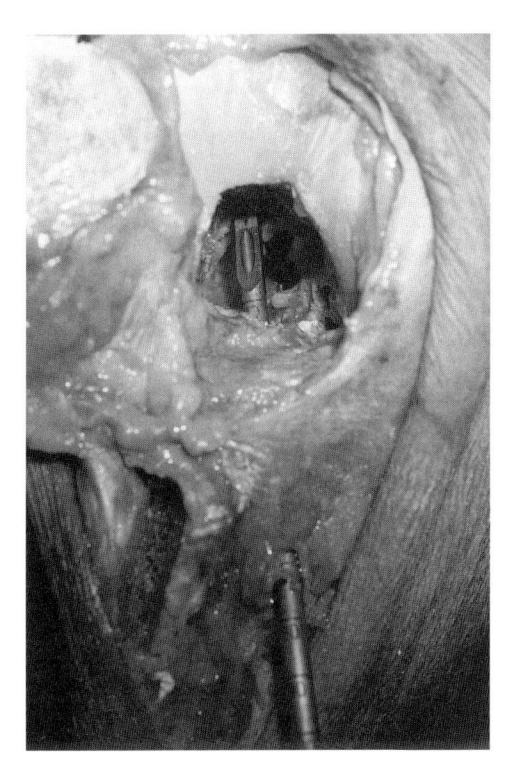

Fig. 9.10. Placement of the 7 mm offset guide for placement of the ACL femoral tunnel. This guide is placed through the tibial tunnel and hooked over the posterior femoral cortex.

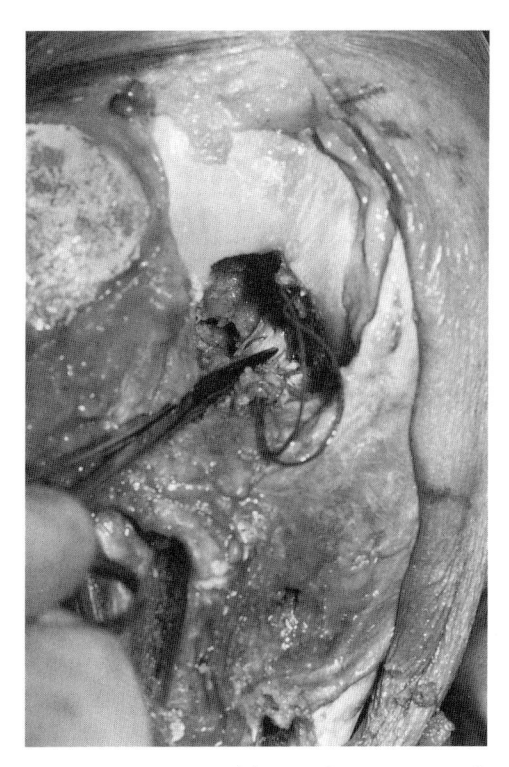

Fig. 9.11. Passage of the quadriceps autograft for reconstruction of the PCL. The tibial plug has already been passed anterograde through the tibial tunnel. Note the two limbs of the autograft: the posteromedial is already through the femoral tunnel, and the anterolateral limb is anterior as identified by the Ethibond whipstitches. (See color plate.)

posteromedial limb is done in extension (Figure 9.11; see color plate). A Nitnol wire is placed anterior to the tibial bone plug in the tunnel, and the sutures are pulled with an anterograde force while a cannulated 9 mm × 30 mm interference screw is placed. Tibial backup fixation can be obtained with a button or post with soft tissue washer anteriorly in the tibia. Then, the anterolateral limb is tensioned in 90° of flexion and secured with a soft tissue screw placed in a retrograde fashions through the femoral notch over a guide pin, restoring the normal tibial step-off (Figures 9.12 and 9.13; see color plates).

Passage and fixation of the ACL graft occur next. A Beath needle is placed through the ACL tibial tunnel up into the femoral tunnel. The bone–patellar tendon–bone autograft is passed into position in a retrograde manner. The femoral side is secured with a cannulated 7 mm × 25 mm interference screw. With the knee in 20° of flexion, the tibial side is secured with a cannulated 9 mm × 30 mm interference screw while an anterograde force is applied on the tibial bone plug sutures (Figure 9.14; see color plate).

Posterolateral corner injuries are addressed next. Low grade posterolateral injuries are successfully managed with nonoperative treatment.[14] Acute repairs of the posterolateral corner can be successful in the first 6 weeks if the tissue quality is good and the injury not profound. Surgical repair should be performed as close to the time of injury as possible, to permit identification of anatomic structures prior to formation of scar and inflammatory

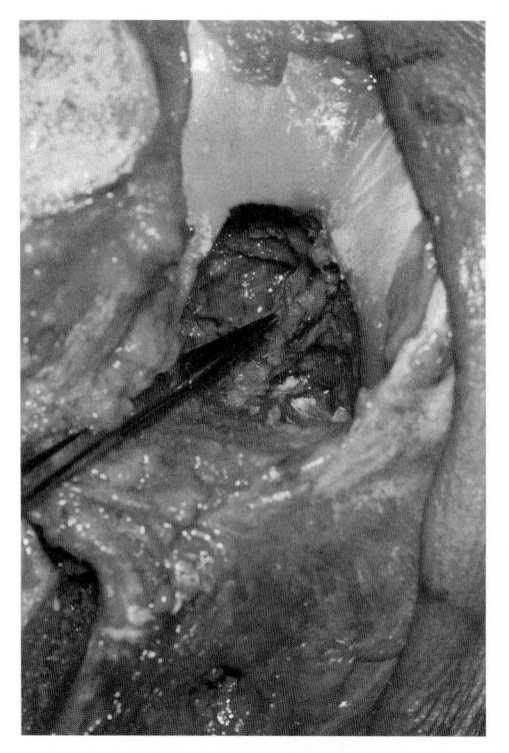

Fig. 9.12. Anterolateral limb of the quadriceps graft being pulled retrograde into the femoral tunnel in front of the posteromedial limb.

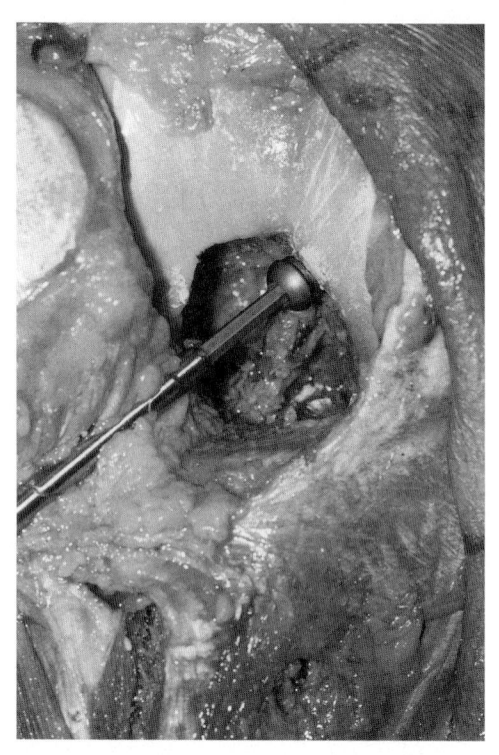

Fig. 9.13. Fixation of the anterolateral limb of the PCL reconstruction with a cannulated soft tissue screw in a retrograde fashion through the notch. (See color plate.)

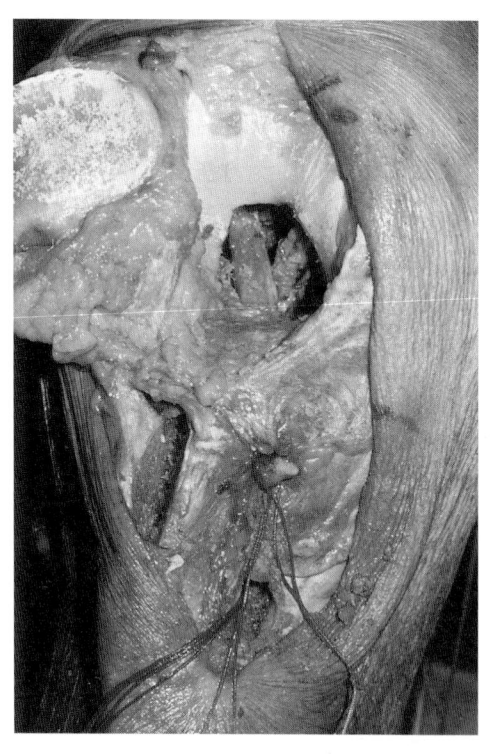

Fig. 9.14. Passage of the PCL and ACL autografts as seen from the anteromedial aspect of the knee. Note position of the femoral grafts and the relationships of the tibial ACL autograft harvest site and the tibial tunnels of the PCL (inferior) and ACL (superior). (See color plate.)

9. Open Surgical Treatment

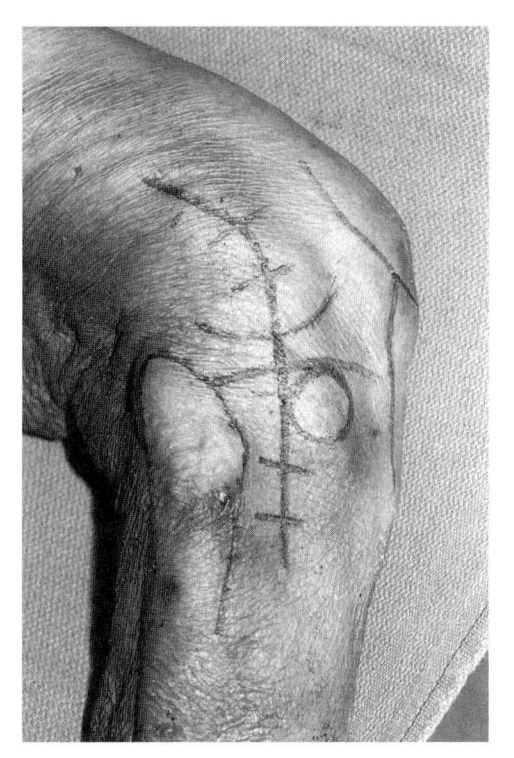

Fig. 9.15. Position of preferred lateral incision for PLC reconstruction.

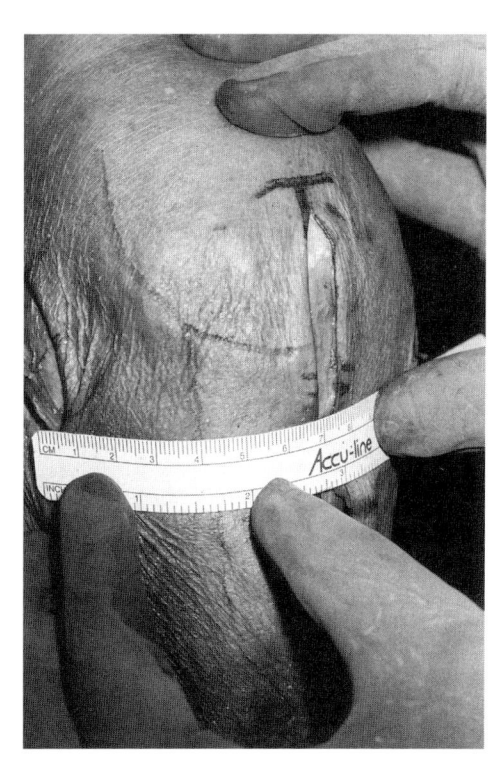

Fig. 9.16. Relationship of the lateral incision to the anterior incision.

tissue.[14] In general, avulsion fractures of the popliteus tendon, the fibular collateral ligament, and the arcuate ligament can be repaired with direct sutures to bone, suture anchors, or soft tissue screws with washers. For both acute and chronic high grade posterolateral corner injuries, the senior author prefers reconstruction with double-hamstring autograft to restore both varus and rotational stability. The vast majority of patients treated with this injury at our institution manifest this form. The technique just described restores the LCL and the popliteus tendon, tightens the posterolateral capsule, and serves to reinforce the posterolateral corner with autogenous tissue. Autogenous graft tissue is preferred owing a high complication rate, such as soft tissue failure and infection, with allograft tissue in our experience.

A no. 10 blade is used to dissect a full-thickness skin flap through a laterally based hockey stick incision (Figure 9.15). Care is taken to preserve a 6 to 8 cm skin bridge from the anterior incision (Figure 9.16). The femoral starting point is just posterior to the lateral epicondyle. The incision courses distally to bisect the fibular head and Gerdy's tubercle (Figure 9.17). The peroneal nerve is identified, dissected free, and protected with a vascular loop throughout the entire procedure (Figure 9.18). Exposure of the lateral femoral condyle is made through a longitudinal incision of the iliotibial band. The proximal aspect of the fibula and the biceps femoris tendon are isolated. Damage to the LCL, popliteus, and arcuate ligament is assessed. Using the footprint of the proximal origin of the LCL and the insertion of the popliteus (Figure 9.19), the femoral fixation site for the posterolateral reconstruction is identified between these two points (Figure 9.20). Once this has been done, the fibula is drilled with a guide pin in an anterior-to-posterior direction, superior to the fibular neck. A 7 mm tunnel is created

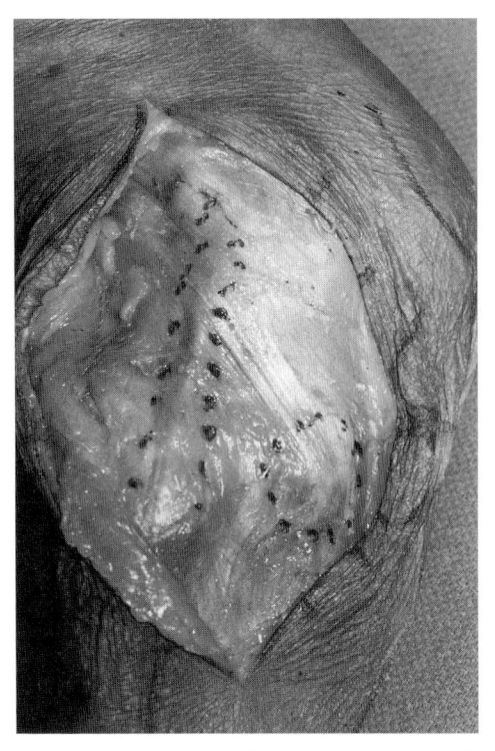

Fig. 9.17. Exposure of the PLC with development of full-thickness skin flaps. Note relationship of the fibular head to Gerdy's tubercle.

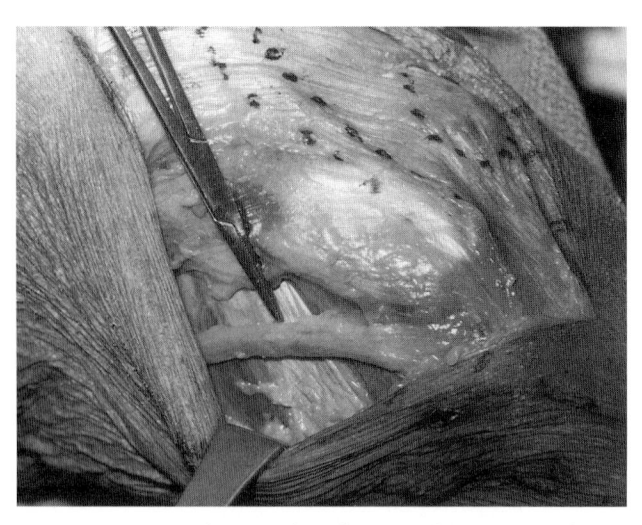

Fig. 9.18. Peroneal nerve identification, dissection, and protection are critical in PLC exposure and reconstruction.

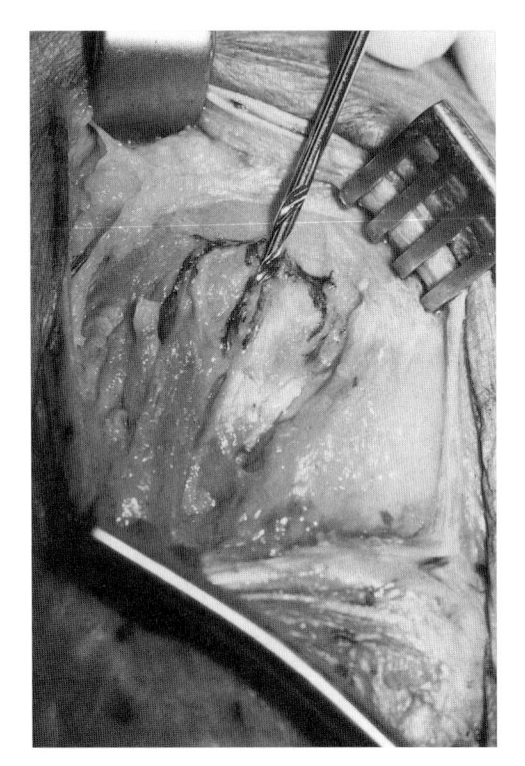

Fig. 9.19. Identification of lateral femoral position for PLC reconstruction between the LCL and the popliteus insertion.

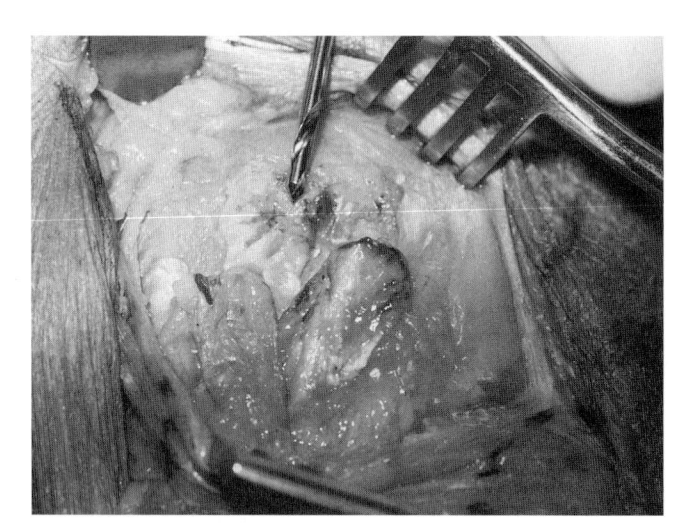

Fig. 9.20. Preparation of the lateral femoral position for PLC reconstruction.

9. Open Surgical Treatment

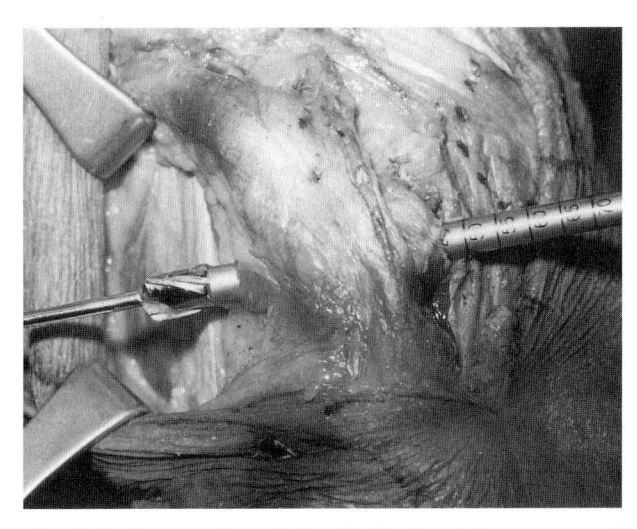

Fig. 9.21. Preparation of the fibular head for passage of double-hamstring autograft. A 7mm reamer is used in an anterior-to-posterior direction over a guide wire. (See color plate.)

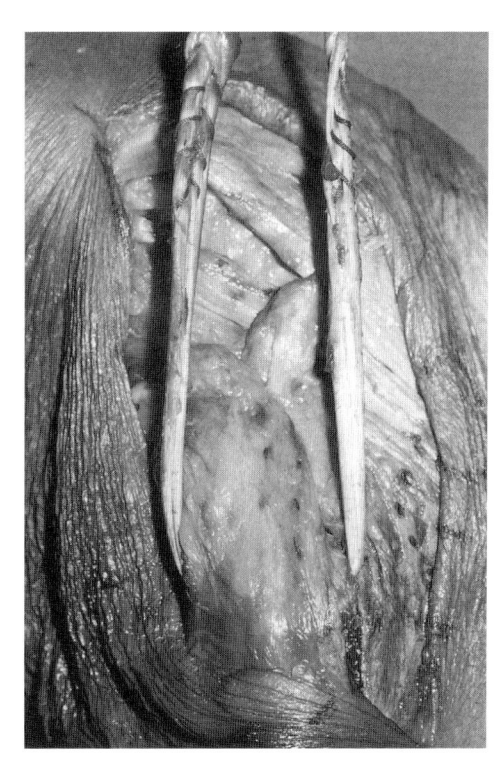

Fig. 9.22. Passage of the double-hamstring autograft through the fibular head. (See color plate.)

with a reamer (Figure 9.21; see color plate). The double-stranded hamstring graft is placed into position by pulling the graft through the fibular head (Figure 9.22; see color plate). Both strands are looped once to produce a figure-of-eight alignment underneath the biceps tendon and iliotibial band (Figure 9.23; see color plate). The posterior loop forms the popliteofibular complex, while the anterior loop forms the LCL. The free ends are wrapped around a 30 to 35mm cancellous AO or Arthrex screw with soft tissue washer. Once the screw has been tightened into place, the remaining posterior loop is placed through the fibular tunnel again, and tied onto the anterior loop with whipstitched sutures (Figure 9.24; see color plate). If necessary, 2.0 Vicryl is used to reinforce the posterior band. The posterolateral complex is tensioned and tightened while the knee is internally rotated in 30° of flexion with a slight valgus force on the knee. The posterolateral capsule is then addressed and secured to the posterior aspect of the construct using no. 2 nonabsorbable sutures.

Medial side injuries need to be addressed in the context of the ACL/PCL/medial side injury pattern. Grade I and II MCL injuries often respond to nonoperative treatment.[34,35,37] The senior author prefers to evaluate the medial complex after the foregoing procedural steps (i.e., placement of the PCL and then the ACL using the operative technique already stated) have been performed. If there is still anteromedial instability or significant valgus opening greater than 5mm, the decision to imbricate the present available tissue versus Achilles tendon allograft augmentation must be made. In the repair or reconstruction of the MCL, in addition to the PCL/ACL, a single anterior incision is utilized slightly biased to the medial side. Soft tissue is undermined to expose the MCL without the need for a

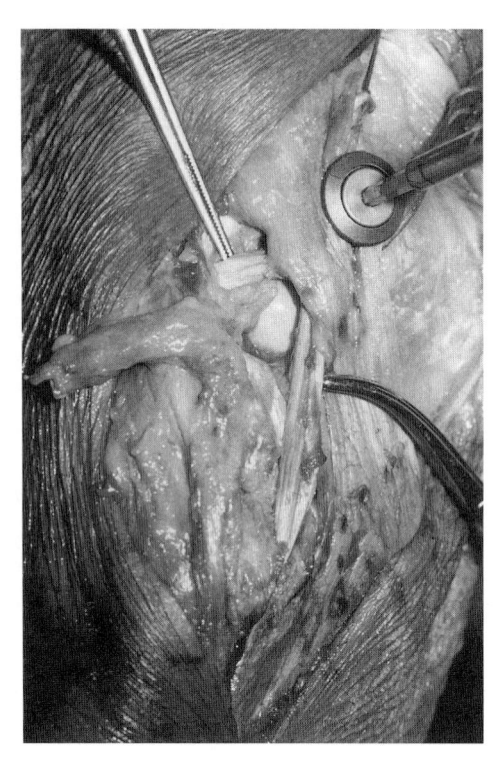

Fig. 9.23. Fixation of the PLC fibular "O" autograft. The graft is passed in a figure-of-eight fashion such that the posterior limb (left) serves as the popliteofibular complex and the anterior limb (right) serves as the reconstructed LCL. (See color plate.)

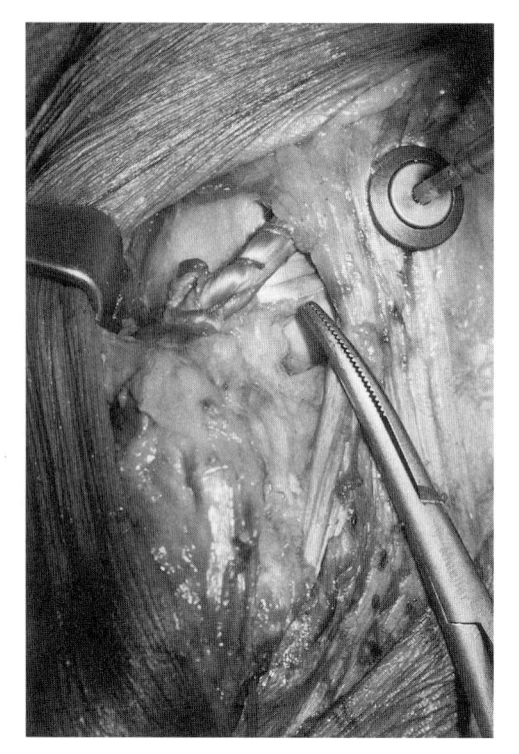

Fig. 9.24. Fixation of the PLC graft often allows for overlapping of the anterior and posterior limbs with extra tendon. Care is taken to ensure that the tendon is captured by the soft tissue washer. (See color plate.)

second medial incision. We have had a very low complication rate with allograft tissue on the medial side. For this reason, we have a low threshold for allograft use in this scenario. There is also concern with the use of hamstring harvest in the already compromised medial side of the knee.

Imbrication of available tissue can be done with a tibial-based repair with Mitek anchor sutures, moving the tibial site of the MCL anteriorly on the tibia. Also, if the MCL is in its appropriate location and its fibers are attenuated, the MCL can be incised in the midpoint and imbricated in a pants-over-vest fashion with no. 2 Ethibond sutures. Further, if there is gross tissue damage, the Achilles tendon allograft is the senior author's preferred graft. The bone plug is placed in the MCL origin on the medial femoral condyle inset at the femoral origin, using 6.5 mm cancellous screws. The tibial end is then secured with suture anchors with the knee in 20 to 30° of flexion.

The incisions are closed over drains with deep 0 Vicryl figure-of-eight interrupted sutures. Subcutaneous skin is closed with 2.0 Vicryl inverted simple sutures. A 3.0 Prolene running suture is used to close the subcuticular layer. The incision is dressed with Steri-Strips, 4 × 4 gauze, soft roll, and Bias wrap. A cryotherapy device is then placed over the Bias wrap. The lower extremity is then placed into a hinged knee brace that is locked in extension and manually bent into a static valgus position. Care is taken not to place the leg in a varus and/or hyperextension position while it is being put into the brace.

Rehabilitation

There is little in the literature about rehabilitation of combined ACL/PCL/PLC/MCL injuries. The goal is to create an environment that fosters controlled arthrofibrosis, since postoperative fibrosis and stiffness is desirable to a point.[41] Avoidance of continuous passive motion, early weight bearing, accelerated rehabilitation, and positions that may lead to subluxation comprise our protocol for the first 2 weeks. Long-leg brace in full extension with touchdown weight bearing for 6 to 8 weeks is the rule. At 2 weeks, the brace can be unlocked with progression to full range of motion as tolerated. Great care is taken to avoid varus stress and valgus stress in PLC and MCL reconstructed patients, respectively. Crutches may be discontinued with appearance of good quadriceps control of the leg at 6 weeks. We start physical therapy for active and passive range of motion as tolerated at 2 weeks. Patients are advised that up to 20% of them will require a manipulation under anesthesia for arthrofibrosis. We consider this to be an acceptable rate in light of the alternative likelihood of recurrent instability with a more aggressive physical therapy program.

At 3 to 6 months, initial strength training can begin with closed-chained exercises. From 6 to 9 months, advanced strength training can be performed, as long as the patient demonstrates functional progression. Return to heavy labor or sports can occur at approximately 9 to 12 months, once strength and range of motion have been found to be appropriate. Loss of 10 to 15° of terminal flexion is expected in reconstructions of multiple ligament injured knees, but this does not usually cause a functional problem for the patient.[14]

Complications

Multiple ligament injuries to the knee are far more devastating than are isolated ligament injuries.[13] There are complications inherent to the operative intervention of these combined injuries. Potential complications include failure to recognize and treat vascular injuries from the trauma itself, along with vascular injury that can result from postoperative subluxation.[13,14] Iatrogenic injuries may range from neurovascular insults to tibial plateau fractures at the time of reconstruction. Failure to understand all instability components may lead to early failure. Motion loss, infection, postoperative knee pain, and painful hardware have also been described.[13,14]

Conclusions

Multiple ligament injuries of the knee present the orthopaedic surgeon with myriad management challenges. We feel that the open surgical approach has several advantages. First, the approach is relatively straightforward and is effective in minimizing operating room time. Second, all structures can be evaluated directly and fixed securely. With these injuries, our goal is to create an environment of controlled arthrofibrosis with a resultant stable and functional knee.

References

1. Shelbourne KD, Klootwyk TE. Low velocity knee dislocation. Treatment principles. Clin Sports Med 2000; 19(3):443–456.

2. Hoover NW. Injuries of the popliteal artery associated with fracture and dislocations. Surg Clin North Am 1961; 47:1099–1112.
3. Jones ER, Smith EC, Bone GE. Vascular and orthopedic complications of knee dislocation. Surg, Gynecol Obstet 1979; 149:554–558.
4. Kannus P, Jarvinen M. Non-operative treatment of acute knee ligament injuries. Am J Sports Med 1990; 9:244–260.
5. Treiman GS, Yellin AE, Weaver FA, et al. Low-velocity knee dislocation. Orthop Rev 1991; 20:995–1004.
6. Walker DN, Hardison RR, Schenck RC. A baker's dozen of knee dislocations. Am J Knee Surg 1994; 7:177–124.
7. Good L, Johnson RJ. The dislocated knee. J Am Acad Orthop Surg 1995; 3:284–292.
8. Stuart MJ. Evaluation and treatment principles of knee dislocations. Oper Techniques Sports Med 2001; 9(2):91–95.
9. Fanelli GC. PCL injuries in trauma patients. Arthroscopy 1993; 9:291–294.
10. Fanelli GC, Edson CJ. PCL injuries in trauma patients. II: Arthroscopy 1995; 11:526–529.
11. Kennedy JC. Complete dislocation of the knee joint. J Bone Joint Surg Am 1963; 45:889-904.
12. Fanelli GC, Giannotti BF, Edson CJ. Current concepts review. The posterior cruciate ligament arthroscopic evaluation and treatment. Arthroscopy 1994; 10:673–688.
13. Klimkiewicz JJU, Petrie RS, Harner CD. Surgical treatment of combined injury to anterior cruciate ligament, posterior cruciate ligament, and medial structures. Clin Sports Med 2000; 19(3):479–491.
14. Fanelli GC. Treatment of combined anterior cruciate ligament–posterior cruciate ligament–lateral side injuries of the knee. Clin Sports Med 2000; 19(3):493–501.
15. Wascher DC, Dvirnak PC, DeCoster TA. Knee dislocation: initial assessment and implications for treatment. J Orthop Trauma 1997; 11:525–529.
16. Wascher DC, Graver JD, Markoff KL. Biceps tendon tenodesis for posterolateral instability of the knee: an in vitro study. Am J Sports Med 1993; 21:400–406.
17. Kleinberg EO, Crites BM, Flinn WR, Moorman CT. The role of arteriography in assessing popliteal artery injury in knee dislocations. Submitted to J Orthop Trauma.
18. Woo SLY, Inoue M, MeGurk-Burleson E, et al. Treatment of the medial collateral ligament injury. II: Structure and function of canine knees in response to differing treatment regimens. Am J Sports Med 1987; 15:22–29.
19. Harner CD, Hoher J. Current concepts: evaluation and treatment of posterior cruciate ligament injuries. Am J Sports Med 1998; 26:471–482.
20. Yu JS, Goodwin D, Salonen D, et al. Complete dislocation of the knee: spectrum of associated soft-tissue injuries depicted by MR imaging. AJR Am J Roentgenol 1995; 164:135–139.
21. Hill JA, Rana NA. Complications of posterolateral dislocation of the knee: case report and literature review. Clin Orthop 1981; 154:212–215.
22. Quinlan AG, Sharrard WJ. Posterolateral dislocation of the knee with capsular interposition. J Bone Joint Surg Br 1956; 40:660.
23. Noyes FR, Barber-Westin SD. Reconstruction of the anterior and posterior cruciate ligaments after knee dislocation: use of early postoperative motion to decrease arthrofibrosis. Am J Sports Med 1997; 25:769–778.
24. Shapiro MS, Freedman EL. Allograft reconstruction of the anterior and posterior cruciate ligaments after traumatic knee dislocation. Am J Sports Med 1995; 23:580–587.
25. Shelbourne KD, Porter CD, Clingman JA, et al. Low velocity knee dislocation. Orthop Rev 1991; 20:995–1004.
26. Wascher DC, Becker JR, Dexter JG, et al. Reconstruction of the anterior and posterior cruciate ligaments after knee dislocation: results using fresh-frozen nonirradiated allografts. Am J Sports Med 1999; 27:189–196.
27. Fanelli GC, Giannotti BF, Edson CJ. Arthroscopically assisted combined anterior and posterior cruciate ligament reconstruction. Arthroscopy 1996; 12:5–14.

28. Fanelli GC, Giannotti BF, Edson CJ. Arthroscopically assisted combined posterior cruciate ligament/posterior lateral complex reconstruction. Arthroscopy 1996; 12:521–530.
29. Dersheid GL, Garrick JG. Medial collateral ligament injuries in football: non-operative management of grade I and grade II sprains. Am J Sports Med 1981; 9:365–368.
30. Ellsaasser JC, Reynolds FC, Omohundro JR. The non-operative treatment of collateral ligament injuries of the knee in professional football players: an analysis of seventy-four injuries treated non-operatively and twenty-four injuries treated surgically. J Bone Joint Surg Am 1974; 56:1185–1190.
31. Indelicato PA. Isolated medial collateral ligament injuries in the knee. J Am Acad Orthop Surg 1995; 3:9–14.
32. Indelicato PA, Hermansdorfer J, Huegel M. Non-operative management of complete tears of the medial collateral ligament of the knee in intercollegiate football players. Clin Orthop 1990; 256:174–177.
33. Inove M, McGurk-Burleson E, Hollis JM, et al. Treatment of the medial collateral ligament injury. I: The importance of the anterior cruciate ligament on varus–valgus knee laxity. Am J Sports Med 1987; 15:15–21.
34. Jones RE, Henley MB, Francis P. Non-operative management of grade III collateral ligament injury in high school football players. Clin Orthop 1986; 213: 137–140.
35. Hillard-Semball D, Daniel DM, Stone ML, et al. Combined injuries to the anterior cruciate and medial collateral ligaments of the knee. J Bone Joint Surg Am 1996; 78:169–175.
36. Paulos LE, Bair BA. Transosseous reconstruction of the posterior cruciate ligament: single- and double-tunnel techniques. Oper Techniques Sports Med 2001; 9(2):60–68.
37. Harner CD, Irrgang JJ, Paul J, et al. Loss of motion after anterior cruciate reconstruction. Am J Sports Med 1992; 20:499–506.
38. Race A, Amis AA. PCL reconstruction: in vitro biomechanical comparison of 'isometric' versus single and double-bundled 'anatomic' grafts. J Bone Joint Surg Br 1998; 80:173–179.
39. Petrie R, Harner C. Double-bundle posterior cruciate ligament reconstruction technique: University of Pittsburgh approach. Oper Techniques Sports Med 1999; 7:118–126.
40. Petrie R, Harner C. Evaluation and management of the posterior cruciate injured knee. Oper Techniques Sports Med 1999; 7:93–103.
41. Cooper DE. Treatment of combined posterior cruciate ligament and posterolateral injuries of the knee. Oper Techniques Sports Med 1999; 7:135–142.

Chapter Ten

Management of Arterial and Venous Injuries in the Dislocated Knee

Peter J. Armstrong and David P. Franklin

Historical Overview

Interest in the diagnosis and treatment of vascular injuries around the knee has coincided with the advances in vascular surgery throughout the past century. Multiple armed conflicts from war, as well as modern trauma series, have clarified the need for expeditious popliteal artery repair and have suggested the need for popliteal venous repair. The World War II experience reported by Debakey and Simone[1] revealed a 72% amputation rate when the injured popliteal artery was ligated. Repair of traumatic popliteal artery injuries in the Korean War reduced the amputation rate to 32%.[2] Despite continued advances in patient evacuation, the amputation rate for popliteal artery injuries in the Vietnam War remained at 32%.[3] As trauma in America has increased, the incidence of popliteal arterial and venous injury has increased as well.

Injuries to the popliteal artery continue to account for a disproportionately high number of lower extremity amputations, accounting for only 10% of vascular trauma but 65% of amputations.[4] In addition, popliteal vascular injury associated with blunt trauma has a higher amputation rate than injuries secondary to missiles or stab wounds.[5] Historically, popliteal artery injuries associated with knee dislocation have resulted in extremely high amputation rates, as shown in Table 10.1.

Knee dislocations continue to be an underdiagnosed injury in more contemporary series. The reported individual hospital experience remains small even in large urban centers, as shown in Table 10.2. The incidence of identified popliteal artery injury with knee dislocation ranges from 10 to 43%.[4,6–20] Recent improvements in the expeditious diagnosis and treatment of popliteal artery injury have decreased amputation rates in some series to 0 to 3%.[21,22]

Anatomy

Embryologically, the popliteal artery is derived from the sciatic artery, which is the axial artery of the lower extremity. As the femoral artery arises from the external iliac artery, it becomes the dominant artery of the lower limb. The femoral artery then joins with the popliteal artery and is responsible for forming the anterior tibial artery and posterior tibial artery. The residual vessels originating as the sciatic artery include the inferior gluteal artery, the popliteal artery, and the peroneal artery.

Table 10.1. Knee dislocation with popliteal artery occlusions: series prior to 1973

Series	Knee dislocations	Popliteal artery occlusion	Resultant amputations
Hoover[6]	14	9	8
Kennedy[7]	22	7	5
Reckling and Peltier[8]	15	3	0
Shields et al.[9]	26	10	5
Myers and Harvey[10]	18	3	1
Taylor et al.[11]	42	3	2
Total	137	35 (25.5%)	21 (60%)

Table 10.2. Series of knee dislocations

City	Knee dislocations	Number of years
Cincinnati[12]	30	10
Los Angeles[13]	32	11
Jacksonville[14]	38	6.5
Phoenix[15]	7	4
Albuquerque[16]	47	8
Atlanta[17]	19	4

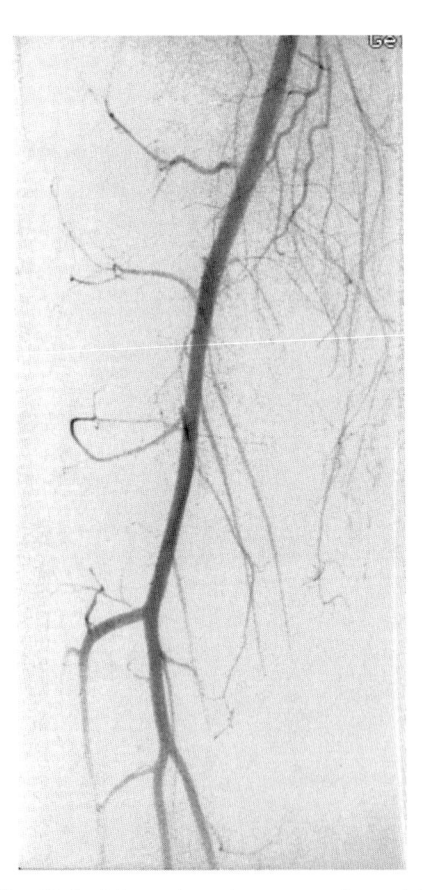

Fig. 10.1. Normal angiogram performed in a patient with knee dislocation. Patent popliteal and tibial arteries without evidence of spasm or injury are demonstrated.

By birth, the popliteal artery is a continuation of the superficial femoral artery as it passes through the tendinous hiatus in the adductor magnus muscle, Hunter's canal. It has several small branches including the medial and lateral superior geniculate, middle geniculate, and medial and lateral inferior geniculate arteries. The popliteal artery then divides into the tibial arteries as it exits the popliteal fossa. A normal angiogram of the popliteal and proximal tibial vessels obtained in a patient sustaining a knee dislocation during professional bicycle motocross (BMX) racing is shown in Figure 10.1.

The popliteal vein forms by the joining of the anterior and posterior tibial veins at the lower border of the popliteus muscle. The vein runs medially and then crosses superficially and laterally over the popliteal artery. The popliteal vein becomes the superficial femoral vein as it traverses the tendinous hiatus in the adductor magnus muscle, Hunter's canal. The popliteal vein is frequently duplicated, being present on both the medial and lateral sides of the popliteal artery. The popliteal vessels are tethered to the femur at Hunter's canal and to the tibia by the soleus muscle.

Exposure of the superior portion of the popliteal vessels is initiated by abducting the thigh with flexion at the hip and knee. A 10 to 12 cm incision is positioned on the anterior border of the lower sartorius or the inferior edge of the femur if palpable (Figure 10.2). The sartorius muscle is retracted posteromedially after separating the fascia. The vessels are located by separating the tendinous fibers of the adductor magnus tendon. The popliteal vein is located laterally to the artery at this level.

The distal portion of the popliteal artery is also approached by abducting the leg while flexing the knee and hip. The 10 to 12 cm incision is made 1 cm posterior to the medial border of the tibia. The deep fascia is incised parallel to the skin incision. The medial head of the gastrocnemius muscle is retracted posteromedially, and the vascular bundle is located. The vascular sheath is incised and contains the popliteal artery, popliteal vein, and the tibial nerve. The popliteal artery is located superolaterally to the vein.

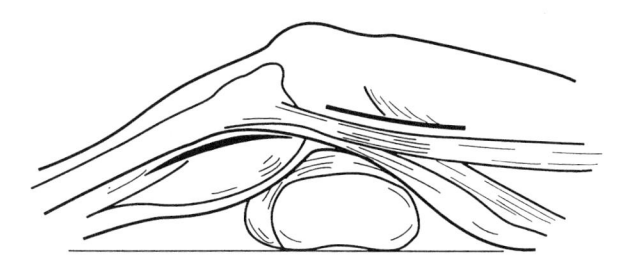

Fig. 10.2. Medial approach to right lower extremity with placement of incisions for proximal and distal popliteal exposure.

The popliteal vein is often paired in this area. Approximately 5 to 6 cm of popliteal artery can be easily isolated down to the origin of the anterior tibial artery.

Posterior exposure of the popliteal artery is favored for cases of localized popliteal artery trauma such as intimal flaps or segmental thrombosis. The posterior approach may assist simultaneous revascularization in bilateral popliteal artery injuries. The patient is placed prone with a pillow under both knees. The incision is S shaped and starts medially with the horizontal component centered in the popliteal skin crease ending laterally as shown in Figure 10.3. Skin flaps are elevated to allow exposure. The lesser saphenous vein is identified and preserved, if possible, after the superficial and deep fascias have been incised. The popliteal vein and deeper popliteal artery will be identified after separation of the popliteal fat (Figure 10.4). Careful dissection must be maintained to prevent injury to the tibial nerve.

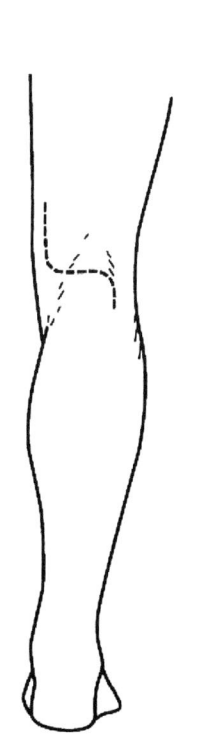

Fig. 10.3. Posterior right popliteal fossa skin incision.

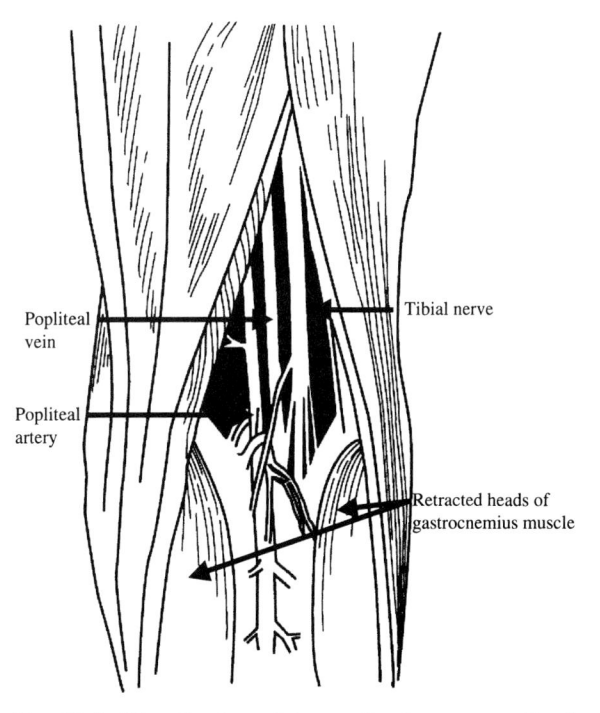

Fig. 10.4. Visualization of the popliteal artery, popliteal vein, and tibial nerve via the posterior approach. The heads of the gastrocnemius muscle have been separated to allow visualization of the anterior tibial artery and tibioperoneal trunk.

Table 10.3. Causes of knee dislocation

Series	Knee dislocations	Distribution of causes (%)				Popliteal injuries
		MVA	Falls	Sports	Other/work	
Kennedy[7]	22	54.5	4.5	49	32	7 (32%)
Roman et al.[12]	30	60	30	7	3	10 (33%)
Dennis et al.[14]	38	64.8	13.5	8.1	16.2	9 (24%)
Wascher et al.[16]	47	74	6	18	2	11 (23%)
Kaufman and Martin[17]	19	42	47	0	11	6 (32%)
Sisto and Warren[19]	20	50	0	30	20	2 (10%)
Treiman et al.[23]	115	64	18	0	18	27 (23%)
Jones et al.[24]	22	82	4.5	9	4.5	10 (45%)
Total	313					82
Average		61.4%	15.4%	10.1%	13.1%	26.2%[a]

[a] Percentage reflects rounding errors.

Mechanism of Injury

The common causes of knee dislocation are well described: motor vehicle accidents, falls, sports injuries, and work-related injuries (Table 10.3).[7,12,14,16,17,19,23,24] The majority of injuries are secondary to motor vehicle accidents including driver and passenger injuries, motor vehicle versus pedestrian injuries (bumper injuries), and motorcycle accidents. Falls from heights are the second most common cause of knee dislocations. However, a series of peripheral vascular injuries due to falls by White et al.[25] described only 1 out of 7 patients with documented knee dislocations (bilateral). Dislocation of the knee during total knee arthroplasty may also cause popliteal artery injury either by direct penetrating injury or by shearing as shown in Figure 10.5. Other interesting reported causes of knee dislocations include trampoline injuries,[26] martial arts injury,[27] and spontaneous knee dislocation in the morbidly obese.[28]

Fig. 10.5. Left lateral angiogram of popliteal artery after total knee replacement showing preexisting atherosclerosis in proximal popliteal artery. Distal popliteal artery and tibioperoneal trunk occlusion is demonstrated.

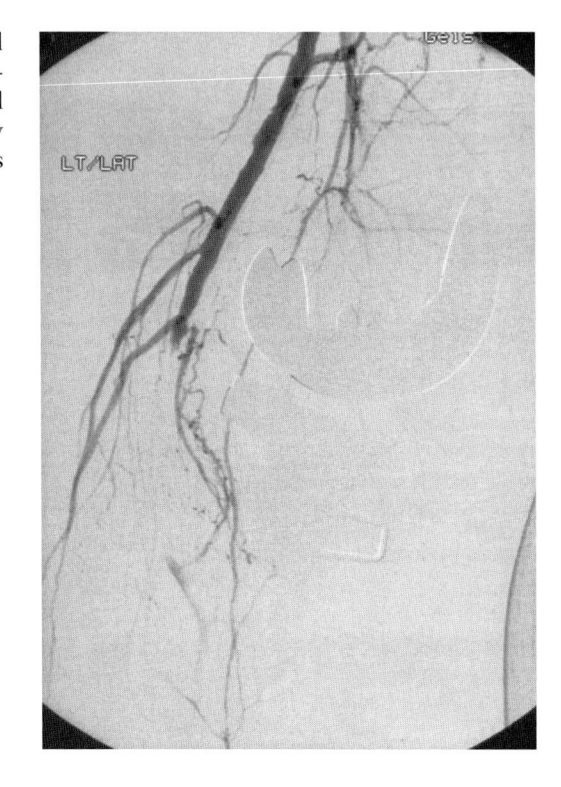

10. Vascular Injuries in the Dislocated Knee

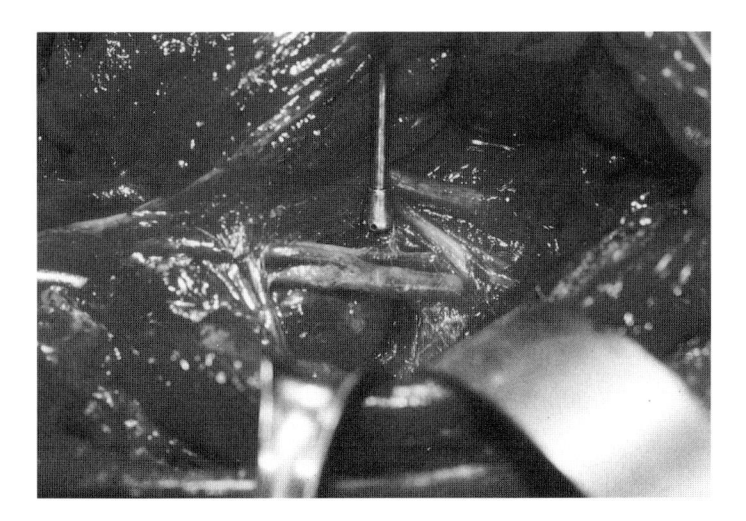

Fig. 10.6. A thrombosed popliteal artery secondary to knee dislocation is shown from a posterior approach. The contused popliteal artery is inferior to the suction tip; the popliteal vein and tibial nerve are also well visualized. (See color plate.)

Kennedy[7] used a stress machine in a cadaver model to investigate the mechanisms of knee dislocation and vascular injury. During anterior knee dislocation, he found that tearing of the posterior capsule occurred at 30° of hyperextension followed by tearing and rupture of the posterior cruciate ligament. He noted that progressive degrees of hyperextension caused considerable stretching of the popliteal artery, with rupture at an average of 50° of hyperextension.

The mechanisms of vascular injury, both artery and vein, include stretching that results in intimal injury, contusion, laceration, transection, or avulsion. Trauma in proximity to a vessel may also cause vascular spasm without actual vascular injury occurring.

Intimal injury is a tear of the inner lining, the intima, of the blood vessel while the remaining layers, media and adventitia, remain intact (Figure 10.6; see color plate). Intimal injuries as well as vessel wall contusion may predispose the vessel to thrombosis or distal embolization with activation of the coagulation cascade (Figure 10.7). A pseudoaneurysm, also known as a false aneurysm, is secondary to a laceration or full-thickness injury to the arterial wall. Initially the blood is focally contained by soft tissue adjacent to the area of injury. Pseudoaneurysms may lead to embolization, compressive symptoms, or rupture. Both intimal injuries and pseudoaneurysms may present with a normal pulse examination.

Anterior knee dislocations are more likely to cause intimal injury from excessive stretch, with or without resultant thrombosis. Posterior knee dislocations are more likely to result in complete transection of the vessel. Both types of knee dislocation have consistently been shown to have an increased association with popliteal artery injury, with each accounting for approximately 40% of popliteal injuries in several combined series reported by one author.[18] Concomitant fractures can also result in direct injury of the popliteal artery or vein as shown in Figure 10.8.

Evaluation

Patients presenting with knee dislocations must be evaluated under a complete trauma protocol. As previously described, the majority of knee dislocations are secondary to motor vehicle accidents and falls. These patients have a significant incidence of coexisting trauma. In the series by Wascher

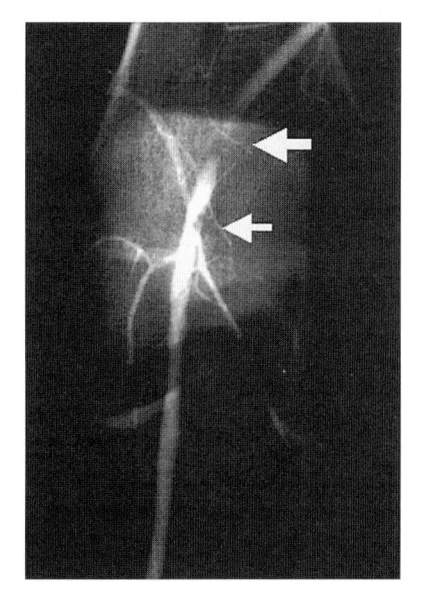

Fig. 10.7. Angiogram of traumatic popliteal artery injury revealing proximal occlusion (top arrow) from intimal injury with embolus (bottom arrow).

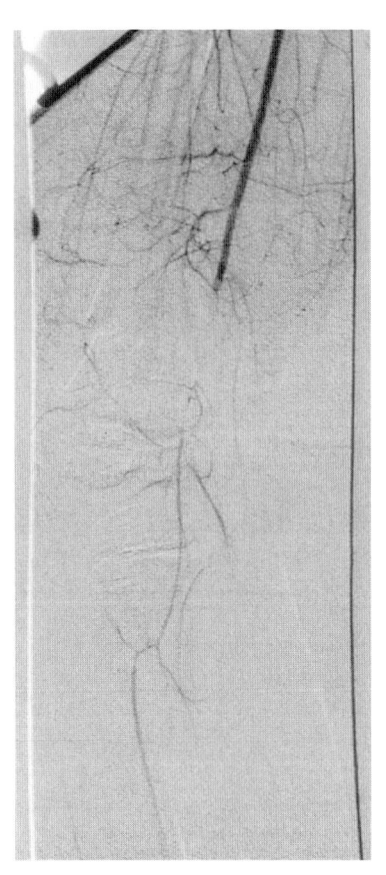

Fig. 10.8. Proximal popliteal artery occlusion at the level of supracondylar femoral fracture.

et al.,[16] a knee dislocation secondary to high energy trauma was associated with a concomitant life-threatening injury in 27% of the cases, with a resulting mortality rate of 5%. In the report by Treiman et al.,[23] 105 of 220 patients with knee dislocation presented with associated life-threatening injuries, ongoing hemorrhage, or a severely ischemic limb, causing these patients to be removed from the authors' study on selective angiography. Therefore, patients presenting with knee dislocations must be evaluated under a stringent trauma protocol.

Trauma patients must be purposefully evaluated for both dislocated knee and multiple ligament injured knee, as well as potential limb ischemia secondary to vascular injury or compartment syndrome. A history of knee dislocation by prehospital personnel or other observers must be taken seriously because as many as 50% of knee dislocations may be reduced prior to presentation at the hospital.[7,29–31] In addition, Varnell et al.[32] showed that the incidence of popliteal artery injury was the same with severe knee ligament disruption and knee dislocation. If a knee dislocation or multiple ligament injured knee is identified, a brief history focusing on the mechanism of injury, preexisting vascular disease, and vascular disease risk factors should be obtained. The limb should be evaluated for hard signs of vascular injury as listed in Table 10.4.

Hard signs are indicative but not diagnostic of arterial injury. Pulselessness and pallor may be secondary to compartment syndrome, arterial spasm, or arterial injury. Paresthesias and paralysis may be secondary to coexisting nerve injury, compartment syndrome, or arterial injury. Poikilothermia may be secondary to hypothermia, compartment syndrome, or arterial injury. When hard signs of ischemia are present, patients should be immediately considered for angiography or surgical exploration. Soft signs should prompt consideration for serial physical examination or adjunctive objective tests such as color flow duplex or angiography.

Complete pulse examination of the limb, including femoral, popliteal, dorsalis pedis, and posterior tibial arteries, should be performed with the initial evaluation and after knee reduction. Comparison with the contralateral limb may assist in revealing subtle pulse discrepancies. A decrement in pulse examination findings after knee reduction is indicative of potential arterial injury. Auscultation for bruits in the popliteal fossa should also be performed. A complete lower extremity motor and sensory exam is important at initial evaluation and after knee reduction to identify potential associated nerve injury, traumatic or ischemic, as well as to document baseline function. The leg should then be serially evaluated for clinical signs of a compartment syndrome.

Multiple studies have shown that a popliteal artery injury may be present despite palpable pulses. Palpable pulses are found in 25 to 55% of patients with popliteal artery injuries. In 6 series with 80 popliteal artery injuries in

Table 10.4. Signs of arterial injury

Hard signs	Soft signs
Pulselessness	Stable hematoma
Pallor	Peripheral nerve deficit
Paresthesias	Unexplained shock
Paralysis	Proximity wounds
Poikilothermia	Fracture dislocation (elbow or knee)
Pain	Decreased distal pulses
Bruit	
Pulsatile bleeding	

Table 10.5. Popliteal artery injuries with normal pulses

Series	Knee dislocations	Popliteal artery injuries	Injuries with normal pulses
Dennis et al.[14]	38	9	5 (55%)
Kaufman et al.[17]	19	6	2 (33%)
Treiman et al.[23]	115	33	9 (27%)
Jones et al.[24]	22	10	3 (30%)
Varnell et al.[32]	30	12	4 (25%)
O'Donnell et al.[33]	10	10	3 (30%)
Total	234	80 (34%)	26 (32%)

234 knee dislocations, palpable pulses were present in 32% of popliteal artery injuries (Table 10.5).[14,17,23,24,32,33] The numerous collateral vessels that provide circulation around the knee are abundant although small in caliber. Frequently, the collateral vessels are also injured secondary to the knee dislocation and are at risk for delayed thrombosis with resultant critical ischemia. Palpable pulses may therefore be present with either intact collateral circulation or nonocclusive popliteal artery injuries. Conversely, diminished or absent pulses may be secondary to arterial spasm without injury of the arterial tree.

Patients with obviously ischemic limbs as shown by the presence of hard signs, as well as patients with life-threatening injuries requiring surgery, are brought immediately to the operating room. Formal angiography in the setting of an obviously ischemic limb has been shown to add a minimum of 2 to 3 h of additional ischemic time, with little benefit compared with intraoperative angiography.[13,34]

Adjunctive tests for patients with knee dislocation and normal pulses include ankle–brachial index (ABI), color flow duplex scan, and angiography. Traditionally, routine formal angiography was advocated for all patients with knee dislocation.[24] In contrast, some recent authors have advocated selective angiography based on serial physical examinations.[14,15,20,23] Frykberg et al.[35] found that routine angiography performed solely for proximity in asymptomatic penetrating extremity wounds yielded a medical cost of $66,000 per identified vascular injury that required surgery. Table 10.5 lists several series that evaluated the need for routine arteriography. Overall, 34% of patients with knee dislocation had identified popliteal artery injuries, with 32% of these patients maintaining palpable pulses despite the arterial injury. Of these 6 studies, 3 reported on patients with normal pulses who eventually required surgery,[23,24,33] whereas in 3 studies patients with normal pulses did not require surgery.[14,17,32] Recently, serial physical examination, ABI, and color flow duplex scan have been evaluated for their ability to detect vascular injuries.

Serial physical examination is performed for 72 h on an inpatient basis for the patient who presents with normal neurovascular examination findings. Any change in vascular status prompts either formal angiography or surgical exploration. This management protocol is predicated on data showing that nonocclusive minimal vascular injuries such as intimal injuries, arteriovenous fistulas, and small false aneurysms will likely heal without adverse clinical sequelae. In an evaluation of 61 nonocclusive arterial injuries in 50 patients in multiple locations, Stain et al.[36] found resolution, improvement, or stabilization in 87% of a subset of 30 patients who had follow-up angiography at 1 to 12 weeks. Furthermore, Stain et al. showed that none of these 50 patients required surgery because of delayed arterial thrombosis, hemorrhage, or ischemia. However, 10 patients had persistent arteriovenous fistulas treated at the time of repeat arteriography. Only 8 of the 10 could be treated successfully using endovascular techniques, and the remaining 2 refused operative therapy.

The evaluation of serial physical examination and nonoperative management for popliteal artery injury secondary to knee dislocation has been reported in 29 patients in the literature. In these seven series of patients with normal pulse examinations, only 2 of the 29 patients required surgery.[14,16,17,20,23,32,37] Of the patients requiring surgery, one was operated on for thrombosis of the popliteal artery during the 72h observation phase, while the other presented at 5 weeks with a ruptured popliteal pseudoaneurysm.[23,37] In summary, serial physical examination will miss the approximately 32% of injuries that present with palpable pulses. The majority of these injuries are presumed to be minor and may not require surgery. However, approximately 6% will require major limb salvage surgery, with some having a delayed presentation. To date, serial observation series with resultant amputations have not been reported.

An ABI is obtained by placing a blood pressure cuff at the ankle and determining the systolic blood pressure of the peroneal, dorsalis pedis, and posterior tibial arteries with the handheld Doppler. The brachial artery systolic pressure is then divided by the highest systolic blood pressure at the ankle. The ABI is normally greater than 1.0, while an ABI less than 0.90 is suggestive of a vascular injury.[38] Lynch and Johansen[39] found that an ABI of less than 0.9 had a sensitivity of 87% and a specificity of 97% for arterial injury, with 94% of patients having positive arteriographic findings. With an ABI greater than 0.9, only 5 minor injuries were found in 79 limbs within 2 weeks of injury by color duplex evaluation.[38] The ABI, however, does not diagnose nonocclusive popliteal artery injuries such as intimal flaps and pseudoaneurysms. The ABI does give more usable objective data than a simple Doppler signal. The presence of a Doppler signal does not rule out vascular injury.

Color flow duplex scan is used extensively in the vascular laboratory, and although it is operator dependent, it has been shown to safely and accurately diagnose nontraumatic arterial pathology. It has the potential ability to detect minor arterial injuries such as intimal flaps, narrowing, arteriovenous fistula and pseudoaneurysms as well as venous injuries.[40] Bynoe et al.[41] evaluated color flow duplex in 198 patients with 319 potential vascular injuries. These injuries were due to penetrating trauma in 79% and blunt trauma in 21% of patients. They found the sensitivity to be 95% with a specificity of 99% and an overall accuracy of 98%. A major limitation of duplex examination in trauma patients is local swelling or hematoma, which precludes complete visualization of the vascular system. Color flow duplex has not been specifically evaluated for a potential role in vascular evaluation of the dislocated knee.

The question of the appropriate vascular evaluation for a patient with a knee dislocation without signs of ischemia and palpable pulses continues to be controversial but with a leaning toward selective rather than routine angiography. Routine angiography does permit diagnoses of occult vascular injury, but many of these injuries may be adequately managed with serial observation. A series by Applebaum et al.[20] found 3 radiographic abnormalities during the performance of routine arteriography in 22 patients with knee dislocation, fracture, or soft tissue injury and palpable pulses. None of these injuries, which included one popliteal intimal defect, required surgery. However, several authors have reported significant arterial pathology requiring surgical repair that was missed upon review of serial physical examinations.[24,33,37] Given the potentially devastating consequence of a missed popliteal artery injury, routine arteriography or duplex examination with serial physical examination is recommended for all patients presenting with knee dislocation.

Indications for operation include limb ischemia, ongoing hemorrhage, compartment syndrome, significant angiographic lesion, or significant arterial lesion by duplex examination.

Operative Technique

The fundamentals of operation on popliteal artery injuries include prompt restoration of pulsatile arterial flow, removal of distal thrombus, systemic heparin therapy if not contraindicated, and treatment of compartment syndrome.

The controversy over whether to perform vascular repair or orthopaedic repair first in combined injuries continues. The appropriate sequence depends on injury time course and ischemic severity. Prolonged ischemic time or significant ischemic severity mandates prompt restoration of arterial flow prior to orthopaedic repair. The concern for disruption of vascular repair secondary to orthopaedic manipulation has not been demonstrated in many large series. Even so, several authors continue to recommend that the vascular surgeon reevaluate the vascular reconstruction at the end of orthopaedic manipulation. Temporary vascular shunts, introduced by Eger et al.[42] in 1971, may be used as a bridge to arterial reconstruction. These shunts may be used to allow arterial perfusion during transport or skeletal fixation. The use of temporary shunts is well established as demonstrated by their use in carotid surgery. Thrombectomy should be performed prior to placement of shunts to prevent distal embolization. Systemic or local heparin therapy should also be considered. In a series by Johansen et al.[43] without the use of systemic heparin therapy, the average shunt dwell time was 3.7h. There were no complications referenced to the use of shunts in this series.

Patient positioning is dependent on the requirement of any coexisting life- or limb-threatening injuries. The popliteal artery reconstruction can be approached using either a medial or a posterior approach. The medial approach is preferred, although the posterior approach may be helpful when focal as well as bilateral limited popliteal artery injuries are being treated. An open knee joint as visualized from the posterior approach is shown in Figure 10.9 (see color plate). Both lower extremities should always be prepped to allow harvest of contralateral greater saphenous vein if required.

The method of vascular repair depends on the nature of the popliteal artery injury. Choices include lateral repair, end-to-end repair, intimal repair with vein patch, or interposition grafting (Figure 10.10). The majority of popliteal artery injuries secondary to knee dislocation require an interposition vein graft secondary to the extent of arterial injury. The popliteal artery must be debrided to normal-appearing artery prior to anastamosis. End-to-end repair may require extensive mobilization of the popliteal artery with sacrifice of collateral vessels to ensure a tension-free repair. Interposition grafting is most commonly performed with the greater saphenous vein from the contralateral limb. Prosthetic grafts, including Teflon and Dacron, have been evaluated for these repairs but have a decreased patency rate and raise the potential concern for increased risk of infection.[44]

The extent of venous repair in association with popliteal artery injuries continues to be controversial. Treatment options include ligation, lateral repair, and interposition vein grafting. An early report of a civilian experi-

Fig. 10.9. Open joint secondary to a knee dislocation shown from the posterior approach during surgery for a popliteal artery occlusion. The extensive amount of tissue injury is evident, as is the large hematoma that was evacuated from the lateral aspect of the wound. (See color plate.)

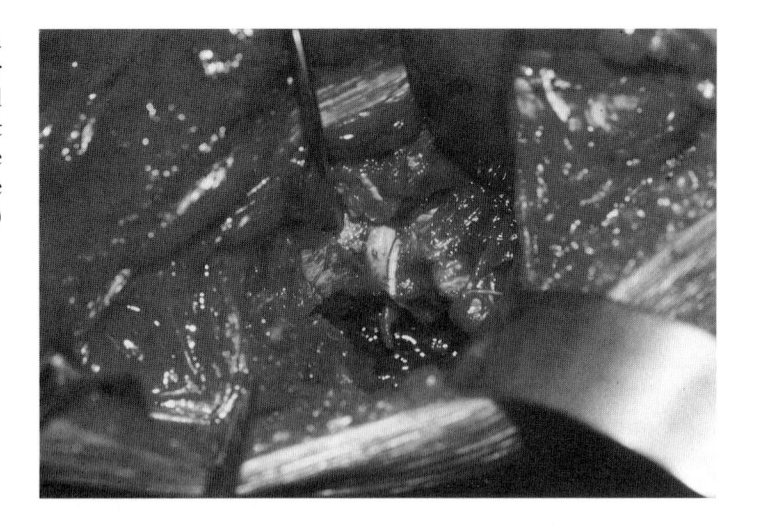

ence with major venous injuries was published in 1960 but included only 4 popliteal venous repairs.[45] The need for venous repair in conjunction with popliteal artery repair was first evaluated in Vietnam by Rich et al.[46] The Vietnam experience revealed several cases of leg amputation secondary to venous hypertension after venous ligation with popliteal artery repair.[47] In an experimental canine hind limb model, Hobson et al.[48] showed that venous ligation caused a 50 to 75% reduction in femoral arterial flow and an increase in femoral venous pressure. The fate of venous repairs was evaluated by Meyer et al.[49] in 36 patients. They found that 40% of the veins had thrombosed by postoperative day 7 and that lateral repair had a statistically significant increased patency rate compared with interposition vein grafting. Noninvasive evaluation that includes physical examination and impedance plethysmography was not found to provide an accurate assessment of venous patency in this setting.

A retrospective analysis of 115 venous injuries in civilians found an increased incidence of lower extremity edema after vein ligation compared

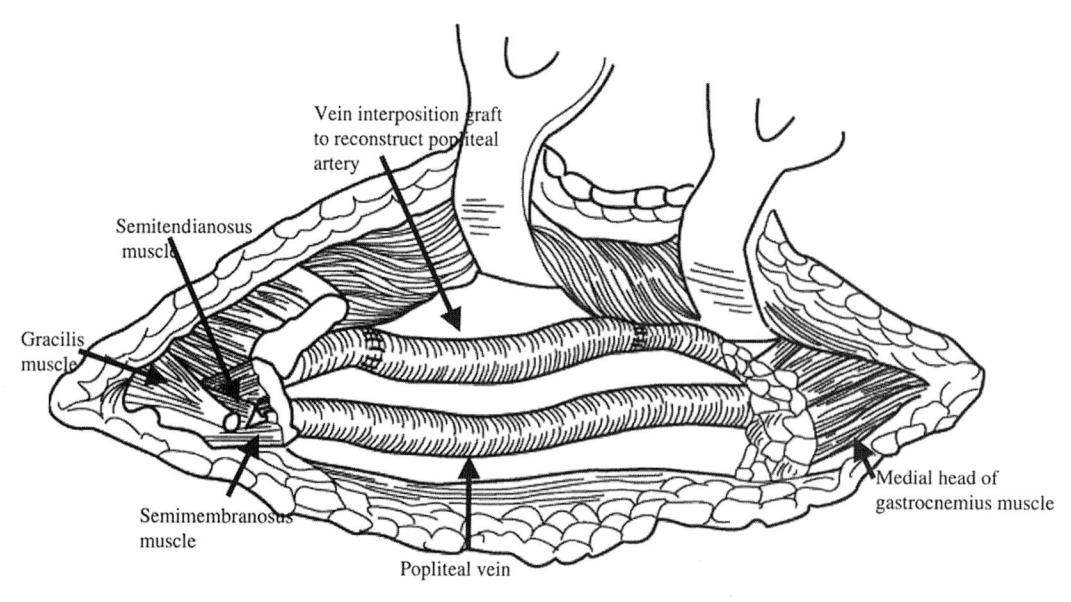

Fig. 10.10. Popliteal artery repair with interposition saphenous vein graft.

with repair.[50] Concern for an increased incidence of pulmonary embolus and thrombophlebitis after venous repair has not been supported by the literature.[49,51] Civilian series of vein ligation versus repair have not shown a statistically significant difference in amputation rates.[52,53] General agreement can currently be reached on the appropriateness of popliteal venous repair by lateral suture in stable patients. The ipsilateral saphenous vein should never be harvested for arterial or venous repair because it maintains superficial venous drainage of the injured leg. Prior to venous repair, all proximal and distal thrombi must be removed. The role of interposition grafting in popliteal venous repair continues to be controversial.

The role for primary amputation in knee dislocations is usually not dependent on vascular injury but rather on the extent of neurologic, soft tissue, and osseous damage. Absolute indications in the literature include complete tibial nerve disruption in the adult and warm ischemia time greater than 6 h in extensive crush injuries.[54]

Adjunctive Measures

Limb salvage after popliteal artery injuries may be affected by small-vessel thrombosis distal to the injury. The use of systemic heparin or local thrombolytics to combat distal small vessel thrombosis has been evaluated. Melton et al.[55] studied factors that may affect limb salvage after popliteal artery trauma. They found that severity of limb injury was highly predictive of amputation. The only controllable factor found to affect amputation rate was the use of systemic heparin or local urokinase. Daugherty et al.[56] found that 75% of patients undergoing systemic anticoagulation versus 43% of patients not undergoing anticoagulation had a satisfactory result after popliteal artery repair. Wagner et al.[53] also found a statistically significant decrease in amputation rate with systemic heparinization. In the absence of contraindications, systemic anticoagulation with heparin is recommended for all patients with popliteal artery injury. Intraoperative thrombolytic therapy should also be considered in patients with distal thrombosis if no contraindication exists.

The use of mannitol to limit reperfusion syndrome after popliteal artery repair is supported by experimental and clinical evaluation. Buchbinder et al.[57] studied the effects of mannitol in the canine hind limb model. Mannitol administration was found to decrease tissue edema, vascular resistance, and the low flow state. These investigators then utilized mannitol in 15 consecutive patients with lower extremity ischemia and none developed graft thrombosis or compartment syndrome. Mannitol is known to be an oxygen free radical scavenger and osmotic diuretic. Reperfusion injury in many organs is mediated by oxygen free radical production, which is known to increase vascular permeability.[58,59] Routine use of mannitol is recommended based on safety and reported efficacy.[53]

Muscular vessels may develop spasm after injury and account for decreased pulses on physical examination. Spasm can clearly be recognized by its traces in angiographic findings (Figure 10.11). Decreased or absent pulses must never be attributed to spasm without objective angiographic evidence. If spasm is noted on angiography, intra-arterial infusion of vasodilators may be performed. Tolazoline has been most effective in improving distal flow secondary to spasm after fracture reduction.[60] Prior to vasodilator therapy, compartment syndrome, which may be responsible for an abnormal pulse exam in the absence of any arterial injury, must be ruled out as a cause of vessel narrowing.

Fig. 10.11. Angiogram reveals diffuse popliteal spasm in association with knee injury, distal femur fracture.

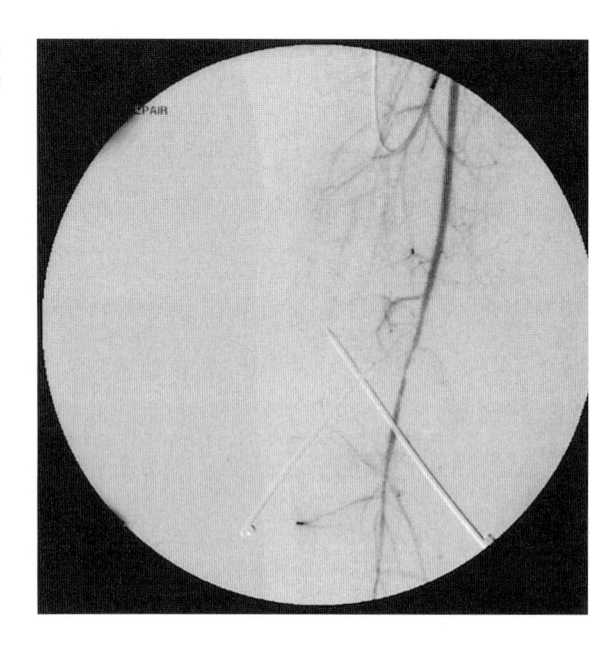

Four-compartment fasciotomy for the treatment of compartment syndrome is required in 50 to 80% of patients with popliteal artery injury.[5,21,52,53,61,62] Fainzilber et al.[61] found fasciotomy to significantly correlate with limb salvage. These authors also found a zero amputation rate in 10 patients when popliteal vein ligation was combined with fasciotomy. Fasciotomy should be performed prior to vascular repair if compartment syndrome is confirmed or suspected. Absolute indications for fasciotomy include confirmed compartment syndrome by compartment pressure measurement or combined arterial and venous repair. Fasciotomy should also be strongly considered in cases of prolonged shock, prolonged ischemia, or extremity swelling.

Conclusions

Vascular injury in the dislocated knee continues to account for significant morbidity. As recently as 1995, a 47% amputation rate for popliteal artery injuries in blunt trauma still existed.[61] Controllable factors that have been found to increase limb salvage include decreased ischemia time, systemic anticoagulation, and four-compartment fasciotomy. The decrease in amputation rates seen in penetrating popliteal artery injuries continues to elude the patients with blunt popliteal artery injury. A high index of suspicion of vascular injury must always be present. Prompt recognition of vascular injury, prompt restoration of flow, and use of proven adjuncts provide the optimal possibility of limb salvage with popliteal artery injuries.

References

1. Debakey ME, Simone FA. Battle injuries of the arteries in World War II. Ann Surg 1946; 123:534–579.
2. Hughes CW. Arterial repair during the Korean War. Ann Surg 1958; 147: 555–561.
3. Rich NM, Baugh JH, Hughes CW. Popliteal artery injuries in Vietnam. Am J Surg 1969; 118:531–534.

4. Daugherty ME, Sachatello CR, Ernst CB. Improved treatment of popliteal artery injuries. Arch Surg 1978; 113:1317–1321.
5. Reynolds R, McDowell HA, Diethelm AG. The surgical treatment of blunt and penetrating injuries of the popliteal artery. Am Surg 1983; 49(8):405–410.
6. Hoover NW. Injuries of the popliteal artery associated with fractures and dislocations. Surg Clin North Am 1961; 41:1099–1112.
7. Kennedy JC. Complete dislocation of the knee joint. J Bone Joint Surg Am 1963; 45(5):889–904.
8. Reckling FW, Peltier LF. Acute knee dislocations and their complications. J Trauma 1969; 9:181–191.
9. Shields L, Mohinder M, Cave EF. Complete dislocation of the knee: experience at the Massachusetts General Hospital. J Trauma 1969; 9:192–195.
10. Myers MH, Harvey JP. Traumatic dislocation of the knee joint: a study of 18 cases. J Bone Joint Surg Am 1971; 53:16–29.
11. Taylor AR, Arden GP, Rainey HA. Traumatic dislocation of the knee: a report of 43 cases with special reference to conservative treatment. J Bone Joint Surg Br 1972; 54:96–102.
12. Roman PD, Hopson CN, Zenni EJ. Traumatic dislocation of the knee: a report of 30 cases and literature review. Orthop Rev 1987; 16(12):917–924.
13. Bryan T, Merritt P, Hack B. Popliteal arterial injuries associated with fractures or dislocations about the knee as a result of blunt trauma. Orthop Rev 1991; 20(6):525–530.
14. Dennis JW, Jagger C, Frykberg ER, et al. Reassessing the role of arteriograms in the management of posterior knee dislocations. J Trauma 1993; 35(5): 692–697.
15. Bunt TJ, Malone JM, Karpman R, et al. Frequency of vascular injury with blunt trauma-induced extremity injury. Am J Surg 1990; 160:226–228.
16. Wascher, DC, Dvirnak PC, DeCoster TA. Knee dislocation: initial assessment and implications for treatment. J Orthop Trauma 1997; 11:525–529.
17. Kaufman SL, Martin LG. Arterial injuries associated with complete dislocation of the knee. Radiology 1992; 184:153–155.
18. Green NE, Allen BL. Vascular injuries associated with dislocations of the knee. J Bone Joint Surg Am 1977; 59:236–241.
19. Sisto DJ, Warren RF. Complete knee dislocation: a follow-up study of operative treatment. Clin Orthop 1985; 198:94–101.
20. Applebaum R, Yellin AE, Pentecost M, et al. Role of routine arteriography in blunt lower-extremity trauma. Am J Surg 1990; 160:221–225.
21. Lim LT, Michuda MS, Flanigan DP, Pankovich A. Popliteal artery trauma: 31 consecutive cases without amputation. Arch Surg 1980; 115:1307–1313.
22. Bishara RA, Pasch AR, Lim LT, et al. Improved results in the treatment of civilian vascular injuries associated with fractures and dislocations. J Vasc Surg 1986; 3:707–711.
23. Treiman GS, Yellin AE, Weaver FA, et al. Examination of the patient with a knee dislocation: the case for selective arteriography. Arch Surg 1992; 127: 1056–1063.
24. Jones RE, Smith EC, Bone GE. Vascular and orthopedic complications of knee dislocation. Surg Gynecol Obstet 1979; 149:554–558.
25. White RA, Scher LA, Samson RH, Veith FJ. Peripheral vascular injuries associated with falls from heights. J Trauma 1987; 27(4):411–414.
26. Kwolek CJ, Sundaram S, Schwarcz TH, Endean ED. Popliteal artery thrombosis associated with trampoline injuries and anterior knee dislocations in children. Am Surgeon 1998; 64(12):1183–1187.
27. Viswanath YKS, Rogers IM. A non-contact complete knee dislocation with popliteal artery disruption, a rare martial arts injury. Postgrad Med J 1999; 75(887):552–553.
28. Hagino RT, DeCaprio JD, Valentine RJ, Clagett GP. Spontaneous popliteal vascular injury in the morbidly obese. J Vasc Surg 1998; 28(3):458–463.
29. Lefrak EA. Knee dislocation. Arch Surg 1976; 111:1021–1024.
30. O'Donoghue DH. Dislocation of the knee. Orthop Rev 1975; 4:19–29.
31. Wascher DC. High-velocity knee dislocation with vascular injury: treatment principles. Clin Sports Med 2000; 19:457–77.
32. Varnell RM, Coldwell DM, Sangeorzan BJ, Johansen KH. Arterial injury complicating knee disruption. Am J Surg 1989; 55(12):699–704.

33. O'Donnell TF, Brewster DC, Darling RC, et al. Arterial injuries associated with fractures and/or dislocations of the knee. J Trauma 1977; 17(10):775–782.
34. Shah DM, Naraynsingh V, Leather RP, et al. Advances in the management of acute popliteal vascular blunt injuries. J Trauma 1985; 25(8):793–797.
35. Frykberg ER, Crump JM, Vines FS. A reassessment of the role of arteriography in penetrating proximity extremity trauma: a prospective study. J Trauma 1989; 29:1041–1052.
36. Stain SC, Yellin AE, Weaver FA, Pentecost MJ. Selective management of non-occlusive arterial injuries. Arch Surg 1989; 124:1136–1141.
37. Gable DR, Allen JW, Richardson JD. Blunt popliteal artery injury: is physical examination alone enough for evaluation? J Trauma 1997; 43(3):541–544.
38. Johansen K, Lynch K, Paun M, et al. Non-invasive vascular tests reliably exclude occult arterial trauma in injured extremities. J Trauma 1991; 31:515–522.
39. Lynch K, Johansen K. Can Doppler pressure measurement replace "exclusion" arteriography in the diagnosis of occult extremity arterial trauma? Ann Surg 1991; 214:737–41.
40. Fry WR, Smith S, Sayers DV, et al. The success of duplex ultrasonographic scanning in diagnosis of extremity vascular proximity trauma. Arch Surg 1993; 128(12):1368–1372.
41. Bynoe RP, Miles WS, Bell RM, et al. Noninvasive diagnosis of vascular trauma by duplex ultrasonography. J Vasc Surg 1991; 14(3):346–352.
42. Eger M, Golcman L, Goldstein A, et al. The use of a temporary shunt in the management of arterial vascular injuries. Surg Gynecol Obstet 1971; 132:67–70.
43. Johansen K, Bandyk D, Thiele B, Hansen ST. Temporary intraluminal shunts: resolution of a management dilemma in complex vascular injuries. J Trauma 1982; 22(5):395–402.
44. Feliciano DV, Bitondo CG, Mattox KL, et al. Civilian trauma in the 1980's: a 1 year experience with 456 vascular and cardiac injuries. Ann Surg 1984; 199:717–24.
45. Gaspar MR, Treiman RL. The management of injuries to major veins. Am J Surg 1960; 100:171–175.
46. Rich NM, Baugh JH, Hughes CW. Popliteal artery injuries in Vietnam. Am J Surg 1969; 118:531–534.
47. Rich NM, Jarstfer BS, Greer RM. Popliteal artery repair failure: causes and possible prevention. J Cardiovasc Surg 1974; 15:340–351.
48. Hobson RW, Howard EW, Wright CB, Collins GJ, Rich NM. Hemodynamics of canine femoral venous ligation: significance in combined arterial and venous injuries. Surgery 1973; 74:824–829.
49. Meyer, J, Walsh J, Schuler J, et al. The early fate of venous repair after civilian vascular trauma. Ann Surg 1987; 206(4):458–464.
50. Agarwal N, Shah PM, Clauss RH, et al. Experience with 115 civilian venous injuries. J Trauma 1982; 22(10):827–832.
51. Rich NM, Collins GJ, Andersen CA, et al. Autogenous venous interposition grafts in repair of major venous injuries. J Trauma 1977; 17:512–520.
52. Peck JJ, Eastman AB, Bergan JJ, et al. Popliteal vascular trauma: a community experience. Arch Surg 1990; 125:1339–1344.
53. Wagner WH, Calkins ER, Yellin AE, et al. Blunt popliteal artery trauma: one hundred consecutive injuries. J Vasc Surg 1988; 7(5):736–743.
54. Lange RH, Bach AW, Habsen ST Jr, et al. Open tibial fractures with associated vascular injuries: prognosis for limb salvage. J Trauma 1985; 25(3): 203–208.
55. Melton SM, Croce MA, Patton JH, et al. Popliteal artery trauma: systemic anticoagulation and intraoperative thrombolysis improves limb salvage. Ann Surg 1997; 225(5):518–529.
56. Daugherty ME, Sachatello CR, Ernst CB. Improved treament of popliteal artery injuries. Arch Surg 1978; 113:1317–1321.
57. Buchbinder D, Karmody AM, Leather RP, Shah DM. Hypertonic mannitol: its use in the prevention of revascularization syndrome after acute arterial ischemia. Arch Surg 1981; 116:414–421.
58. McCord JM. Oxygen-derived free radicals in postischemic tissue injury. N Engl J Med 1985; 312:159–163.

59. Bulkley GB. The role of oxygen free radicals in human disease processes. Surgery 1983; 94:407–411.
60. Dickerman RM, Gewertz BL, Foley DW, et al. Selective intra-arterial tolazoline infusion in peripheral arterial trauma. Surgery 1977; 81(5):605–609.
61. Fainzilber G, Roy-Shapira A, Wall M, Mattox K. Predictors of amputation for popliteal artery injuries. Am J Surg 1995; 170:568–571.
62. McCabe CJ, Ferguson CM, Ottinger LW. Improved limb salvage in popliteal artery injuries. J Trauma 1983; 23(11):982–985.

Chapter Eleven

Management of Acute and Chronic Nerve Injuries

Timothy J. Monahan

Dislocation of the knee is a serious and potentially limb-threatening injury. Associated ligamentous injuries, fractures, and vascular and nerve injuries are common. Prompt recognition of a knee dislocation and appropriate treatment of associated injuries are necessary to minimize the complications of this severe and potentially devastating injury. Peroneal nerve injury occurs in about 28% of knee dislocations and cases of multiple ligament injury. Despite numerous advances in nerve repair techniques, the prognosis for nerve injuries following knee dislocation remains poor, with overall recovery of 40%. This chapter provides a review of current recommendations for evaluation, treatment, and management of complications associated with nerve injury in knee dislocation, as well as areas for future study to improve prognosis and treatment.

Incidence

The incidence of peroneal nerve injury following knee dislocation is up to 50%,[1] with an overall incidence of 108/379 (28%) in the English language literature.[1-14] Despite evolving treatment methods, recovery remains sporadic, with an overall rate of 44/110 (40%).[1,2,4,5,7-12,15-18]

Although popliteal vessel and common peroneal nerve injuries are common in knee dislocation, tibial nerve injuries have not been reported except in patients in whom amputation was required.[4,15,18]

Mechanism

Platt described the association of common peroneal nerve injury with an adduction force to the knee, resulting in avulsion of the fibular styloid by the biceps tendon and knee joint dislocation.[19] He later reported 9 cases of the "ligamentous peroneal nerve syndrome," with peroneal nerve injuries ranging from stretching in continuity to complete rupture (Figure 11.1).

Highet and Holmes reported 8 more cases of common peroneal (lateral popliteal) nerve traction injuries and noted complete paralysis in 16 of 17 cases.[20] Nerve exploration was performed, and considerable variation in the degree of nerve disruption was found. Damaged nerve tissue was excised and cross sections were examined. Findings included abundant scar tissue in the connective tissue structure; even where the nerve trunk appeared in the microscopic and the Schwann tubes in microscopic continuity, the regen-

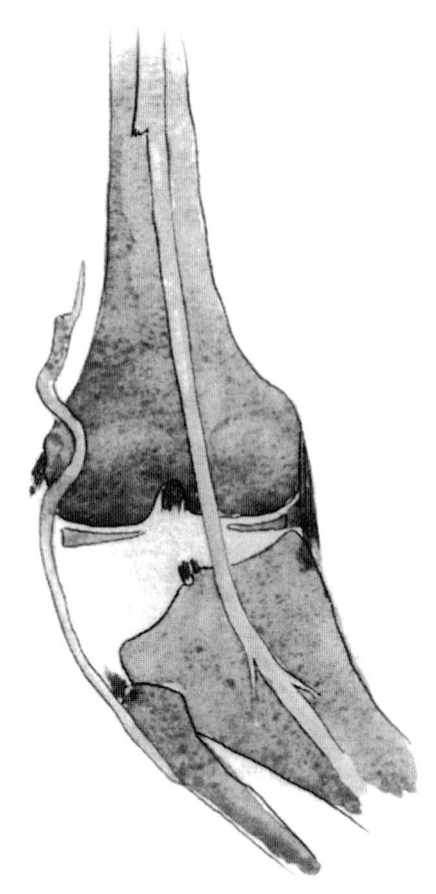

Fig. 11.1. The ligamentous peroneal nerve syndrome. (Reprinted with permission from White J. The results of traction injuries to the common peroneal nerve. J Bone Joint Surg Br 1968; 50:346–350.)

erating nerve fibers were small in diameter and unmyelinated. Changes were attributed to inflammation and later scarring of the connective tissue portion of the nerve.[20]

The peroneal division, in contrast to the tibial division of the sciatic nerve, is more likely to be compromised for a given injury mechanism and less likely to regenerate to a level of useful function.[21] Many anatomic factors may account for this difference. The peroneal division contains a smaller amount of epineural connective tissue protecting the impulse-conducting fascicular tissue. The peroneal division courses superficially over the proximal fibula, where it is poorly protected; it passes through a fibrous arcade, resulting in distal tethering by nerve branches, and has a relatively poor blood supply.[21,22] Further, recovery of the relatively long anterior compartment muscles innervated by the peroneal nerve appears to require coordinated input to multiple sites along the muscles to obtain a functional motor response. Therefore, noncoordinated input resulting from disordered or incomplete reinnervation may be insufficient to produce useful dorsiflexion of the foot or toes.[21]

Anatomy

The sciatic nerve arises from the posterior divisions of the L4, L5, S1, S2, and S3 nerve roots. Branching into the posterior tibial and peroneal divisions occurs at the level of the mid- to distal thigh. The common peroneal nerve passes inferolaterally, gives off a sural communicating branch, and courses deep to and innervates the short head of the biceps femoris. It is then separated from the lateral femoral condyle by the upper portion of the gastrocnemius and plantaris muscles. It continues posterior to the popliteus tendon and the tendinous attachment of the soleus muscle to the fibular head. It passes around the neck of the fibula, remaining adjacent to the periosteum, during which its internal fascicular arrangement rotates 180°.[23] After passing around the fibular neck, the common peroneal nerve passes through a tunnel, the roof of which is formed by the origin of the peroneus longus and intermuscular septum, with arches of fibrous tissue that complete the structure by attachment to the fibular head and shaft. The common peroneal nerve usually divides into three branches: an articular branch to the knee capsule, and the deep and superficial peroneal nerves. The superficial peroneal nerve innervates the peroneus longus and brevis muscles and supplies sensation to the lateral aspect of the leg and dorsum of the foot. The deep peroneal nerve passes through another fibro-osseus tunnel formed by the origin of the extensor digitorum longus muscle and enters the anterior compartment, where it innervates the tibialis anterior, extensor digitorum longus, extensor hallucis longus, and extensor digitorum brevis and supplies sensation to the dorsal first web space (Figure 11.2).

Seddon[24] classified nerve injuries in order of increasing severity as neuropraxia, axonotmesis, and neurotmesis. Neuropraxia is demyelination of large nerve fibers without axonal degeneration. Axonotmesis involves disruption of the axons while axonal sheaths remain intact, resulting in interruption of nerve function. Neurotmesis is complete nerve disruption.[24]

Sunderland[25] further classified nerve injuries as first- through fifth-degree injuries based on neural anatomy. First-degree injury involves demyelination only (neuropraxia). Second-degree injury involves axonal disruption only. Third-degree injury involves axonal and endoneurial tube disruption. Fourth-degree injury involves epineurium rupture, leaving only the peri-

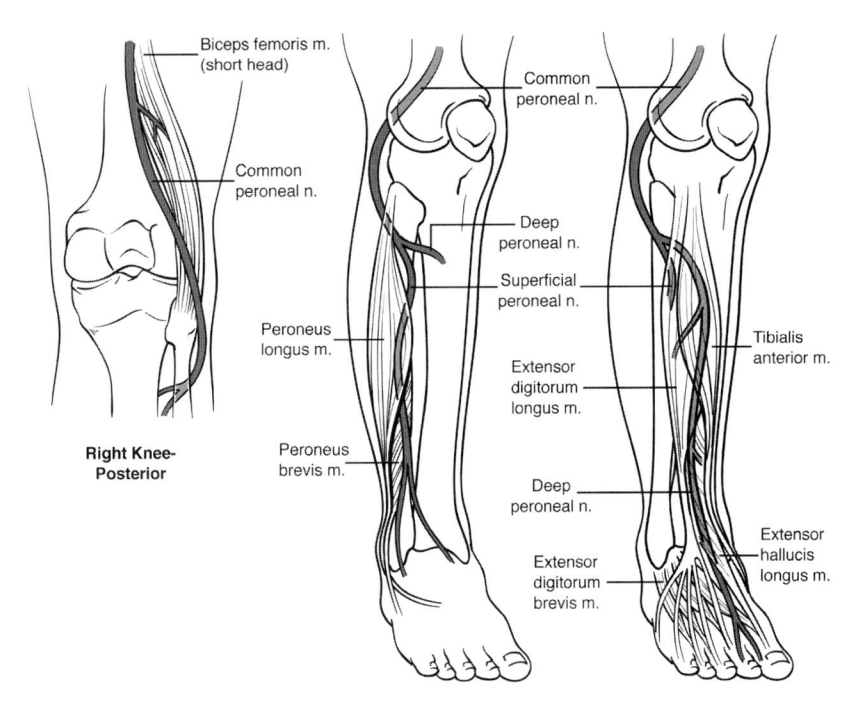

Fig. 11.2. Anatomy of the peroneal nerve. *Left*: muscles innervated by the peroneal nerve above the knee. *Center*: muscles innervated by the superficial peroneal nerve. *Right*: muscles innervated by the deep peroneal nerve.

neurium intact. Fifth-degree injury represents complete anatomic disruption (neurotmesis).[25]

Neuropraxia may be distinguished clinically and by electromyelography (EMG) from more severe injuries. Clinically, sensation remains largely intact without signs of motor atrophy in neuropraxia, while EMG shows nerve conduction to remain intact distal to the injury site despite the absence of voluntary action potentials. In axonotmesis or neurotmesis, sensation is not spared and EMG testing shows complete interruption of nerve conduction. It is impossible to distinguish between axonotmesis (second- through fourth-degree injury) and neurotmesis (fifth-degree injury) by initial clinical evaluation or EMG testing. Long-term observation is therefore required.

Initial Evaluation

An attempt should be made to elicit mechanism of injury during history taking or by report, and a high degree of suspicion is required in evaluating knee instability for associated injuries. While most multiple ligament injuries and dislocations are sustained in high energy trauma or in lower velocity athletic events, these injury complexes, termed "ultra-low velocity knee dislocations,"[15] have been observed in obese individuals during activities of daily living. Despite the differing mechanisms, the rates of neurologic injury, neurologic recovery, and vascular injury are remarkably similar. In ultra-low velocity injuries, 7 of 17 patients (41%) sustained popliteal vascular injury, 7 of 17 sustained neurologic injury (5 with isolated peroneal nerve, 2 with peroneal and tibial nerve injury), and 2 required above-knee amputation. Of those available to follow-up, 50% (2 of 4) neurologic recovery was observed.[15]

Careful physical examination is mandatory because severe and possibly limb-threatening injuries may be masked by a benign appearance. Obvious deformity may not be apparent, since a knee dislocation may present in the reduced position and associated capsular rupture may allow swelling to diffuse into adjacent tissues. Therefore, a pattern of soft tissue injury that suggests dislocation, such as a three-ligament knee injury,[6,26] should be considered to be a potential dislocation, necessitating careful examination for related nerve, vascular, and other soft tissue injuries. Peroneal palsy may also occur in association with an avulsion of the fibular styloid process and lateral knee instability without dislocation.

A thorough ligamentous examination is necessary to assess stability, though care should be taken to not place further strain on neurovascular structures. For example, varus stress should be carefully applied during examination, and hyperextension should be avoided in reduction of an anterior dislocation. If the knee joint is dislocated, immediate reduction should be obtained and not delayed to obtain prereduction radiographs.[4] This is because recovery of peroneal injury was noted following initial reduction in some cases,[1,10] and vascular compromise may be corrected with reduction.

Posterolateral knee dislocation is almost always accompanied by buttonholing of the medial femoral condyle through the medial joint capsule and invagination of the medial collateral ligament (MCL) into the joint surface. Clinically, at the medial joint line the skin will have a puckered appearance, which becomes more pronounced when attempts are made to reduce the dislocation. Open reduction is therefore required. Radiographically, the medial–tibial condyle is displaced posteriorly owing to rotation of the femur on the tibia. Peroneal nerve exploration should be carried out along with open reduction, with awareness that locating the proximal end of the ruptured nerve may be difficult.[10]

A thorough neurologic and vascular examination should be performed, both pre- and postreduction. Motor examination of peroneal innervated muscles should be carried out, remembering that radiculopathy of L4 or L5 may be another cause of footdrop. Radiculopathy may be evaluated by checking quadriceps function (femoral nerve, L4), hip adductor function (obturator nerve, L4), and gluteus medius function (superior gluteal nerve, L5).[27] Sensory examination should also be performed, remembering that sensation may be spared in incomplete lesions, particularly in the case of neuropraxia.

Vascular injury is common in multiple ligament injured knees and is a potentially limb-threatening complication. Interruption of popliteal artery flow leaves insufficient collateral circulation to maintain viability of the leg.[28] Clinical examination should evaluate any evidence of ischemia, diminished pulses, or a compartment syndrome, both pre- and postreduction. Warm skin at the foot may be present in cases of complete arterial occlusion and should not be considered to be evidence of intact blood supply.[29] The presence of normal pulses, likewise, does not rule out an arterial injury, particularly since traction injuries may result in an intimal tear, resulting in thrombus formation within a few hours to several days.[9,29-31] Any sign of diminished pulses or ischemia on postreduction examination warrants immediate vascular reconstruction, addressing both arterial and venous injury,[32] at which time fasciotomy should be performed. Common peroneal nerve exploration should also be considered at this time, unless lateral ligament reconstruction is planned later, allowing exploration to be performed concurrently. If postreduction vascular examination is normal, sequential physical examination of vascular status is required, and although controversial, arteriography is a justifiable postreduction study in potential knee dislocations and is recommended based on this review.

Arteriography has been recommended if ligament reconstruction is to be performed, other surgeries requiring tourniquet application to the extremity are required, or any concern exists for vascular compromise.[9,33] Arteriography, however, should not in any case delay vascular reconstruction in an ischemic limb.

Immobilization of the knee in 15 to 20° of flexion is recommended to stabilize the knee and prevent any further neurologic or vascular injury. Circumferential casting should be avoided to allow monitoring of neurologic, vascular, and compartment status and to avoid any potentially constrictive effect.[4] Decreased sensation and paralysis in the extremity noted on serial examination may result from neurologic or vascular insults, and differentiating between the two may be difficult. For this reason, and because delayed diagnosis of nerve injury may be confused with limb ischemia, initial neurologic deficits should be carefully documented.[34] A gradual loss of cutaneous sensation over the digits suggests critical ischemia.[4,35] Stocking paresthesia more commonly results from compartment syndrome than from simultaneous injury to both common peroneal and tibial nerves.[36]

History of Treatment

Throughout the spectrum of studies reviewed, many different recommendations are made, based on limited experience and sometimes without explanation or justification. Comparison of results across different studies is difficult owing to the variability in extent and severity of peroneal nerve traction injuries. Less favorable results have been observed with lengthy extent of damage to the nerve trunk. This may be due to several factors: severity of initial injury, extensive fibrosis preventing ordered reinnervation, large gaps between injured nerve trunks after removal of damaged tissue, and lengthy delay in exploration.

Highet and Holmes[20] recommended that neurolysis be performed if the nerve was normal in appearance. If, however, the nerve was abnormal in appearance or on palpation, despite preservation of macroscopic continuity, these authors advised examining trial sections starting at the center of the lesion, with resection performed until normal tissue is encountered. They performed nerve resection and end-to-end suture repair as described, with only 1 of 5 cases showing partial recovery. Additional factors contributing to these poor results were identified: postoperative injury inflicted during stretching of the knee joint; delay in nerve exploration, as inflammation and resulting vascular and fibrotic changes appear to be progressive from the time of injury; and large (>10cm) defects. Large defects required excessive mobilization of the nerve stumps and immobilization in excessive knee flexion to allow primary nerve repair.

Platt and Lond recommended exploration of peroneal nerve injuries within 3 to 4 weeks following injury based on 3 patients who underwent nerve suture repair and had decreased recovery with longer delays prior to repair.[37]

Gurdjian et al. recommend peroneal nerve exploration 4 to 6 weeks postinjury if no recovery is present.[38] Towne, Blazina, and their colleagues state that early exploration is important, with definitive repair to be made as soon as possible.[39] Neither set of authors offers any explanation to support these recommendations.

White, who believed that the best time for exploration is between 3 and 5 months postinjury, when the extent of intraneural fibrosis is most easily assessed, argued that results for lesions in continuity in Platt's series might have been poor because assessment of nerve damage had been made too early.[40] It should be noted that White's results showed significantly better recovery than previous reports. He described 6 traction injuries of the common peroneal nerve. In 2, the nerve was disrupted and suture repair led to functional recovery. Three of the 4 remaining lesions in continuity were explored, and the fourth was observed. All patients recovered fully. While it is not possible to dogmatize on the basis of White's small number of cases, his conclusions appear to logically follow based on available evidence. Additionally, most other authors recommend exploration if no recovery is present at 3 to 4 months.[41–43]

Disparities in findings and recommendations continue to be widespread in the literature. For example, Seddon had come to the conclusion that "owing to the great longitudinal extent of the damage in the nerve trunk, surgical repair of these injuries is hardly ever worth attempting in any situation."[40] Myers et al. stated that "exploration of the nerve in four patients in this series was of no value,"[8] while Sisto and Warren observed markedly increased function in two complete peroneal nerve lesions in continuity following delayed exploration and neurolysis.[9]

Given the wide variety of injury extent, treatments instituted, and recovery observed, it becomes clear that adequate guidance and clinical judgment require knowledge of the physiology and natural history of traction injuries to the common peroneal nerve.

Natural History of Common Peroneal Injury

Nerve regeneration occurs at a rate of 1 mm/day after an initial latency period. Target muscle motor endplate absorption begins approximately 12 to 16 months after denervation,[44] and associated degenerative changes such as muscle atrophy, shrinkage, deformation, and replacement by fibrous and fatty tissue necessitate reinnervation by 24 months for optimal function of most muscles.[45] Some authors even suggest that reinnervation must occur within 9 to 12 months for useful function.[46] The average distances from the lateral femoral epicondyle to the tibialis anterior and peroneus longus muscles are 103 to 189 mm and 94 to 150 mm, respectively.[25] Therefore, 3 to 6 months may elapse before the first signs of reinnervation are detected in axonotmesis and neurotmesis injuries,[47] and even longer times may be expected if the injury extends to the division of the sciatic nerve at the mid- to distal thigh level, as is described by many investigators. Clinically, a Tinel's sign may be observed at the level of injury with advancement of 1 mm/day as recovery proceeds. The order of recovery is usually peroneal muscles, tibialis anterior, followed by extensor hallucis longus.[21]

In neuropraxia (first-degree injury), recovery is commonly observed within 1 to 4 months.[47] In second- and third-degree injuries, Terranova et al. state that good functional recovery is expected and that any surgical procedure or further disturbance of the nerve would lessen the functional return. In more severe traction injuries, minimal recovery or plateau at an inadequate level will be observed.[47] A complete peroneal palsy results in loss of ankle dorsiflexion, foot eversion, and toe extension. Equinovarus deformity of the foot results with a peroneal palsy in the presence of a functioning tibialis posterior. Sensory loss on the dorsum and lateral foot do not present a significant functional deficit, but footdrop and resulting gait impairment result in a 30 to 35% disability of the limb according to Bateman.[23]

For nerve lesions in continuity that have not recovered, a small window of opportunity exists between the onset of ability to distinguish the extent of the lesion and the degenerative changes in motor endplates and muscle that preclude recovery. Therefore, selection of the timing of nerve exploration and repair is very important.

Recommendations for Follow-Up Observation

An ankle–foot orthosis or other brace should be used to keep the affected ankle and great toe at neutral flexion to prevent a fixed equinus contracture due to the deficient anterior compartment muscle function. At 3 weeks EMG testing should be obtained, to attempt to determine whether the nerve lesion is a neuropraxia or a more severe disruption. Clinical examination should note whether the lesion is complete or incomplete, and any recovery that is observed, including the presence and advancement of a Tinel's sign, should be described. In an incomplete lesion, electric testing is unnecessary, and the lesion may be followed clinically to assess recovery. In complete lesions, follow-up EMG testing and careful clinical examination are warranted 3 to 4 months postinjury to assess for signs of recovery (e.g., polyphasic waveforms on EMG testing imply muscle reinnervation). If no recovery is observed, peroneal nerve exploration is warranted at 3 to 5 months, when fibrosis will be visible and progressive and degenerative changes will continue to narrow the window of opportunity for recovery. Wilkinson and Birch showed that the quality of recovery was most influenced by the nature of the injury and the delay between injury and repair.[48] The recommendation of Berry and Richardson is therefore reiterated: "When the continuity of the (peroneal) nerve is in doubt, it is probably unreasonable to wait for evidence of recovery beyond 6 months."[49]

Surgical intervention for injuries associated with dislocation may be emergently required or otherwise desirable prior to the observation timetable above. For example, vascular repair, open reduction due to irreducible dislocation or open injury, compartment syndrome, and ligament reconstruction, particularly of the lateral structures, may warrant concurrent nerve exploration. The following guidance is offered regarding nerve exploration.

1. Irreducible dislocation requiring open reduction is commonly seen in posterolateral dislocations. Shields et al. reported that the posterolateral mechanism is most likely to cause severe and permanent peroneal nerve injury.[10] These authors reported complete nerve rupture with inability to locate the proximal nerve stump in 2 of 4 cases. It therefore seems warranted to perform common peroneal nerve exploration concurrent with open reduction if nerve function is absent. Except in cases of nerve discontinuity, however, it may be that the full extent of damage to the nerve cannot be assessed at this early stage.

2. Injury to the vascular structures and the peroneal nerve would be expected from a similar type of injury and are frequently seen together. Further, the approach to exploration and reconstruction of popliteal vascular structures allows access to a significant portion of the common peroneal nerve course. It seems reasonable, therefore, to assess the continuity of the nerve at the same time.

3. Compartment syndrome can cause additional nerve injury from ischemia and compression. In addition to fasciotomy, it is probably warranted to release the overlying arch of connective tissue formed by the interosseus membrane and the origin of the peroneus longus, which contains the common peroneal nerve just past the fibular neck, since this arch may serve as a compression site in the presence of severe swelling. Just as ligamentous reconstruction is not recommended with open fasciotomies

owing to increased risk of infection, it is probably unwise to perform a complete nerve exploration and attempt repair at this time.

4. If lateral ligament reconstruction is planned within a few weeks of open reduction or vascular repair, it may be warranted to delay exploration of the entire nerve course, because with the resulting delay, the extent of damage may be better assessed in conjunction with the lateral reconstruction procedure. Exploration is readily performed concurrently with lateral ligament reconstruction, since the common peroneal nerve is identified over a significant portion of its course to prevent iatrogenic injury. In any of the foregoing cases, repair probably should be limited to correcting neurotmesis and surrounding grossly abnormal tissue, since it is likely that the extent of nerve damage has been inadequately assessed. Intraoperative EMG may be helpful, both to establish a baseline and to assess the extent of injury. Transmitted nerve action potentials indicate continuity, and tissue should be preserved and observation continued if transmitted potentials are present.

5. Regarding timing of lateral ligament reconstruction, Terranova et al. had recommended delaying repair until the Tinel's sign moved beyond the fibular head.[47] This approach is strongly discouraged because recognition of the lateral compartment anatomy and repair are much easier in the acute setting, and restoration of stability may minimize the possibility of subsequent traction injury to the nerve.

When exploration of the common peroneal nerve is performed, the surgeon must be mindful that traction injuries may result in variable degrees of injury over an extensive length, possibly extending from the sciatic nerve bifurcation to its branching distal to the fibular head. Bateman states that the usual injury occurs in the vicinity of the fibular head, and identification of the distal segment may be difficult, because the injury may be at the level of the terminal branches. He therefore recommends first locating the nerve proximally and dissecting distally, remaining subperiosteal at the level of the fibular head and neck. The tissue flap may then be retracted laterally without damaging the nerve, and the distal branches may be seen through the elevated periosteum.[23] It is strongly emphasized that exploration of the entire course of the common peroneal nerve, including the proximal portion, is required to determine the entire extent of injury so prompt appropriate treatment may be selected.[50]

Clinical judgment is required to assess the severity of lesions in continuity and should be supplemented by intraoperative EMG testing if possible, to gain additional information about the location and extent of injury. The following general guidance is provided to aid in treatment of nerve injury, which may consist of: neurolysis alone or in some combination with direct suture repair, with or without excision of a nerve segment, or vascularized or nonvascularized nerve grafting.

1. Peroneal nerve vascular supply is compromised by traction injury to the vessels and hematoma inside and outside of the nerve sheath. Excessive mobilization of the nerve should be avoided, since this might further degrade already compromised circulation to the healing nerve tissue.

2. Direct suture repair is preferable if healthy nerve ends may be approximated without tension in a position of function.[51] If resection of abnormal tissue is required, and tension at the suture site results when the nerve ends are approximated, a nerve graft should be used. Excessive tension on a nerve repair may result in fibrosis at the suture line, which may impede ordered reinnervation,[51] or ischemia at the repaired ends, which may produce a neuroma in continuity.[44]

3. Vascularized nerve graft should be considered in long-nerve defects and in a tissue bed that has been severely scarred owing to the resulting poor surrounding blood supply for regenerating nerve. Hems and Glasby have reported that, in rabbits, larger fiber diameters are present distal to the vascularized grafts, suggesting that more potential exists for functional connections to be made. Regeneration is also faster in vascularized as opposed to free nerve grafts,[52] a property that may have value in minimizing end organ atrophy, particularly for large defects.

4. Sural nerve is a good routine graft source. Contralateral sural nerve should be considered if the sural nerve is functional on the injured side, to preserve as much protective sensation as possible over the lateral aspect of the foot. If the ipsilateral sural nerve is not functioning, it should be used as the graft source to avoid creating additional disability.[22]

5. Nerve grafting is performed in a cable fashion because of the size mismatch between common peroneal and sural nerves. In addition, the 180° rotation of the internal fascicular arrangement of the nerve fibers as the common peroneal passes around the fibular neck must be accounted for in grafting.

6. Sedel and Nizard reported poor results of nerve grafting in all 3 patients with vascular trauma and stated that vascular damage, even if adequately repaired, appears to be a contraindication to nerve grafting.[53]

In cases of complete nerve disruption, direct repair or nerve grafting is required. It is advisable, based on the observations of Highet and Holmes, to examine nerve cross sections starting at the discontinuity and advancing proximal and distal until normal-appearing nerve tissue is encountered, to avoid including damaged fibrotic tissue in the repair.[53] The most difficult judgment is required in the management of a lesion in continuity. An incomplete injury or neuropraxia may be distinguished clinically and by EMG from more severe injuries and warrants observation rather than exploration.

Differentiating between second- and third-degree injuries, which will not likely be improved by resection and repair, and fourth-degree lesions, which will likely have inadequate recovery unless surgical repair is performed,[46] is a difficult task based on subjective judgment. The decision is further complicated by varying degrees of injury throughout a long segment of affected nerve. Further, reported results are small in number and often cite contradictory information. For example, Sisto and Warren reported good recovery in 2 cases in which neurolysis was performed for nerve injuries in continuity at 5 weeks and 9 months postinjury, respectively.[9] In contrast, Highet and Holmes observed little functional recovery, abnormal axon regeneration, and progressive fibrosis resulting from lesions in continuity.[20] In general, it appears that nerve tissue that is grossly abnormal in appearance and to palpation requires resection and repair or grafting in an attempt to achieve ordered reinnervation of the long anterior compartment muscles required for useful dorsiflexion of the foot and toes. Again, examination of tissue cross sections starting at the lesion and extending outward is probably useful to avoid the resection of healthy tissue, or the inclusion of injured fibrotic scar tissue, which could compromise the repair.

New techniques for bridging segmental nerve defects are being studied, such as nerve guides, stimulation with cytokines, use of laminin, and nerve transplants. Trumble et al. reported that overall regeneration with these techniques has not been superior to results from autogenous sural nerve grafts.[44]

Regardless of the repair method used, observation should be implemented until it is certain that functional recovery will not occur before a reconstructive procedure to compensate for anterior or lateral compartment deficiency is attempted.[50] In the interim, an ankle–foot orthosis should be fitted to prevent equinus contracture, flexion contracture of the great toe, or fixed deformity. During follow-up examinations to assess recovery, it should be noted that scarring in the surrounding nerve bed may cause a compression neuropathy in addition to the traction injury and may require additional exploration and neurolysis.[47] It should also be noted and communicated to the patient that even with the best known treatments for traction injury to the peroneal nerve, functional recovery has been observed in only 40% of cases.

Reconstruction Options for Failed Nerve Repair or Regeneration

Several procedures have been described for the correction of footdrop resulting from peroneal nerve palsy or other causes of paralysis. In 1923 Campbell described a posterior bone block of the ankle joint to correct dropfoot deformity.[54] Although effective in paralytic dropfoot, the effectiveness of this measure declined when strong unopposed plantar flexors were present. In 1933 Ober described a transfer of the posterior tibial tendon around the medial border of the tibia to the dorsum of the foot.[55] Barr's technique, which involves passing the transposed posterior tibial tendon through the interosseus membrane, was first described by Watkins et al. in 1954.[56] Lambrinudi arthrodesis of the talocalcaneal, calcaneocuboid, and talonavicular joints, with removal of a bone wedge to correct equinus, was also commonly performed to correct footdrop. Although it was successful in controlling footdrop in 80% of cases, only 25% of the patients were satisfied with the result and felt that function was much better than it had been when they were wearing a brace.[57] Also, recurrent equinus was observed due to stretching of the anterior capsule of the ankle joint.[58] Anterior tibial tenodesis had been unsuccessfully used to correct footdrop in children and was attempted in adults to quickly return men to military service, as described by Clawson and Seddon.[57] Tibialis anterior and peroneus longus tendons were fixed into the tibia with poor results. Four of 5 tenodeses stretched out, resulting in recurrence of dropfoot.[57] Sharrard postulated that tenodesed tendons either stretch out or, more likely, elongate by growth in the presence of active plantar flexors.[59]

Based on the experience above, most of the recent reports have involved tendon transfers alone or in combination with triple arthrodesis and tenodesis. A brief summary of reported procedures and results follows.

Lipscomb and Sanchez described 10 cases of posterior tendon transfer by the Ober method, modified to place the tendon subcutaneously to the midline of the foot rather than through the anterior tibial tendon sheath, combined with triple arthrodesis.[60] They stressed that triple arthrodesis contributes immeasurably to the results but offered no explanation. Presumably, triple arthrodesis corrects the subtalar joint instability that may result from removing the stabilizing posterior tibial tendon in the absence of peroneal tendon function.

Carayon et al. described combined transfer of the posterior tibial tendon to the anterior tibial tendon, and the flexor digitorum longus to the extensor hallucis longus (EHL) and extensor digitorum longus (EDL) tendons, through a window in the interosseus membrane.[61] Encouraging results were obtained in 26 cases of leprosy and 5 cases of traumatic peroneal palsy.

Loop fixation of the tendons shortened the time of immobilization to 15 days, and transfer of two tendons increased dorsiflexion power. The importance of a large proximally extending opening in the interosseus membrane is emphasized as necessary to prevent adhesions.

Spreafico et al. reported on 16 cases using the Barr technique and stressed that it is necessary to make an ample opening in the interosseus membrane and to avoid damage to the periosteum overlying the tibia or fibula. Transfer of the tendon to the third cuneiform is preferred for secure fixation. If the transferred posterior tibial tendon is too short, suture to the tibialis anterior tendon is performed.[62] Peroneus longus transfer should be avoided because it results in changes in the plantar arch.

Pinzur et al. reported that posterior tibial tendon transfer results for traumatic peroneal palsy are not as uniformly successful as for footdrop due to other etiologies. These authors theorized that the decreased excursion of the posterior tibial muscle relative to the anterior compartment muscles is inadequate to move the ankle from normal plantarflexion to dorsiflexion. They reported a series of 9 cases of interosseus posterior tibial tendon transfer combined with anterior tibial tendon tenodesis. A normal gait pattern was observed and stretching out of the tenodesis was not observed at a minimum follow-up of 24 months.[63]

Richard reported a series of 39 interosseus posterior tibial tendon transfers with a split tail attached to both EHL and EDL tendons.[64] Adequate active dorsiflexion at follow-up examination was reported in 82% of cases, but mean plantar flexion was reduced, indicating that the transfer acted partly as a tenodesis. These findings are corroborated by Hall, who found that the circumtibial route (Ober) has 25 to 30° of ankle motion, compared with 17° in the interosseus route.[65] Hall also noted that an average of 10° of dorsiflexion was lost at 2-year follow-up when an Achilles tendon lengthening was not performed. Richard tensioned the tendon transfer at 20° of dorsiflexion and found that the amount of postoperative dorsiflexion achieved was 10° less than when the transfer was tensioned.[64] Richard prefers split attachment to EHL and EDL, as described by Srinivasan et al.,[66] to osseous tunnel attachment in the cuneiform for two reasons: it is easier to adjust tension to control inversion/eversion deformity by tensioning than by selecting a single fixation point, and split attachment minimizes the likelihood and severity of neuropathic arthropathy, particularly in those predisposed to this condition owing to leprosy.

Ninkovic et al. reported 6 cases of transposition of the lateral head of the gastrocnemius muscle to the tibialis anterior, EHL, and EDL tendons, with concurrent transposition of the proximal deep peroneal nerve stump to the motor nerve of the lateral head of the gastrocnemius muscle.[67] Prerequisites for the procedure include a viable proximal portion of the common peroneal nerve, in which the deep peroneal nerve component can be located at its branching from the tibial nerve, and permanent peroneal nerve posttraumatic paralysis (no recovery 18 months after injury or the last surgical procedure). Advantages include avoiding use of an antagonist muscle, which otherwise requires retraining, and retaining full motion in active plantar flexion. One limitation may be the inability to locate the deep peroneal branch proximally in a severe traction injury, with resultant scarring following the observation period.

Direct comparison of the reported results is not feasible owing to the varying mechanisms, extent, and etiology of injury in the reports just discussed.[60–67] The following guidance is offered, however, to assist in treatment selection.

1. Turner and Cooper report on a patient whose traumatic peroneal nerve injury had showed no recovery after one year, at which time posterior tibial tendon transfer was performed. Tibialis anterior function subsequently regained normal strength, creating a calcaneovalgus deformity.[68] This complication underscores the need to observe for an adequate time to ensure that no recovery of anterior compartment muscles has occurred before a tendon transfer is attempted. Available data on nerve regeneration suggest that 18 months after injury or the last surgical procedure should be adequate.[67]

2. Excursion of tibialis anterior and EHL tendons ranges from 3 to 5 cm, while tibialis posterior has an excursion of only 2 cm.[69] The tibialis posterior muscle is capable of generating strong dorsiflexion of the foot,[60] as expected from an average muscle–tendon unit weight of 78 g, compared with 122 g of the tibialis anterior.[70] Failures of the transfer to function adequately were much more common from loss of fixation than from weakness of a previously normally functioning tibialis posterior.[61,62] Considering the transferred posterior tibial tendon's adequate strength and the previously described decreases in ankle motion due to its decreased excursion, efforts should be made to attach the tendon transfer closer to the axis of rotation to allow more ankle motion for a given tendon excursion. Routing the transfer through a tendon sheath as opposed to subcutaneously would help in this regard.

3. Ober's technique of advancing the posterior tibial tendon distally such that the muscle fibers, rather than tendon, are in contact with the tibia, should be carefully followed to obtain maximum strength and excursion.

4. Success of the Barr technique requires a generous interosseus membrane window and care not to disturb the tibial or fibular periosteum. Both conditions are crucial to minimize adhesions of the transferred tendon.

5. Tendon transfer cannot be expected to correct a fixed deformity. Fixed deformity, most commonly Achilles contracture causing equinus, must be corrected by lengthening prior to the transfer.[56] Richard lengthened the Achilles tendon if unable to achieve 20° of dorsiflexion,[64] and Hall observed a decrease in dorsiflexion of 10° in all cases in which the Achilles was not lengthened, even in the absence of fixed contracture.[65] Malayvia correlated gait with objective measurements of active dorsiflexion and found that patients with a normal heel–toe gait had average dorsiflexion of 5°, while those who had an abnormal gait achieved only 5° short of neutral flexion.[71] Therefore, passive dorsiflexion of at least 20° should be obtained preoperatively to achieve a satisfactory postoperative result.

6. Cozen emphasizes that bracing for dropfoot must include the toes to avoid contracture due to the unopposed flexors.[58] The literature says little about whether it is necessary to address the unopposed flexors when the patient is ambulatory. Specifically, is it beneficial or necessary to use flexor hallucis longus as a tendon transfer to the extensors to remove a potentially deforming force, as suggested by Carayon et al.,[61] to incorporate the toe extensors only into a single repair, as in the method of Srinivasan et al.,[66] to include all extensors into a single repair, as in the method proposed by Nincovic et al.,[67] or to route the transfer to a bony tunnel in the lateral cuneiform? Clawson and Seddon stated that it has yet to be decided whether it is best to attach the tendon to the mid-dorsum of the foot or to the toe extensors.[57] The evidence seems to indicate that better balance of inversion and eversion forces may be obtained by using the extensors, as long as reliable tensioning and a solid repair are obtained.

Future Directions

Tomiano et al. stated that "Although advances in microneural surgery have improved the results of reconstruction following brachial plexus injury, there are few if any reports in the sports literature which address similar advances in the treatment of peroneal nerve palsy following knee dislocation."[50] It would be desirable to improve the functional outcome in these injuries, or at the very least, to widen the window of opportunity between the onset of ability to accurately determine the extent of injury in traction lesions and the time at which repair must be conducted to allow a chance of functional reinnervation, before irreversible atrophy of muscle and motor endplates occurs. The time for diagnosis of the extent of damage is relatively well established. Delaying motor endplate resorption and fibrous changes in the target muscle would potentially result in a significant treatment advance.

Grimby et al. compared firing properties in anterior tibial motor units with EMG in normal subjects with footdrop due to acute common peroneal nerve injury, both during initial injury and recovery.[72] Results fell into two distinct groups: one group maximally used remaining motor units until they became fatigued; the other had force reserves that were not recruited at all. In other words, one group appeared to have the ability to prevent footdrop but did not use it in prolonged walking. This finding raises the question of whether stimulation of the nerve below the point of injury may help function in the short term and possibly delay degenerative changes in the muscle and motor endplates. Another finding was that the high firing rate signals, required to cause remaining motor units to function, actually blocked the electric signal propagation from the newly reinnervated and developing motor units. This raises the question of whether electric stimulation of existing motor units may actually be harmful to the development of newly reinnervating motor units.

The use of peripheral nerve stimulators was studied to improve the gait of stroke patients, and it was noted that in these subjects, the devices may cause exaggerated ankle dorsiflexion with varying subtalar eversion, depending on how well the device is mounted. Voight and Sinkjaer studied whether any joint or soft tissue damage results from long-term use of the stimulators.[73] The bone on bone forces were not increased by the stimulator and were low compared to normal subjects. Therefore, the authors concluded that no harmful effects to the ankle joint or to surrounding tissues are caused by use of the stimulator.[73]

Several additional findings may affect current treatment for acute and chronic nerve injuries:

1. Goldspink et al. found that denervated muscles immobilized in a lengthened position adapted to their new length by adding sarcomeres.[74] Herbison et al. found that elongation of denervated rat muscle resulted in increased muscle weight,[75] with resulting sparing of motor atrophy. Ability of the muscle–tendon unit to generate force was not adversely affected by the elongated state.[76]

2. Nerve root neurectomy was performed in rats, causing partial denervation of a muscle or muscle group. Large myelinated axons were found to increase in response to denervation and increased even more as the remaining muscle was subjected to overwork by tenotomizing synergistic muscle groups. It was proposed that nerves adapt to injury that causes enlargement of the motor unit by undergoing axonal hypertrophy.[77]

3. Evidence also exists that direct current stimulation of repaired rat sciatic nerves increases distal fiber size, myelin sheath thickness, and function.[78]

4. Electric current stimulation was found to increase the number of crossing fibers and function when applied across a delayed nerve lesion (neuroma).[79]

The application of these findings to acute nerve injury may be that exercise of the reinnervating muscle–tendon unit may increase the effectiveness of remaining or regenerated nerve axons to restore function. If exercise is impossible due to interruption of nerve continuity, then outside stimulation distal to the nerve defect may preserve integrity of the motor unit until reinnervation occurs. Stimulation by electric current proximal to the defect may also have a role in improving results of nerve regeneration.

Further study appears to be warranted to determine whether peripheral nerve stimulation or muscle group stretching may aid in the recovery of nerve injury, particularly in the case of traction injuries in the lower extremity, where long distances for reinnervation contribute to a poor prognosis for recovery.

Conclusions

Owing to the relatively low incidence of knee dislocation and the variability in associated injuries, particularly the variability in extent and severity of peroneal nerve injury, a controlled study of outcomes is probably an impractical way to attempt to advance treatment effectiveness. It is clear, however, that prompt recognition of a knee dislocation and appropriate treatment of associated vascular, neurologic, ligamentous, and soft tissue envelope injuries is necessary to minimize the complications of this severe and potentially devastating injury. Despite numerous advances in nerve repair techniques, the prognosis for nerve injuries following knee dislocation remains poor.

References

1. Thomsen PB, Rud B, Jensen UH. Stability and motion after traumatic dislocation of the knee. Acta Orthop Scand 1984; 55(3):278–283.
2. Montgomery TJ, Savoie FH, White JL, et al. Orthopaedic management of knee dislocations: comparison of surgical reconstruction and immobilization. Am J Knee Surg 1995; 8(3):97–103.
3. Kennedy JC. Complete dislocation of the knee joint. J Bone Joint Surg Am 1963; 45(5):889–904.
4. Roman PD, Hopson CN, Zenni EJ. Traumatic dislocation of the knee: a report of 30 cases and literature review. Orthop Rev 1987; 16(12):33–40.
5. Jones RE, Smith EC, Bone GE. Vascular and orthopaedic complications of knee dislocation. Surg Gynecol Obstet 1979; 149:554–558.
6. Shelbourne KD, Porter DA, Clingman JA, et al. Low velocity knee dislocation. Orthop Rev 1991; 20(11):995–1004.
7. Myers MH, Harvey JP Jr. Traumatic dislocation of the knee joint. J Bone Joint Surg Am 1971; 53(1):16–29.
8. Myers MH, Tillman MM, Harvey, JP. Follow-up notes on articles previously published in the Journal on Traumatic Dislocation of the Knee Joint. J Bone Joint Surg Am 1975; 57(3):430–433.
9. Sisto DJ, Warren RF: Complete knee dislocation: a follow-up study of operative treatment. Clin Orthop 1985; 198:94–101.
10. Shields L, Mital M, Cave EF. Complete dislocation of the knee: experience at the Massachusetts General Hospital. J Trauma 1969; 9(3):192–215.
11. Taylor AR, Arden GP, Rainey HA. Traumatic dislocation of the knee. J Bone Joint Surg Br 1972; 54(1):96–102.

12. Siliski JM, Plancher K, Ribbans W. Traumatic dislocation of the knee: complications and results of operative and nonoperative treatment. Paper no 117 presented at: Annual Meeting Scientific Program of the American Academy of Orthopaedic Surgeons; 1989.
13. Malizos KN, Xenakis T, Mavrodontidis AN, et al. Knee dislocations and their management: a report of 16 cases. Acta Orthop Scand 1997; (suppl 275):80–83.
14. Towne LC, Blazina ME, Marmor L, et al. Lateral compartment syndrome of the knee. Clin Orthop 1971; 76:160–168.
15. Azar FM, Brandt JC, Phillips BB, et al. Ultra-low velocity knee dislocations. Paper no 70 presented at: the 15th Annual Meeting of the Orthopaedic Trauma Association; October 1999.
16. Kline DG. Operative management of major nerve lesions of the lower extremity. Surg Clin N Am 1972; 52(5):1247–1265.
17. Chaing, YH, Chang MC, Liu Y, et al. Surgical treatment for peroneal nerve palsy. Chin Med J Free China Ed 2000; 63(8):591–597.
18. Ottolenghi CE, Traversa CH. Vascular and nervous complications in injuries of the knee joint. Reconstr Surg Traumatol 1974; 14:114–135.
19. Platt H. On the peripheral nerve complications of certain fractures. J Bone Joint Surg 1928; 10:403–414.
20. Highet WB, Holmes W. Traction injuries to the lateral popliteal nerve and traction injuries to peripheral nerves after suture. B J Surg 1942; 30:212–233.
21. Kline DG, Kim D, Midha R, et al. Management and results of sciatic nerve injuries: a 24-year experience. J Neurosurg 1998; 89:13–23.
22. Wood MB. Peroneal nerve repair, surgical results. Clin Orthop 1991; 267:206–210.
23. Bateman JE. Trauma to Nerves in Limbs. Philadelphia: WB Saunders; 1962.
24. Seddon H. Three types of nerve injury. Brain 1943; 66:237.
25. Sunderland S. Nerves and Nerve Injuries. 2nd ed. Edinburgh: Churchill Livingstone; 1978; 974.
26. O'Donoghue DH. Dislocation of the knee. Orthop Rev 1975; 4(5):19–29.
27. Pickett JB. Localizing peroneal nerve lesions. Am Fam Phys 1985; 31(2):189–196.
28. Cohn SL, Taylor WC. Vascular problems of the lower extremity in athletes. Clin Sports Med 1990; 9(2):449–470.
29. Morton JH, Southgate WA, Deweese JA. Arterial injuries of the extremities. Surg Gynecol Obstet 1966; 123:611–627.
30. Bassett FH, Silver D. Arterial injury associated with fractures. Arch Surg 1966; 92:13–19.
31. Klingensmith W, Oles P, Martinez H. Arterial injuries associated with dislocation of the knee or fracture of the lower femur. Surg Gynecol Obstet 1965; 120:961–964.
32. Cone, JB. Vascular injury associated with fracture-dislocations of the lower extremity. Clin Orthop 1989; 243:30–35.
33. Snyder, WH. Vascular injuries near the knee: an updated series and overview of the problem. Surgery 1982; 91:502–506.
34. Ghalambor N, Vangsness T. Traumatic dislocation of the knee: a review of the literature. Bull Hosp Joint Dis 1995; 54(1):19–24.
35. Montgomery JB. Dislocation of the knee. Orthop Clin N Am 1987; 18(1):149–156.
36. Schenck RC. The dislocated knee. Instructional Course Lect 1994; 43:127–136.
37. Platt H, Lond MS. Traction lesions of the external popliteal nerve. Lancet 1940; 2:612.
38. Gurdjian ES, Hardy WG, Lindner W, Thomas LM. Nerve injuries in association with fractures and dislocations of long bones. Clin Orthop 1963; 27:147–150.
39. Towne LC, Blazina ME, Marmor L, Lawrence JF. Lateral compartment syndrome of the knee. Clin Orthop 1971; 76:160–168.
40. White J. The results of traction injuries to the common peroneal nerve. J Bone Joint Surg Br 1968; 50(2):346–350.
41. Mont MA, Dellon AL, Chen F, et al. The operative treatment of peroneal nerve palsy. J Bone Joint Surg Am 1996; 78(6):863–869.
42. Demuynck M, Zuker RM. The peroneal nerve: is repair worthwhile? J Reconstr Microsurg 1987; 3(3):193–197,199.

43. Aldea PA, Shaw WW. Management of acute lower extremity nerve injuries. Foot Ankle 1986; 7(2):82–94.
44. Trumble TE, Vanderhooft E, Khan U. Sural nerve grafting for lower extremity nerve injuries. J Orthop Trauma 1995; 9(2):158–163.
45. Dubuisson A, Kline D. Indications for peripheral nerve and brachial plexus surgery. Neurol Clin 1992; 10(4):935–951.
46. Hudson AR, Kline DG. Nerve Injuries. Philadelphia: WB Saunders; 1995.
47. Terranova WA, McLaughlin RE, Morgan RF. An algorithm for the management of ligamentous injuries. Orthopaedics 1986; 9(8):1135–1140.
48. Wilkinson MCP, Birch R. Repair of the common peroneal nerve. J Bone Joint Surg Br 1995; 77(3):501–503.
49. Berry H, Richardson PM. Common peroneal nerve palsy: a clinical and electrophysiological review. J Neurol Neurosurg Psychiatr 1976; 39:1162–1171.
50. Tomiano M, Day C, Papageorgiou C, Harner C, et al. Peroneal palsy following knee dislocation: pathoanatomy and implications for treatment. Knee Surg Sports Traumatol Arthrosc 2000; 8(3):163–165.
51. Terzis J, Faibisoff B, Williams B. The nerve gap: suture under tension vs graft. Plast Reconstr Surg 1975; 56(2):166–170.
52. Hems TEJ, Glasby MA. Comparison of different methods of repair of long peripheral nerve defects: an experimental study. Br J Plast Surg 1992; 45:497–502.
53. Sedel L, Nizard RS. Nerve grafting for traction injuries of the common peroneal nerve, a report of 17 cases. J Bone Joint Surg Br 1993; 75(5):772–774.
54. Campbell WC. An operation for the correction of "drop-foot." J Bone Joint Surg Am 1923; 5:815–825.
55. Ober FR. Tendon transposition in the lower extremity. N Engl J Med 1933; 209:52.
56. Watkins M, Jones B, Ryder CT, et al. Transplantation of the posterior tibial tendon. J Bone Joint Surg Am 1954; 36:1181–1189.
57. Clawson DK, Seddon HJ. The late consequences of sciatic nerve injury. J Bone Joint Surg Br 1960; 42(2):213–225.
58. Cozen L. Management of foot drop in adults after permanent peroneal nerve loss. Clin Orthop 1969; 67:151–158.
59. Sharrard WJW. Paralytic deformity in the lower limb. J Bone Joint Surg Br 1967; 49(4):743.
60. Lipscomb PR, Sanchez JJ. Anterior transplantation of the posterior tibial tendon for persistent palsy of the common peroneal nerve. J Bone Joint Surg Am 1961; 43(1):60–66.
61. Carayon A, Bourrel P, Bourges M. Dual transfer of the posterior tibial and flexor digitorum longus tendons for drop foot. J Bone Joint Surg Am 1967; 49(1):144–148.
62. Spreafico G, Morelli A, Cavallazzi RM, et al. Palliative surgery in irreparable lesions of the peroneal nerve. Ital J Orthop Traumatol 1985; 11(2):185–191.
63. Pinzur MS, Kett N, Trilla M. Combined anteroposterior tibial tendon transfer in posttraumatic peroneal palsy. Foot Ankle 1988; 8(5):271–276.
64. Richard BM. Interosseus transfer of tibialis posterior for common peroneal nerve palsy. J Bone Joint Surg Br 1989; 71(5):834–837.
65. Hall G. A review of drop foot corrective surgery. Lepr Rev 1977; 48:185–192.
66. Srinivasan H, Mukhergee SM, Subramaniam RA. Two-tailed transfer of tibialis posterior for correction of drop foot in leprosy. J Bone Joint Surg Br 1968; 50:623–628.
67. Ninkovic M, Sucur Dj, Starovic B, et al. A new approach to persistent traumatic peroneal nerve palsy. Br J Plast Surg 1994; 47:185–189.
68. Turner JW, Cooper RR. Anterior transfer of the tibialis posterior through the interosseus membrane. Clin Orthop 1972; 83:241–244.
69. Biesalski K, Mayer L. Die physiologische Sehnenverpflanzung. Berlin: Verlag von Julius Springer; 1916.
70. Milgram JE. The reconstruction of some extensor mechanisms in the extremities. Instructional Course Lect 1956; 13:121–134.
71. Malaviya GN. Surgery of foot drop in leprosy by tibialis posterior transfer. Lepr J India 1981; 53:360–368.
72. Grimby L, Holm K, Sjøstrom L. Abnormal use of remaining motor units during locomotion in peroneal palsy. Muscle Nerve 1984; 7:327–331.

73. Voight M, Sinkjaer T. Kinematic and kinetic analysis of the walking pattern in hemiplegic patients with foot-drop using a peroneal nerve stimulator. Clin Biomech 2000; 15:340–351.
74. Goldspink G, Tabary C, Tabary JC, et al. Effect of denervation on adaptation of sarcomere number and muscle extensibility to functional length of muscle. J Physiol 1974; 236:733–742.
75. Herbison GJ, Jaweed MM, Ditunno JF Jr. Synergistic tenotomy: effect on chronically denervated slow and fast muscles of rat. Arch Phys Med Rehabil 1975; 56:483–487.
76. Kinney CL, Jaweed MM, Herbison GJ. Overwork effect on partially denervated rat soleus muscle. Arch Phys Med Rehabil 1986; 67:286–289.
77. Jaweed MM, Herbison GJ, Ditunno JF Jr. Overwork-induced axonal hypertrophy in soleus nerve of rat. Arch Phys Med Rehabil 1987; 68:706–709.
78. Shen N, Zhu J. Experimental study using a direct current electrical field to promote peripheral nerve regeneration. J Reconstr Microsurg 1995; 11(3):189–193.
79. Beveridge JA, Politis MJ. Use of exogenous electric current in the treatment of delayed lesions in peripheral nerves. Plast Reconstr Surg 1988; 82(4):573–579.

Chapter Twelve

The Role of Osteotomy

Annunziato Amendola and Michelle Wolcott

Reconstruction of the multiple ligament injured knee can be challenging owing to the many factors necessary to achieve a stable, functional joint. The task of assessing limb alignment and malalignment has been largely ignored in the multiple ligament injured knee, and reconstruction has focused on soft tissue constraints. Although it has been shown that joint alignment plays a critical role in the development of arthritis and overload syndromes, osteotomy to control instability has been a controversial subject. Recent evidence suggests that joint alignment may be just as important in maintaining joint stability, particularly in cases of chronic ligamentous injury. Over time, untreated malalignment can worsen ligamentous laxity and lead to symptomatic chronic instability. In the case of the ACL-deficient knee, for example, varus malalignment can be overemphasized as internal rotation of the tibia places more stress on the lateral structures. This deformity can then be manifested as a posterolateral thrust upon ambulation. Malalignment in the coronal or sagittal plane may be a significant contributing factor in the success of reconstruction of the anterior cruciate ligament (ACL). This chapter discusses the role of osteotomy in these unstable knees as a means of ensuring success in the long-term outcome of ligamentous reconstruction.

Limb Alignment

Normal Alignment

It is first necessary to define the primary tibiofemoral geometry based on both bony and ligamentous anatomy. Meniscal or cartilage loss of either the medial or the lateral compartment will lead to increased varus or valgus alignment, respectively. Normal anatomic knee alignment is somewhat variable but falls within a certain normative range. The posterior tibial slope is the measured bony slope, and perhaps the soft tissues (i.e., cartilage and meniscus) functionally alters the bony slope.

Preexisting Alignment

Individuals with predisposing malalignment, either varus or valgus, and a significant ligamentous injury may not do well with surgical stabilization alone. The reason for this is that theoretically, prior to injury, the neuromuscular or proprioceptive control of the joint was provided by the soft

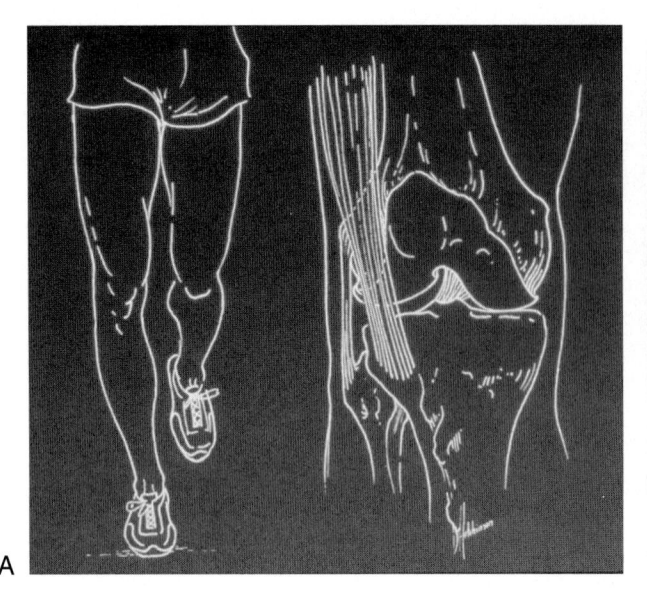

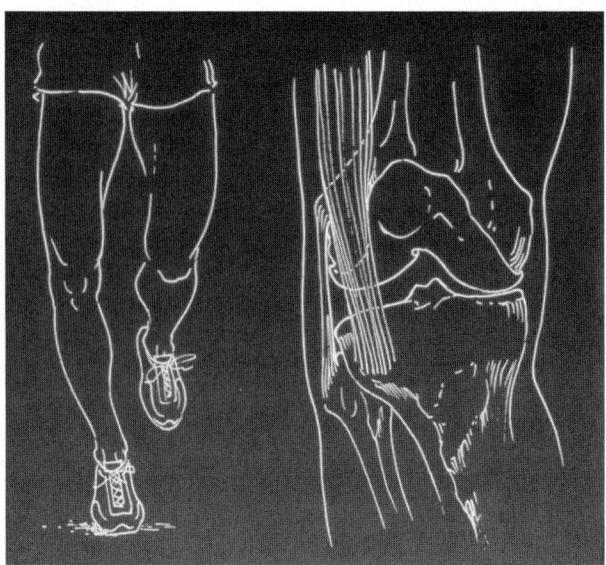

Fig. 12.1. (A) With preexisting physiologic varus, the knee remains stable with ligamentous stability and neuromuscular control. (B) With ACL disruption, knee is unable to maintain normal control, leading to increased varus, lateral collateral laxity, and thrust.

tissue structures, in particular the ligaments. This neuromuscular control may be hindered when ligamentous disruption occurs. Loss of this control may then exacerbate the malalignment, leading to clinical symptoms of instability (Figure 12.1). In this situation, an osteotomy can provide bony stabilization to augment ligamentous reconstruction and improve overall joint function. Although it is clear when malalignment is the culprit in the chronic or failed situation, it may be beneficial then to perform ligamentous reconstruction and osteotomy early to minimize progressive deformity and loss of proprioceptive function and to enhance neuromuscular control.

Triple-Varus Knee

In the ACL-deficient knee, varus malalignment can develop over time as a result of preexisting varus deformity, progressive medial compartment osteoarthrosis, or medial meniscal injury. As the medial compartment narrows, the weight-bearing line shifts medially, leading to primary varus. With progressive narrowing, the posterolateral soft tissue restraints become lax, leading to double varus. As the malalignment becomes more chronic, excessive lateral stress may lead to a hyperextension recurvatum deformity, referred to as triple varus.[1-3] In this situation, ACL reconstruction will decrease anterior tibial translation but will not correct the underlying varus deformity, placing increased stress on the reconstructed ACL. Continued stress on the posterolateral structures will lead to increased laxity and a sensation of giving way. By combining ACL reconstruction with a valgus osteotomy, tension on the ACL can be minimized and stability enhanced.

Acute injury to the posterolateral complex in combination with ACL deficiency with preexisting varus simulates a triple-varus knee. Additional injury to the posterior cruciate ligament (PCL) augments hyperextension deformity. Combined ACL, PCL, and posterolateral corner injuries can further magnify hyperextension varus and external rotational deformities. Therefore, it is important to distinguish osseous as well as ligamentous deformity prior to planning surgical reconstruction.

Tibial Slope (Sagittal Tibial Alignment)

Malalignment in the sagittal plane can also affect knee stability in the setting of ligamentous injury. Increased tibial slope allows increased anterior tibial translation because the femur tends to slide posteriorly along the tibial slope.[4-6] In cases of ACL deficiency, anterior tibial translation can be magnified in the presence of an increased slope. In contrast, PCL-deficient knees are stabilized by increasing tibial slope by reducing the posterior translation (Figure 12.2).[7]

Unicompartmental Degeneration with Malalignment

In the chronic situation, particularly in the presence of meniscal or articular cartilage injury, chronic ligamentous laxity may present with malalignment with unicompartmental joint overload and degeneration.[8] The indication for osteotomy in these conditions may be the need to unload the degenerative compartment to help with instability or thrust. These conditions are most commonly associated with chronic PCL or ACL deficiency. Therefore surgery may be staged or combined, depending on the symptomatology, age, and activity level of the patient. Numerous algorithms exist in the literature for dealing with combined knee laxity and arthrosis.[8]

Indications for Tibial Osteotomy in the Unstable Knee

Our indications for osteotomy are listed in Table 12.1. In all cases of instability, arthrosis, or combined instability and arthrosis, the need for realignment should be deliberately assessed. Varus or valgus deformity should be addressed in the coronal plane, and the need to adjust the sagittal plane or tibial slope should be determined based on the cruciate status. Indications for valgus opening wedge osteotomy include primarily pain relief and correction of mechanical axis. In the presence of unilateral medial compartment degenerative symptoms, osteotomies have been routinely performed with good results.[9-11] More recently, however, these indications have been

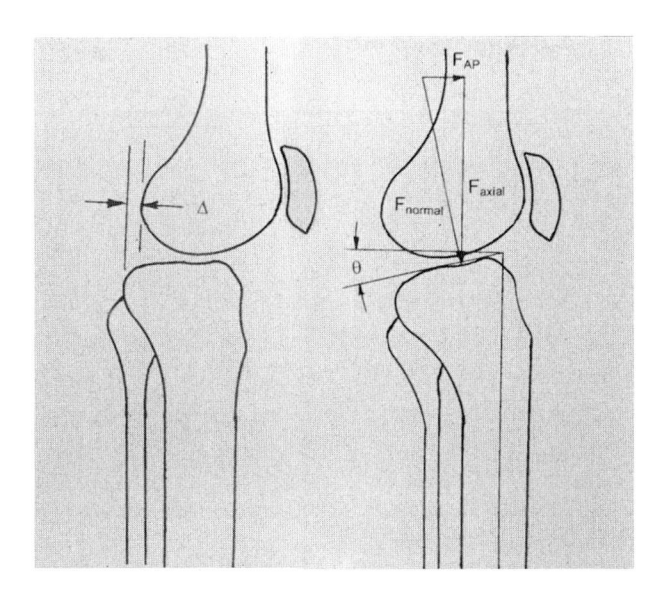

Fig. 12.2. In the case of posterior instability or subluxation (left), increasing the sagittal slope will cause anterior tibial translation, reducing the posterior sag or instability (right).

Table 12.1. Indications for osteotomy

Medial compartment
  Arthrosis
  Arthrosis + varus alignment + varus thrust
  PL instability + varus hyperextension thrust
  Cruciate deficiency + varus alignment ± thrust
  Combined ligamentous laxity + varus, valgus, or PL thrust
  Meniscus/cartilage transplantation with compartment overload

expanded to include posterolateral laxity and varus hyperextension thrust, ACL deficiency and varus thrust or alignment, and combined ligamentous laxity with varus or posterolateral thrust. Osteotomy has also been used when necessary to protect the medial compartment (following meniscal or cartilage transplantation/resurfacing) from excessive loading.[8]

Operative Technique

Although many techniques are available, the opening wedge osteotomy is preferred. Its advantages include multiplanar correction, avoidance of the proximal tibiofibular joint and peroneal nerve, and ease of intraoperative adjustment. In the collateral ligamentously lax knee, distraction by opening wedge osteotomy may provide some tightening and improve the laxity. Disadvantages include possible need for bone graft and difficulty in correcting severe deformity. In these unstable knees, the correction required is often a mild to moderate one, from 5 to 15°, so that an acute opening wedge is acceptable.

Preoperative Planning

Preoperative planning is necessary to achieve an adequate correction. Anteroposterior single long-leg weight-bearing films should be obtained. True lateral films as well as skyline and tunnel views should also be obtained. For correction of coronal deformity, the method of measurement of correction of Dejour et al. is used to determine the size and location of the osteotomy (Figure 12.3).[12] The width of the tibial plateau is measured and marked at 62% from the medial side. A line is drawn from the center

Fig. 12.3. Measuring coronal alignment and planning correction to the 62 to 66% point from medial to lateral compartment. (Courtesy of Frank R. Noyes.)

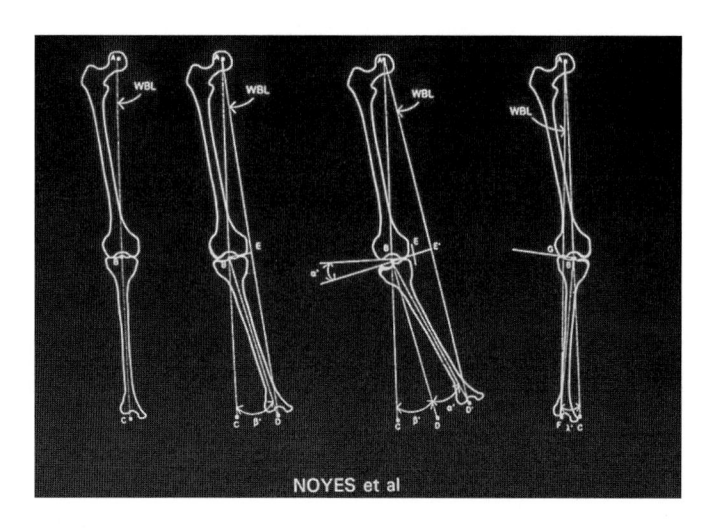

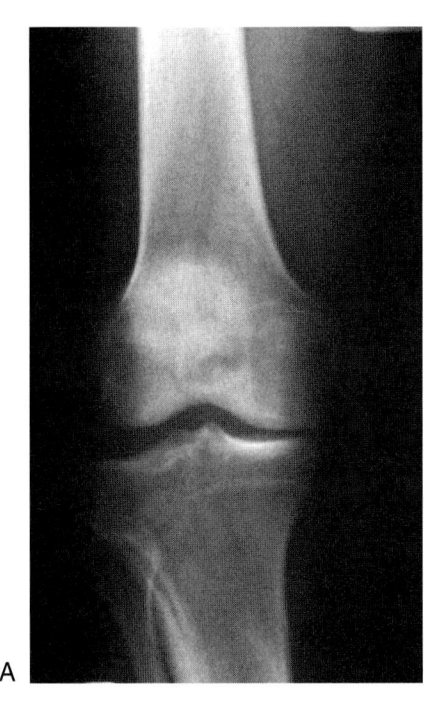

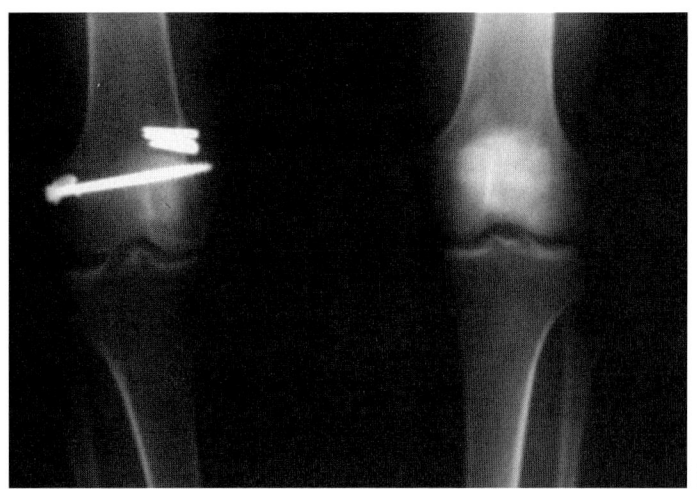

Fig. 12.4. A 20-year-old female whose chronic PCL and posterolateral instability and thrust resulted from a motor vehicle accident. (A) Standing AP demonstrates varus and lateral gapping. (B) Post-PCL reconstruction and biceps tenodesis, standing anteroposterior view demonstrates continued varus with posterolateral instability. (C) Post-osteotomy: realigned, and knee is functionally stable.

of the femoral head to this mark. In a similar fashion, a line is drawn from the center of the talus to this mark. The angle that is created becomes the angle of correction.

To correct any sagittal deformity, the lateral film and tibial slope are assessed. If recurvatum or hyperextension is the problem, then the wedge needs to be positioned anteromedially causing an increase in slope and obliterating the hyperextension (Figure 12.4). If anterior translation or chronic ACL deficiency needs to be addressed, anterior closing is necessary; therefore, the opening wedge needs to be as far posterior as possible.

Surgical Technique

The surgical technique is carried out under fluoroscopic guidance and tourniquet control. The patient is positioned supine with the involved extremity prepped and draped. If ipsilateral iliac crest autograft is to be used, this area is also prepared. The osteotomy is performed through a medial incision halfway between the tibial tubercle and the posteromedial border of the tibia. Dissection is carried down to the level of the sartorius fascia. The fascia is incised in line with the pes anserinus tendons. The pes anserinus tendons are identified and retracted medially, exposing the superficial medial collateral ligament. An elevator is used to release the superior portion of the medial collateral ligament (MCL) attachment and expose the posteromedial border of the tibia. Anteriorly, the fascia is dissected to the level of the patellar tendon attachment at the tibial tubercle. The most superior fibers of the patellar tendon insertion are released, exposing the anterior proximal tibial surface. Blunt retractors are placed under the MCL and patellar tendons, respectively, to allow adequate exposure of the osteotomy site.

A guide pin is placed under fluoroscopic control, beginning 4cm distal to the medial joint line to a point approximately 1cm below the lateral joint line (approximately at the level of the fibular head and crossing proximal to the tibial tubercle). The orientation of the osteotomy is marked, taking into consideration any increase or decrease in tibial slope. An oscillating saw placed below the guide pin is used to begin the osteotomy through the medial and posteromedial cortex. This minimizes the risk of intra-articular fracture. Thin flexible osteotomes are then used to complete the osteotomy, ending approximately 1cm short of the lateral tibial cortex. Once the osteotomy has been completed in this manner, larger osteotomes may be passed through the site and used to gently wedge the osteotomy open. A calibrated wedge osteotome is then used to open the osteotomy to the desired correction. A four-hole Puddu plate (Arthrex, Inc., Naples, FL) with a wedged intraosseous bridge is placed at the most posteromedial position in the osteotomy. This creates a slight decrease in tibial slope (if this is the desired correction). The knee is held in extension while the holes are drilled. Then 6.5mm cancellous screws are placed in the proximal holes, taking care to avoid the articular surface; 4.5mm cortical screws are placed in the distal holes. Bone grafting is often necessary and is commonly performed to ensure bony union. Autograft as well as allograft or synthetic bone matrix may be used. Larger pieces should be placed posteriorly to allow further tibial slope correction, saving smaller pieces for the anterior portion of the osteotomy. Wounds are irrigated and closed.

The osteotomy is protected in a brace for 6 weeks allowing partial weight bearing. Radiographs should then be obtained and weight bearing advanced as consolidation and union are confirmed, generally by 12 weeks.

Results

The high tibial osteotomy (HTO) has increased in popularity in the multiple ligament injured knee for a variety of reasons. Although the procedure was once thought to be contraindicated in this setting, recent evidence has suggested that in cases of varus malalignment with ACL or PCL deficiency, good functional results can be expected. In his study on HTO in ACL-deficient knees, Noyes reported reduction of pain in 71%, elimination of giving way in 85%, and resumption of light recreational activities in 66%.[2] Dejour's earlier results demonstrated a 91% satisfaction rate; however, there was only a 65% rate of return to leisurely sports activities.[12] Both these studies examined the effect of a closing wedge osteotomy in the chronically ACL-deficient knee.

In the PCL-deficient knee the effect of the opening wedge osteotomy is thought to stabilize the knee by decreasing posterior tibial translation. In a biomechanical study Naudie et al. reported that the opening wedge osteotomy led to anterior tibial translation in the normal and ACL-deficient knee at all flexion angles.[13] They demonstrated in the PCL-deficient knee that anterior opening wedge osteotomy caused anterior tibial translation, potentially restoring normal knee biomechanics.[13–15] In the clinical setting, Naudie et al. demonstrated that HTO in the setting of posterior instability improved subjective feelings of instability in 16 of 17 patients at minimum follow-up of 2 years. These patients all had a posterolateral thrust corrected by anteromedial opening wedge osteotomy.[7] All these patients were young and active, returning to a higher activity level postoperatively.

Although experience with this technique is limited, early results of the correction of underlying malalignment in the setting of chronic knee instability are encouraging. In the acute setting there may also be a role for correction of malalignment; however, this has not yet been explored. The multiple ligament injured knee represents a complicated situation in which long-term results of reconstruction have been inconsistent. In some of these cases, superimposed malalignment may be a contributing factor that should not be overlooked. The role of osteotomy in this setting has shown promising early results but will need longer term evaluation before definitive recommendations can be made.

References

1. Markoff KL, Bargar WL, Shoemaker SC, et al. The role of joint load in knee stability. J Bone Joint Surg Am 1988; 70:977–982.
2. Noyes FR, Barber-Westin SD, Hewett TE. High tibial osteotomy and ligament reconstruction for varus angulated anterior cruciate ligament–deficient knees. Am J Sports Med 2000; 28(3):282–296.
3. Hughston JC, Jacobsen KE. Chronic posterolateral rotatory instability of the knee. J Bone Joint Surg Am 1985; 67:351–359.
4. Dejour H, Walch G, Chambat P, et al. Active subluxation in extension: a new concept of study of the ACL deficient knee. Am J Knee Surg 1988; 1:204–211.
5. Dejour H, Neyret P, Bonnin M. In: Fu F, ed. Knee Surgery. Baltimore, MD: Williams & Wilkins; 1994:859–875.
6. Amendola AS, Giffin JR, Sanders DW. Osteotomy for knee stability: the effect of increasing tibial slope on anterior tibial translation. Paper presented at: American Association for Orthopaedic Sports Medicine, Specialty Day; March 2001; San Francisco.
7. Naudie D, Amendola A, Fowler P. Opening wedge high tibial osteotomy for chronic posterior instability. Proceedings of the meeting of the American Association for Orthopaedic Sports Medicine; July 2001; Keystone, CO.
8. Clatworthy M, Amendola AS. The anterior cruciate ligament and arthritis. Clin Sports Med 1999; 18:173–198.
9. Coventry MB. Upper tibial osteotomy for osteoarthritis. J Bone Joint Surg Am 1985; 67:1136–1140.
10. Morrey BF. Upper tibial osteotomy for secondary osteoarthritis of the knee. J Bone Joint Surg Br 1989; 71:554–559.
11. Coventry MB. Osteotomy of the upper portion of the tibia for degenerative arthritis of the knee: a preliminary report. J Bone Joint Surg Am 1965; 47: 984–990.
12. Dejour H, Neyret P, Boileau P, et al. Anterior cruciate reconstruction combined with valgus tibial osteotomy. Clin Orthop 1994; 299:220–228.
13. Naudie D, Roth S, Dunning C, Amendola AS, Giffin JR, Johnson JA, Chess D, King GJW. The effect of opening wedge high tibial osteotomy in the posterior cruciate ligament deficient knee. Paper presented at: 56th Annual Meeting of the Canadian Orthopaedic Association; June 1–4, 2001.
14. Amendola A. The effect of opening wedge high tibial osteotomy in the PCL deficient knee. Proceedings of the meeting of the American Association for Orthopaedic Sports Medicine; July 2001; Keystone, CO.
15. Brown G, Amendola A: Radiographic evaluation and preoperative planning for high tibial osteotomies. Oper Techniques Sports Med 2000; 8(1):2–14.

Chapter Thirteen

Management of Chronic Posterior Tibial Subluxation

Steven C. Chudik, Peter T. Simonian, and Thomas L. Wickiewicz

Chronic fixed posterior tibial subluxation in the multiple ligament injured knee, although extremely rare, is a difficult problem that requires complex management. There are two opposing goals after catastrophic ligamentous knee injury: stability and range of motion. Achieving both of these goals can be very difficult.[1-8] Multiple ligamentous reconstructions are currently the recommended method of dealing with acute unstable knee injuries.[1-4,9-11] Despite modern techniques, recurrent knee laxity or stiffness can be problematic.[1-3,5-8,11,12] These problems are amplified in the case of a chronic posterior tibial subluxation.

To reduce the chronic posterior tibial subluxation, complete releases of scar tissue and capsule are required. Unfortunately, the instability created by this extensive release places increased stresses on the reconstruction. In an attempt to decrease stress on the newly reconstructed ligaments and still allow knee motion, an appropriate form of postoperative protection should be utilized. A limited period of a skeletally fixed knee hinge has been used successfully for this complex problem and can be helpful in reestablishing stable motion and may best achieve the goals of stability and range of motion.

Incidence

Knee dislocations, in general, are rare with an incidence ranging from 0.001% to 0.013%; an orthopaedic surgeon is likely to encounter only a handful of knee dislocations during a career.[3,7,9] Knee dislocations with chronic posterior tibial subluxation are even more rare, and only a small number of case reports have been written about the presentation and management of this problem.[13-17]

Clinical Presentation

Chronic posterior tibial subluxation usually presents itself in limited number of clinical settings. It is a preventable problem that occurs secondary to a delay in diagnosis or inappropriate management. Knee dislocations are not always obvious and can be easily overlooked in the initial assessment of a multiply injured patient with other life-threatening injuries. In one study, Laasonen and Kivioja analyzed the care of 340 trauma patients in the intensive care unit at a single center.[18] These authors found that the physicians initially missed 45 (4.2%) out of 1071 fractures and dislocations of the pelvis and lower extremities. The most severe of the missed injuries were dislocations of the hip and knee. Physicians preoccupied with more life-threatening injuries, and seeing no overt signs of multiple ligament injuries to knees, sometimes overlook these conditions. The overt nature of these injuries is related to their tendency to spontaneously reduce and to the associated disruption of the capsule that allows the acute effusion to escape. The delay in diagnosis is a potentially limb-threatening situation that can lead to chronic posterior tibial subluxation if the delay is significant and the knee is allowed to heal in a malreduced position.

Sometimes, despite an accurate and timely diagnosis, the use of an inappropriate form of initial stabilization can lead to the same result of chronic posterior tibial subluxation. Again, in the case of the multiply injured patient, definitive surgical reconstruction of a knee dislocation often must be postponed while other medical personnel address the patient's more life-threatening injuries. During the period between the injury and surgical reconstruction, the knee dislocation should be reduced and appropriately positioned in full extension and stabilized. Depending on the situation, plaster splints, postoperative braces, and skeletal fixation can all be reasonable methods to stabilize the knee as long as the reduction can be maintained. Chronic posterior tibial subluxation occurs when the chosen method of stabilization is inadequate and there is loss of reduction, which goes unnoticed for some time. Initial and early repeated radiographs should be taken to prevent this occurrence; if at any time the reduction cannot be maintained, a more reliable form of stabilization must be utilized.

Chronic posterior tibial subluxation can also occur following inadequate reconstruction of an acute multiple ligament injured knee. If the knee is never fully reduced, the ligaments are insufficiently reconstructed, or the postoperative protection of the reconstruction is inadequate, residual posterior subluxation can persist and become fixed.

Still, chronic posterior tibial subluxation most commonly occurs after conservative treatment of a multiple ligament injured knee with inadequate immobilization and monitoring. Specifically, this has been most frequently reported after a multiple ligament injured knee has been reduced, placed in a cast, and not monitored appropriately to ensure the reduction.[13-17]

Patients with chronic posterior tibial subluxation may present with complaints of pain, stiffness, and instability. As with any other joint with normal sensory capacity, the malreduced knee causes much pain and disability for the patient. Because of the pain, scarring, and joint incongruity, patients can have significant limitations in knee range of motion and function. However, in addition to the decreased range of motion and stiffness, instability of the knee can be present, contributing to the disability. Inadequate healing of the cruciate ligaments and the posterolateral structures often occurs and can result in persistent anterior, posterior, varus, and rotational instability.

Physical Examination

The physical examination of patients with chronic posterior tibial subluxation is quite remarkable. Gait, if possible, is usually antalgic and significantly affected by either or both the limited range of motion and instability. Grossly, the femoral condyles are very prominent beyond the anterior crest of the tibia secondary to the chronic posteriorly subluxed tibia (Figure 13.1). The range of motion in the flexion and extension arc is greatly reduced. The ligamentous examination usually reveals concomitant instability, especially

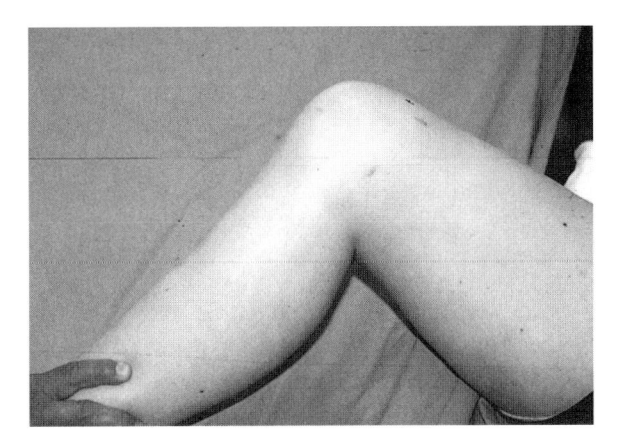

Fig. 13.1. Clinical photograph of chronic fixed posterior tibial subluxation demonstrating the prominence of the femoral condyles beyond the anterior crest of the tibia.

to varus, external rotation, and posterior stresses. A thorough neurologic examination is also important because if coexisting deficits, which usually involve the peroneal nerve, are present, these can both affect prognosis and treatment outcome. The vascular examination is not as crucial as in the acute situation, but chronic vascular insufficiency following the original injury may require further investigation before an extensive reconstruction is considered.

Radiographic Analysis

Radiographic analysis can be helpful to confirm the fixed posterior tibial subluxation and evaluate the knee for other injuries that may affect the treatment and prognosis. In cases of chronic posterior tibial subluxation, the plain lateral radiograph is most striking and will reveal the obvious posterior position of the tibia relative to the femur (Figure 13.2). The deformity is usually more obvious with knee flexion. The anteroposterior radiograph is also important to detect any medial or lateral displacement. Plain radiographs are also helpful to identify any associated fractures, retained hardware, degenerative joint changes, and other bony abnormalities that may

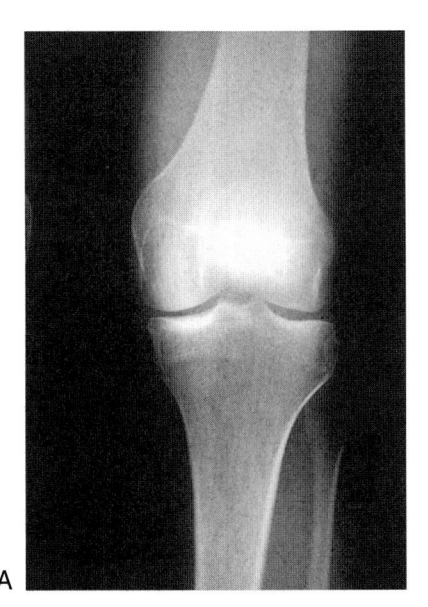

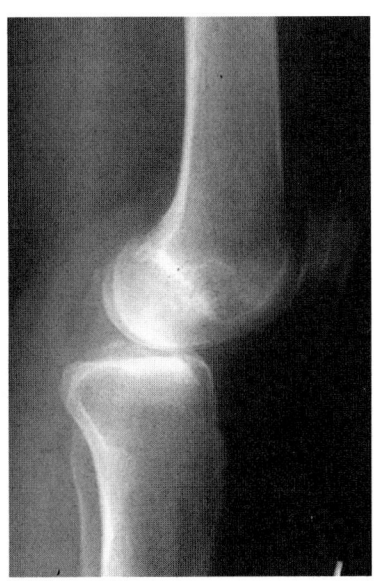

Fig. 13.2. Plain (A) anteroposterior and (B) lateral radiographs demonstrate chronic posterior tibial subluxation. (A From Ref. 17 by permission of *Sports Medicine and Arthroscopy Review*.)

Fig. 13.3. Radiographs demonstrating chronic posterior tibial subluxation 3 months after injury and 10 weeks after surgery: (A) lateral radiograph and (B) anteroposterior radiograph. There is significant posterolateral displacement of the tibia relative to the femur, suggesting gross insufficiency of the posterior cruciate ligament and the posterolateral corner structures. The radiographs also demonstrate some retained hardware in the region of the tibial insertion of the anterior cruciate ligament, representing an attempt by the previous surgeon to primarily repair a tibial avulsion of the anterior cruciate ligament. The patient's previous surgery involved reattachment of the avulsed ACL with suture anchors, repair of the posterior and anterior horns of the medial meniscus, reattachment of the anterior and central portions of the lateral meniscus, and repair of the posterolateral corner including the arcuate and fabellofibular ligaments and the lateral capsule. The patient's leg was in a cast for 5 weeks after surgery, and the reduction was lost (From Ref. 17 by permission of *Sports Medicine and Arthroscopy Review*.)

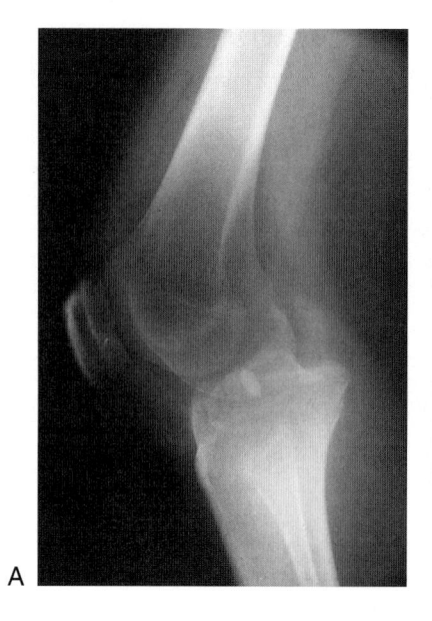

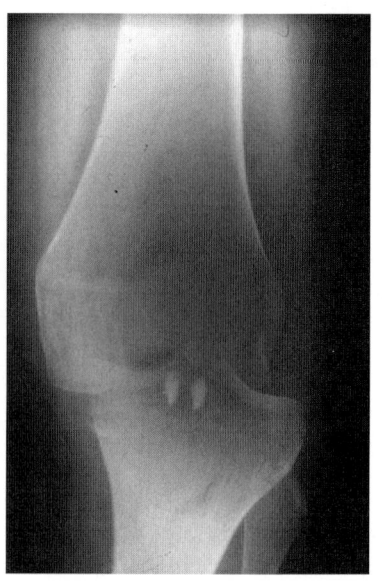

affect treatment (Figure 13.3). For example, evidence for the pattern of injury and help in directing surgical treatment can be provided by avulsion fractures (e.g., of the tibial spine), posterior cruciate ligament (PCL) insertion, medial collateral ligament (MCL) origin, lateral capsule (Segond's fracture), and the head of the fibula. Magnetic resonance imaging (MRI) provides an excellent assessment of the ligamentous, bony, meniscal cartilage, and articular cartilage injuries (Figure 13.4). A thorough knowledge of all the injuries, especially that of the articular cartilage, is essential before surgical treatment is begun. Other subtle findings, such as residual bone contusions, can be detected on the MR image and may help the surgeon decipher the pattern of injury and better plan his or her approach.

Treatment Options

The options for treatment include nonoperative management with or without bracing, amputation, arthrodesis, total knee replacement, and open reduction with or without ligament reconstruction. Nonoperative treatment

Fig. 13.4. A sagittal MR image demonstrating chronic posterior tibial subluxation in another patient. Six months prior to this study, the patient had stepped off a curb and sustained an acute posterior dislocation. She was initially treated with a closed reduction and cast immobilization. (From Ref. 17 by permission of *Sports Medicine and Arthroscopy Review*.)

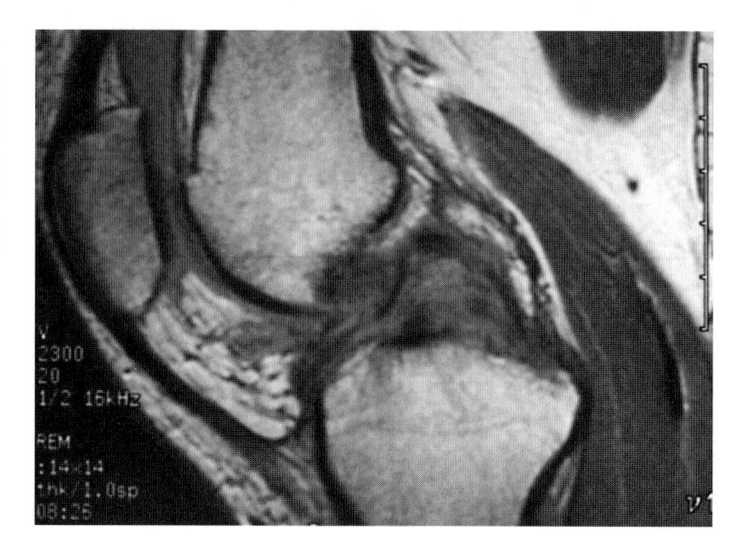

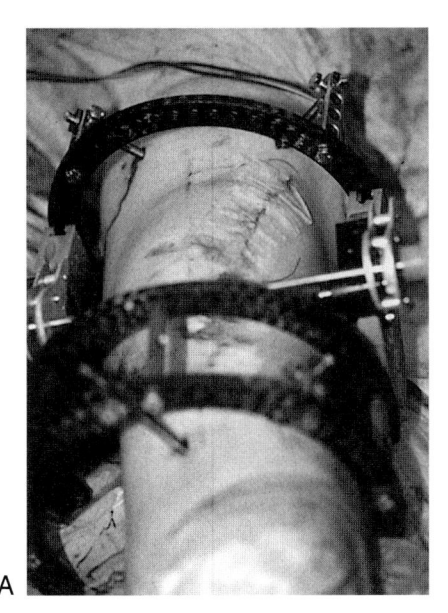

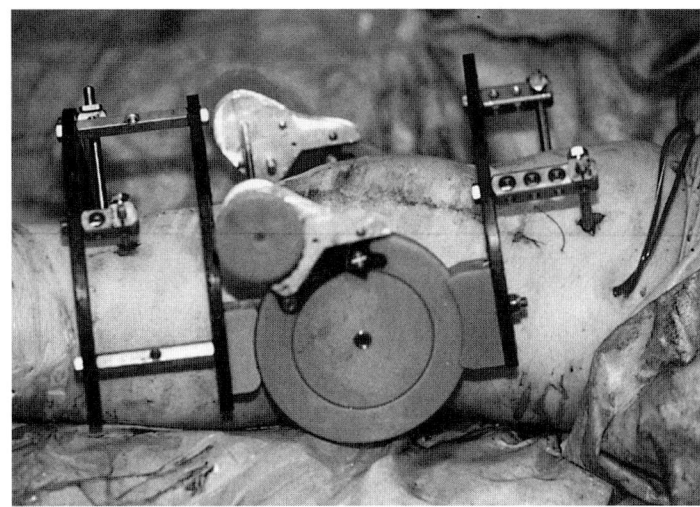

Fig. 13.5. (A,B) Intraoperative photographs of placement of the hinge. (Courtesy of Compass Elbow Hinge; Smith & Nephew Orthopaedics Inc., Memphis, TN.)

Use of Hinges

Hinge Description

The original surgically emplaced hinge was designed for use on the elbow (Compass Elbow Hinge; Smith & Nephew Orthopaedics Inc., Memphis, TN) (Figure 13.5). Since that time, the same company has developed a prototype for universal application to the ankle, elbow, or knee. This version has a poly (ether imide) body with 7° of fixed valgus angulation to accommodate the anatomic valgus alignment of the patient. The hinge can be used for either the right or the left knee by simply inverting the device and reversing its superior and inferior ends. When applied to the knee, the hinge allows 0 to 120° of flexion. Stainless steel rings allow many different sites for skeletal fixation as well as enough clearance for the anterior soft tissues of the thigh in most patients. The hinge also has a single-axis design with a centering hole for easy application.

Hinge Application

Placement of an external hinge must be accurate to allow the most anatomic knee motion (Figure 13.6). To achieve optimal position for the hinge, the placement of an axis or centering pin is critical. The placement of the centering pin is dependent on finding the most isometric point on the medial and lateral femoral condyles. This is done by placing a pin in the middle of both the medial and lateral collateral ligament insertions on the tibia and fibula, respectively, 3cm distal to the joint line. One end of a suture can be placed around each of these pins, while the other end is placed proximally on the medial and lateral femoral condyles. The specific point is then identified on both the medial and lateral femoral condyles where the suture does not lengthen or shorten through a range of knee motion. Once these points have been identified and marked on the femoral condyles, the centering pin is placed from lateral to medial through both of them. The hinge's centering holes are then placed over the centering pin to ensure optimal placement of the hinge. Two 5.0mm Schantz pins are placed in both the femur and

Fig. 13.6. Lateral radiographs of the knee in (A) extension and (B) flexion demonstrate how accurate positioning of the hinge allows for flexion and extension of the knee. This hinge was applied following an open release, reduction, and reconstruction of the ACL, PCL, and posterolateral corner. (From Ref. 17 by permission of *Sports Medicine and Arthroscopy Review*.)

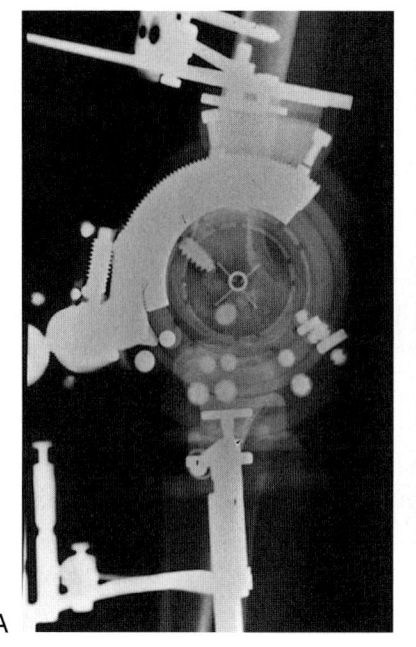

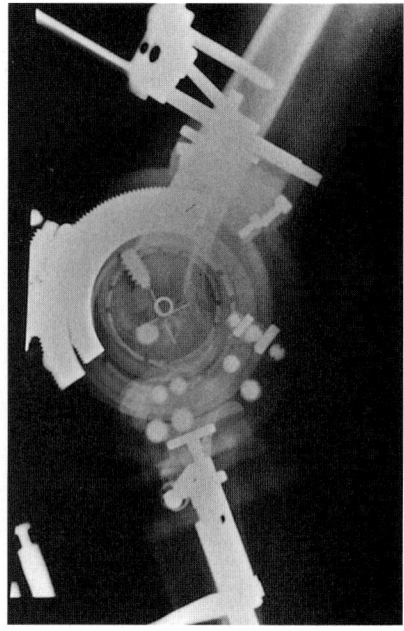

the tibia through the semicircular rings of the hinge to secure it to the bones. The semicircular rings allow for multiple choices for Schantz pin placement; pin placement through the quadriceps and its extensor mechanism should be avoided. The hinge is always applied with the knee in full extension because the hinge allows a normal range of motion for only a limited arc.

Hinge Biomechanics

In an attempt to study the function of this hinge design, a biomechanical examination was conducted (Figure 13.7).[20] The hinge was applied to fresh cadaveric knee specimens. Radiopaque reference markers were placed on the tibia and femur, and each knee was taken through a range of motion from 0 to 100°. Fluoroscopic images were taken at different positions of flexion to quantify changes in anterior and posterior tibial translation and changes in joint compression and distraction. Two experimental interventions were

Fig. 13.7. The hinge applied to a fresh cadaveric knee specimen. With femoral and tibial reference markers, fluoroscopy was used to measure motion between the distal femur and proximal tibia with flexion of the knee specimen. (From Ref. 20 by permission of the *American Journal of Knee Surgery*.)

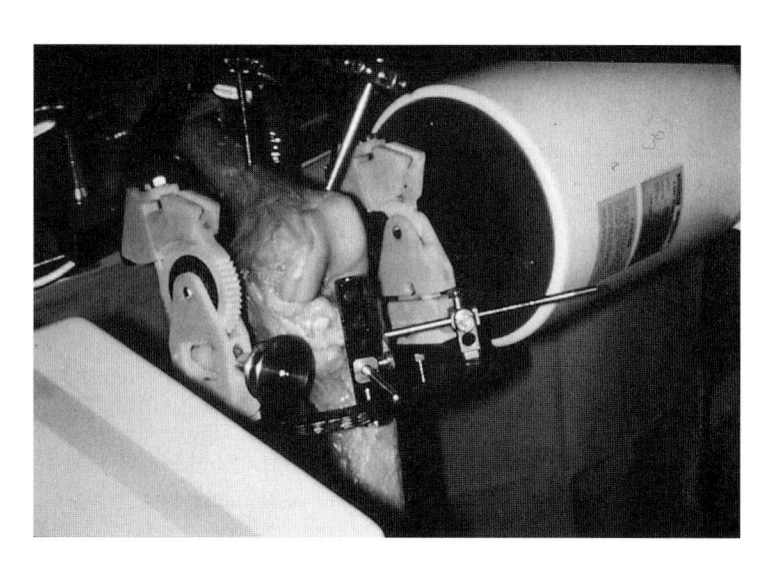

13. Management of Chronic Posterior Tibial Subluxation

Table 13.1. *x*-Axis motion (compression–distraction): differences from the control (the contralateral knee with intact ligaments and no hinge)

Knee position in flexion (degrees)	Knee with intact ligaments and hinge (mm)[a,b]	Knee with disrupted ligaments and hinge (mm)[a,c]
0	0.50 (3.12)	−0.88 (2.85)
20	0.88 (3.44)	−1.62 (3.74)
40	1.38 (2.45)	−0.62 (3.46)
60	1.62 (1.97)	−0.25 (3.92)
80	1.88 (2.30)	0.12 (3.00)
100	1.50 (2.20)	0.50 (2.51)

[a] Numbers in parentheses are standard deviations.
[b] Positive values, joint compression.
[c] Negative values, joint distraction.
Source: Data from Ref. 20.

studied that consisted of an intact knee with the hinge and a knee with multiple ligament disruptions and a hinge. The experimental specimens were compared in pairs against the contralateral knee as a control. The control knee remained intact and without a hinge.

Tables 13.1 and 13.2 list the mean differences and standard deviations of motion mismatch between knee and hinge motion for both interventions, hinge placement with ligaments intact, and hinge placement with the ligaments disrupted, at different angles of flexion. None of the compression–distraction values were statistically significant for knee and hinge mismatch; this is probably a result of the large standard deviations. However, a trend is evident. With the ligaments intact, addition of the hinge resulted in increasing amounts of joint compression with knee flexion (Figure 13.8). When the ligaments were cut, there was some degree of distraction with 0° of knee flexion, which seemed to gradually decrease and became compressive at 80° of flexion (Figure 13.9).

In contrast, the anterior–posterior translation values were statistically significant for knee and hinge mismatch. With the ligaments intact, addition of the hinge resulted in increased amounts of posterior translation, which became statistically significant at 80° of flexion (Figure 13.10). Similarly, when the ligaments were cut with a hinge in place, there was an increasing amount of posterior tibial translation, which became statistically significant at 60° of flexion. There was also a significant amount of anterior tibial translation at 0° in this group (Figure 13.11).

All in all, these results indicate that the hinge allows only a limited range of motion that does not significantly alter tibial translation or joint

Table 13.2. *y*-Axis motion (posterior–anterior tibial translation): differences from the control (the contralateral knee with intact ligaments and no hinge)

Knee position in flexion (degrees)	Knee with intact ligaments and hinge (mm)[a,b]	Knee with disrupted ligaments and hinge (mm)[a,b]
0	0.00 (1.07)	−2.62[c] (2.88)
20	−0.38 (1.92)	−0.75 (2.60)
40	1.25 (2.44)	1.88 (3.36)
60	1.38 (0.96)	4.25[c] (4.50)
80	3.38[c] (2.39)	7.00[c] (5.29)
100	4.62[c] (2.97)	9.88[c] (4.39)

[a] Numbers in parentheses are standard deviations.
[b] Positive values, posterior tibial translation; negative values, anterior tibial translation.
[c] $P < 0.05$.
Source: Data from Ref. 20.

Fig. 13.8. Mean trends for distal femoral motion mismatch in the *x*-axis (compression–distraction) plane between the knee and the hinge with the ligaments intact. Positive values represent increases in joint compression, and negative values represent increases in joint translation (distraction) for each of the differing degrees of knee flexion. None of the *x*-axis values were statistically significant; this is likely because of the large standard deviation. However, a trend is evident: joint compression increased with increasing amounts of flexion. (Adapted from Ref. 20, by permission of the *American Journal of Knee Surgery*.)

Fig. 13.9. Mean trends for distal femoral motion mismatch in the *x*-axis (compression–distraction) plane between the knee and the hinge with the ligaments disrupted. Positive values represent increases in joint compression, and negative values represent increases in joint translation (distraction) for each of the differing degrees of knee flexion. When the ligaments were cut, there was some degree of distraction with 0° of knee flexion, which seems to gradually decrease and became compressive at 80° of flexion. (Adapted from Ref. 20, by permission of the *American Journal of Knee Surgery*.)

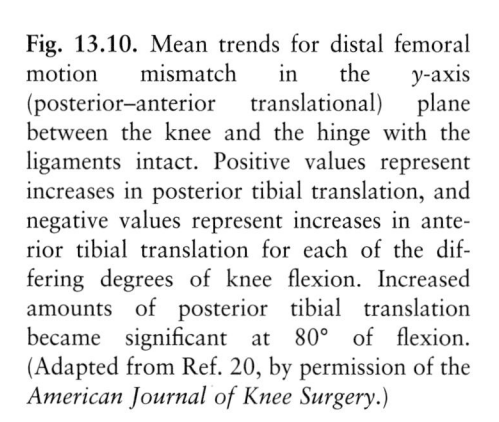

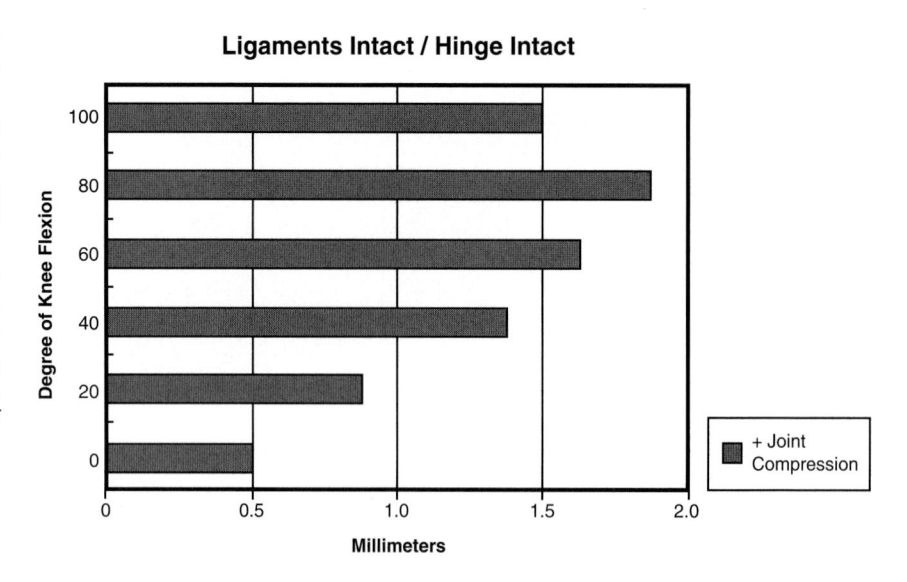

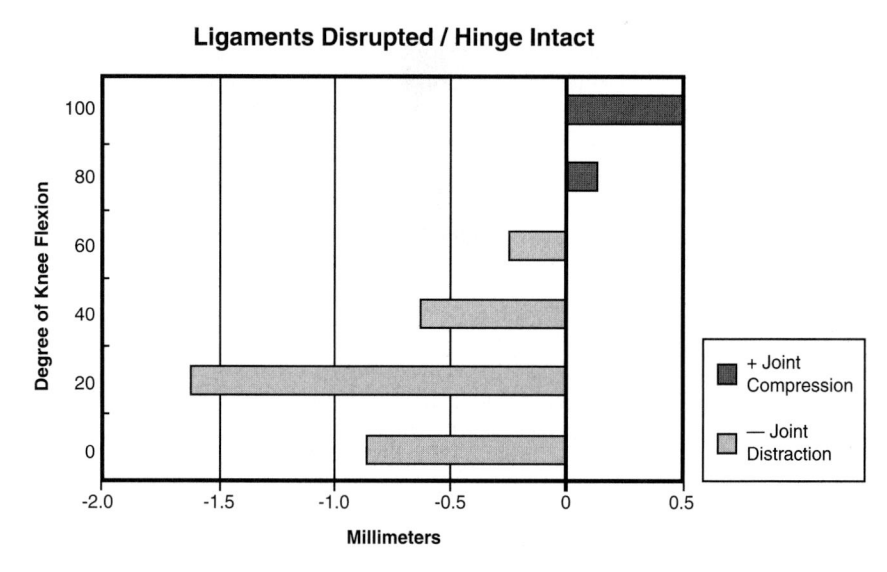

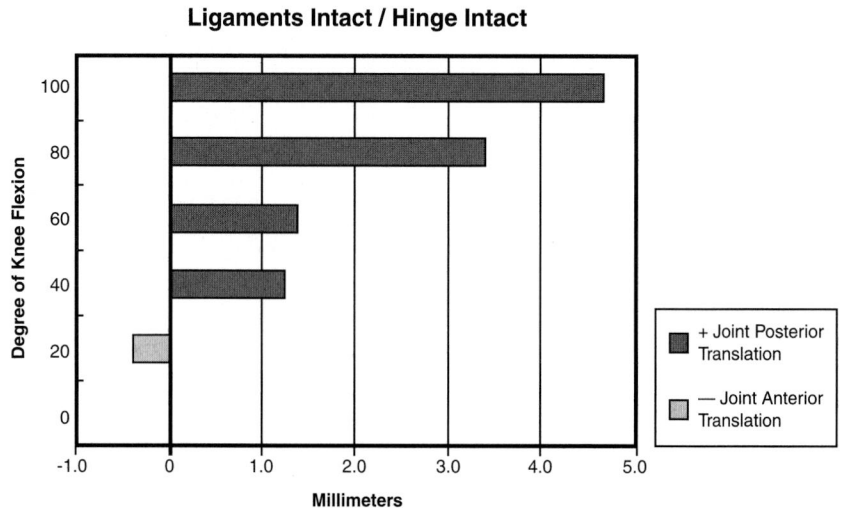

Fig. 13.10. Mean trends for distal femoral motion mismatch in the *y*-axis (posterior–anterior translational) plane between the knee and the hinge with the ligaments intact. Positive values represent increases in posterior tibial translation, and negative values represent increases in anterior tibial translation for each of the differing degrees of knee flexion. Increased amounts of posterior tibial translation became significant at 80° of flexion. (Adapted from Ref. 20, by permission of the *American Journal of Knee Surgery*.)

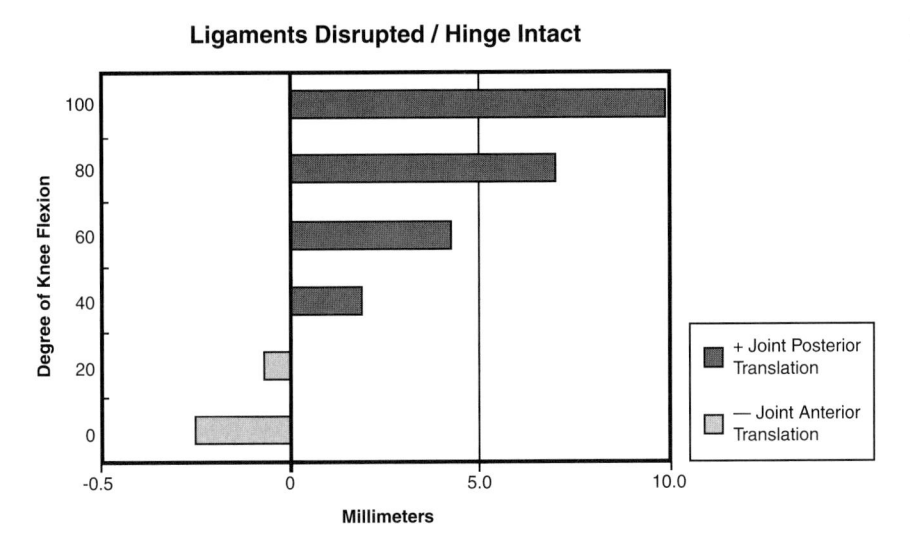

Fig. 13.11. Mean trends for distal femoral motion mismatch in the y-axis (posterior–anterior translational) plane between the knee and the hinge with the ligaments disrupted. Positive values represent increases in posterior tibial translation, and negative values represent increases in anterior tibial translation for each of the differing degrees of knee flexion. There was an increasing amount of posterior tibial translation, which became significant at 60° of flexion. There was also a significant amount of anterior tibial translation at 0° of flexion in this group. (Adapted from Ref. 20, by permission of the *American Journal of Knee Surgery*.)

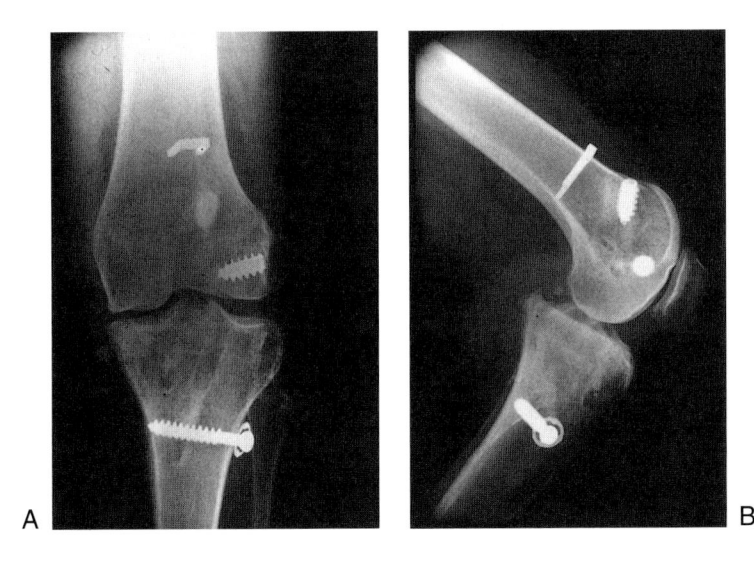

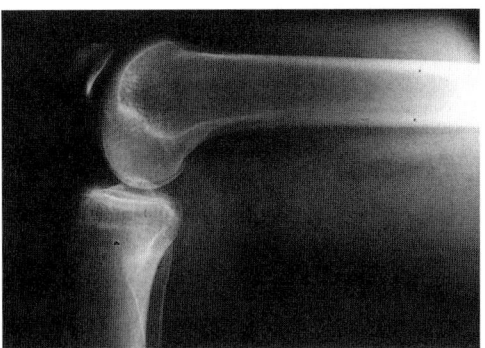

Fig. 13.12. Fourteen months after reduction and reconstruction with hinge application, the anteroposterior radiograph (A) reveals symmetric reduction with a slight reduction in the medial joint space. Comparison lateral radiographs reveal symmetric centering of the joint with the tibia slightly anterior to the femur at 90° of flexion between the injured (B) and noninjured (C) knees. (From Ref. 17, by permission of *Sports Medicine and Arthroscopy Review*.)

compression and distraction. Whether this amount of motion is sufficient to improve the outcome of the grossly unstable knee is unknown.

Clinical Results of Using the Hinge

Clinically, the hinge has been successful in the limited number of cases for which it has been utilized.[15,17] Successful use of the hinge was originally described in a report on two patients from Simonian et al.[16] and supported by a case report by Richter and Lobenhoffer.[15] Each report described using the hinge for only the first 6 weeks following surgical release and allogenic ligament reconstruction for patients with intact articular surfaces presenting with chronic fixed posterior tibial subluxation. After 1-year follow-up, Simonian et al. reported a return of a functional range of motion (−5 to 105° and 0 to 120°), stability (symmetric to the contralateral limb and 5 mm of anteroposterior translation with the anterior surface of the tibia flush with the femoral condyles at 90° of flexion), function (ability to participate in moderate level sporting activities), and an excellent radiographic outcome (Figure 13.12). Recent 6-year follow-up for 1 of the 2 patients

Fig. 13.13. Six-year postoperative radiographs of the patient with chronic posterior tibial subluxation described in Figures 13.3; 13.6; and 13.11: (A) anteroposterior and (B) lateral.

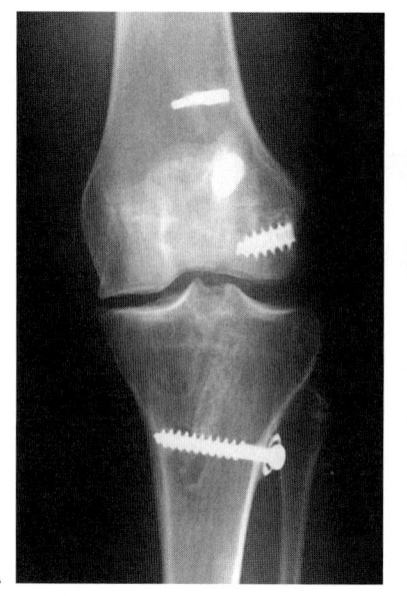

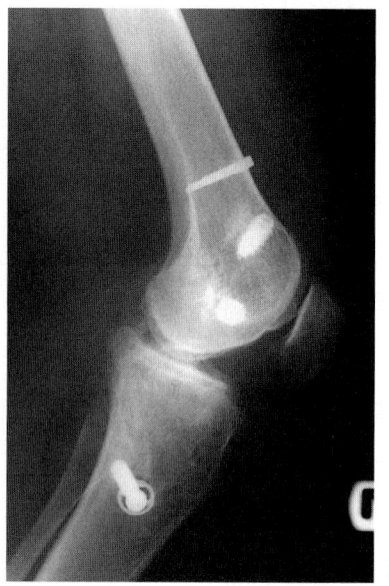

revealed occasional knee soreness, no limitations or change in function, but some radiographic signs of arthritis (Figure 13.13). At 1-year follow-up, Richter and Lobenhoffer reported no pain or impairments with activities of daily living and a return to volleyball, a Lysholm score of 94 points, a Tegner activity score of 4 points, posterior translation of 6 mm by KT 1000 arthrometer, and a lateral radiograph without posterior sag at 30° of flexion.

Discussion

Chronic fixed posterior tibial subluxation in the multiple ligament injured knee, although extremely rare, is a difficult and entirely avoidable problem that requires complex management. Unfortunately, it presents itself after mismanagement. Chronic posterior tibial subluxation is most easily treated by maintaining a high clinical suspicion, providing appropriate management, and properly ensuring reduction for acute multiple ligament knee injuries. Patients with chronic posterior tibial subluxation present with pain, limitations of motion and function, and instability. Proper treatment depends on an accurate diagnosis of the limits to motion, ligamentous insufficiencies, and the other associated injuries such as neurovascular compromise and meniscal and articular cartilage lesions. In patients not having unsalvageable articular cartilage and neurovascular injuries, surgical treatment for chronic posterior tibial subluxation has the two main objectives of reduction of the tibia under the femur and reconstruction of all of the ligamentous deficiencies. Achieving a reduction often requires surgical release of all soft tissues, with the exception of the skin, the extensor mechanism, and the neurovascular structures. To restore stability, all ligamentous deficiencies should be addressed. Since the instability created from this extensive release places increased stresses on the ligamentous reconstruction, the importance of the postoperative protection and monitoring of the reduction should not be underestimated. Appropriate postoperative protection should attempt to optimize early range of motion while maintaining an adequate reduction. In a limited number of cases reported in the literature, surgical release to attain a reduction followed by ligamentous reconstruction with allografts and a limited 6-week period of hinged skeletal fixation has allowed a successful outcome for patients with the complex problem of chronic posterior tibial subluxation.

References

1. Almekinders LC, Logan TC. Results following treatment of traumatic dislocations of the knee joint. Clin Orthop 1992; 284:203–207.
2. Almekinders LC, Dedmond BT. Outcomes of the operatively treated knee dislocation. Clin Sports Med 2000; 19:503–518.
3. Dedmond BT, Almekinders LC. Operative versus nonoperative treatment of knee dislocations. Am J Knee Surg 2001; 14(1): 33–38.
4. Fanelli GC. Treatment of combined anterior cruciate ligament–posterior cruciate ligament–lateral side injuries of the knee. Clin Sports Med 2000; 19:493–503.
5. Frassica FJ, Sim FH, Staeheli JW, Pairolero PC. Dislocation of the knee. Clin Orthop 1991; 263: 200–205.
6. Roman PD, Hopson CN, Zenni EJ. Traumatic dislocation of the knee: a report of 30 cases and literature review. Orthop Rev 1987; 16:917–924.
7. Shields L, Mital M, Cave EF. Complete dislocation of the knee: experience at the Massachusetts General Hospital. J Trauma 1969; 9:192–215.
8. Thomsen PB, Rud B, Jensen UH. Stability and motion after traumatic dislocation of the knee. Acta Orthop Scand 1984; 55:278–283.
9. Myers MH, Moore TM, Harvey JP. Traumatic dislocation of the knee joint. J Bone Joint Surg Am 1975; 57:430–433.
10. Sisto DJ, Warren RF. Complete knee dislocation. A follow-up study of operative treatment. Clin Orthop 1985; 198:94–101.
11. Stayner LR, Coen MJ. Historic perspectives of treatment algorithms in knee dislocation. Clin Sports Med 2000; 19:399–413.
12. Montgomery JB. Dislocation of the knee. Orthop Clin North Am 1987; 18: 149–156.
13. Henshaw RM, Shapiro MS, Oppenheim WL. Delayed reduction of traumatic knee dislocation. Clin Orthop 1996; 330:152–156.
14. Petrie RS, Trousdale RT, Cabanela ME. Total knee arthroplasty for chronic posterior knee dislocation. J Arthroplasty 2000; 15:380–386.
15. Richter M, Lobenhoffer P. Chronic posterior knee dislocation: treatment with arthrolysis, posterior cruciate ligament reconstruction and external fixation device. Injury 1998; 29:546–549.
16. Simonian PT, Wickiewicz TL, Hotchkiss RN, et al. Chronic knee dislocation: reduction, reconstruction, and application of a skeletally fixed knee hinge. Am J Sports Med 1998; 26:1–5.
17. Simonian PT, Shafer BL, Wickiewicz TL. Management of chronic posterior tibial subluxation in the multiligament-injured knee. Sports Med Arthrosc Rev 2001; 9:239–246.
18. Laasonsen EM, Kivioja A. Delayed diagnosis of extremity injuries in patients with multiple injuries. J Trauma 1991; 31:257–260.
19. Montgomery TJ, Savoie FH, White JL, et al. Orthopedic management of knee dislocations: comparison of surgical reconstruction and immobilization. Am Knee Surg 1995; 8:97–103.
20. Simonian PT, Sussman PS, Wickiewicz TL, et al. The skeletally fixed knee hinge for the grossly unstable knee. Am J Knee Surg 1998; 11:181–187.

Chapter Fourteen

Postoperative Rehabilitation

Craig J. Edson

Rehabilitation of the multiple ligament injured knee presents several challenges to the rehabilitation specialist. A thorough understanding of the surgical procedure, the biomechanics of the knee, and the manner in which exercises and daily activities affect the involved structures is imperative. This chapter outlines the exercise protocols currently in place at our facility, as well as the scientific rationale behind the exercises that comprise these postoperative regimens.

Scientific Basis of Exercise

Before specific treatment programs can be established, to ensure that the patient is not engaging in any activity that may place excessive or detrimental forces on the reconstructed ligaments, the effects of exercises and activities of daily living (ADLs) on the knee must be considered. This is best accomplished by controlling the translation forces within the tibiofemoral joint. In addition, the effects of exercises on the patellofemoral joint should be considered.

Terms such as "open chain" and "closed chain" have been adopted over the past few years to describe various exercise techniques and their effects on the knee. This is largely a result of several studies[1-9] that have examined these exercises as they relate to the postoperative course following reconstruction of the anterior cruciate ligament (ACL). These terms are discussed with emphasis on their effects on the tibiofemoral joint, the patellofemoral joint, proprioception, and the primary ligaments of the knee.

Open Versus Closed Chain Exercises

Kinetic chain terminology was originally used to describe the linkage analysis in mechanical engineering. Steindler[10] was the first to apply this principle to human movement when he described a closed kinetic chain activity as the events that occur when the terminal or distal segment is fixed. During closed chain exercises, movement at one joint results in simultaneous movement of all other joints in a predictable manner.[11] Closed kinetic chain exercises involving the lower extremities, such as squats or leg press, incorporate some degree of weight bearing. There are unique physiologic events that occur at the joints when the lower extremity bears weight. For example, Lutz and associates[12] noted a decrease in shear forces at the tibiofemoral joint during closed chain exercises. They attributed this decrease to axial orientation of the applied forces as well as muscular cocontraction. Wilk and associates[13] reported that posterior shear force was generated during the entire motion of closed chain exercises; however, maximal posterior shear force occurred between 88 and 102° of knee flexion. In addition, the maximal electromyographic (EMG) activity for the hamstrings was noted during the extending phase of closed kinetic chain squat exercises. Although these two findings would indicate that closed chain exercises are safe during ACL rehabilitation, they may be detrimental during rehabilitation following reconstruction of the posterior cruciate ligament (PCL).

During open chain exercises of the knee, the distal segment is free, resulting in isolated motions of flexion and extension. These motions have varying effects on the tibiofemoral joint and, subsequently, the ligamentous structures of the knee. For example, several investigators[14-17] have shown that knee extension produces anterior tibial translation between 0 and 60° of flexion. Beyond 60°, quadriceps activity results in minimal tibial translation until approximately 70 to 75° of flexion. The point at which quadriceps contraction produces neither anterior nor posterior tibial translation has been termed the quadriceps neutral angle.[18] At flexion angles greater than the quadriceps neutral angle, quadriceps activity will produce posterior translation of the tibia that is due to the posterior orientation of the quadriceps tendon. Conversely, open chain knee flexion produces posterior translation, although this has been calculated as less than 1 times body weight (BW) during the initial 50° of flexion.[18] Beyond 50°, this force increased to 1.7 times body weight and was further increased when resistance was applied. In practical terms, open chain knee exercises from 0 to 60° may be indicated during PCL reconstruction but not during the initial phase of ACL reconstruction. Open chain flexion exercises should not be used during the initial phase of PCL rehabilitation. For medial collateral ligament (MCL) and lateral collateral ligament (LCL) reconstruction, the goal is to control varus and valgus forces. Therefore, depending on the patient's physiologic alignment, closed chain exercises could be more detrimental during the early phases of healing.

Patellofemoral Joint Forces

In 1979 Hungerford and Barry[19] found that peak patellofemoral joint reaction forces occurred at 36° of knee flexion during open chain knee extension against a 9 kg boot. They determined that these forces, since they were dispersed over a relatively small area of the joint, were injurious to the patellofemoral joint. As knee flexion increases, so does the contact area within the patellofemoral joint, thus distributing the forces over a greater surface area. Recently, Cohen and associates[20] challenged this theory. Utilizing computer simulation, they found little difference in the patellofemoral contact forces during open and closed chain exercises. In addition, they determined that the forces within the patellofemoral joint were not supraphysiologic, regardless of the type of exercise employed. Nonetheless, during the early phases of rehabilitation, complaints of patellofemoral pain should be monitored during open and closed chain exercises, since immobilization and deficits in quadriceps strength might compromise tracking and mobility.

Stress on the Posterior Cruciate Ligament

From the discussion on open and closed chain exercises, one can see that these exercises create distinct and contrasting effects on tibial translation and ligamentous load. Although much has been written about the effects of various exercises and activities on the ACL, there have been limited studies regarding their effect on the PCL. Ohkoshii and associates[21] reported increased posterior shear forces with increasing angles of trunk flexion secondary to heightened activity of the hamstrings. These posterior directed forces were magnified during active knee flexion at all angles beyond 30°. Dahlkuits and colleagues[22] calculated a posterior force of three times BW during squatting activities. These findings were similar to those of Wilk and associates,[13] who found significantly greater posterior shear forces during closed kinetic chain exercises.

Given these findings, it would appear that closed chain exercises are contraindicated during rehabilitation of the PCL. However, during closed chain activities muscular cocontraction occurs and helps to minimize the posterior shear forces and stress on the PCL. Wilk[23] analyzed the outcomes of several studies and determined that quadriceps and hamstring muscle ratios are similar during the first 60° of knee flexion. Kvist and Gillquist[24] also found less tibial translation during closed chain exercises, although they found the coactivation to occur between the quadriceps and gastrocnemius muscles, while hamstring activity was reported as low.

Other studies that examined the effects of various activities on posterior translation and PCL stress have shown varying results. For example, Ericson and Nisell considered the effect of cycling on the PCL and found a posterior shear force of only $0.05 \times BW$ at 105° of knee flexion.[25] Level walking also produced a relatively low posterior shear force of $0.4 \times BW$.[26] Conversely, ascending stairs produced a posterior shear force of $1.7 \times BW$; this reportedly occurred at 45° of knee flexion.[27] This finding appears to contradict previously discussed studies that showed tibial translation was primarily anterior at 45° during closed chain activities. In addition, Smidt[28] found a posterior shear force of only $1.1 \times BW$ with open chain (isometric) knee flexion at this same angle of 45°.

The deleterious effects of open chain knee extension on the ACL have been well documented.[12,17,29-31] This is secondary to the anterior shear force produced by the quadriceps activity, especially at flexion angles of 60° and continuing to full extension. Conversely, in the case of PCL rehabilitation, the same exercises can be performed safely, since no posterior shear forces are produced. Nonetheless, these exercises should be employed judiciously secondary to the potential damaging effects on the articular cartilage of the patellofemoral joint, as discussed earlier. Open chain extension exercises should also be avoided at flexion angles greater than 60°, since as already noted, posterior shear force is produced by the patellar tendon. Open chain flexion exercises should be avoided following PCL reconstruction until healing adequate to withstand this force has occurred.

Rehabilitation Following Multiple Ligament Reconstruction

Since knee dislocation routinely results in complete disruption of the primary stabilizing ligaments of the knee, reconstruction of all structures involved is necessary. Subsequently, the clinician needs to consider the effects of all activities and exercises on all ligaments concerned. The following regimen has been used successfully and is based on the experience accrued over the past 10 years while treating patients with multiple ligament reconstruction (Table 14.1).[32,33]

Postoperative Protocol Following Multiple Ligament Reconstruction

Weeks 1 to 6

During the first 6 weeks after multiple ligament reconstruction (MLR), the emphasis is on graft protection. With injuries of this magnitude, Achilles tendon allograft tissue is utilized for reconstruction of the ACL, PCL, and MCL if necessary. This allows the surgeon to construct a graft of significant diameter and length to simulate the dimensions of the native tissue. Nonetheless, there are insufficient data in the literature that examine the tensile strength of these grafts when implanted simultaneously. Given the likelihood that implanted grafts are most susceptible to the forces applied to them during the early phase of healing, a conservative approach is warranted during this time.

Immediately postoperatively, patients are placed in a long-leg hinged brace locked in full extension, which minimizes tibiofemoral shear force due to the small moment arm of the hamstrings.[11] A continuous cold unit is applied postoperatively to control pain and hemarthrosis. The pads for these units are incorporated into the postoperative dressings but do not directly contact the skin. Protective, antibacterial liners are available to minimize the risk of infection and to protect the dressings from becoming damp. Strict non–weight bearing is enforced during this time period. Keeping the foot off the ground minimizes muscle activity and subsequently, forces on the grafts. Despite some support in the literature for early range-of-motion (ROM) exercises in the early stages following MLR,[34,35] we have found that this early motion can be detrimental to the final outcome. Attempts to incorporate early ROM have resulted, in some instances, in elongation of the PCL and subsequent grade I–II posterior laxity. Another potential complication of early ROM concerns the posterolateral corner (PLC). A split biceps tendon tenodesis is commonly employed to reconstruct the PLC, and fixation is with a screw and washer. Repetitive motion could potentially result in splintering or fragmentation secondary to microtrauma, compromising the integrity of the repair. The biggest risk with immobilization is arthrofibrosis. However, in our population, the number of patients that have required manipulation or other intervention due to loss of motion with this protocol has been less than 3%.

During the initial 6 weeks, quadriceps strengthening is encouraged; this is accomplished through isometrics and low intensity electric stimulation. In addition, aggressive patella mobilization is instituted to minimize restrictions and any motion loss that could be associated with limited patella mobility. Patients may experience hamstring tightness and posterior knee discomfort as a result of maintaining the knee in full extension. Therefore, stretching of the hamstring and the gastrocnemius–soleus complex is encouraged, although vigorous stretching is discouraged to minimize posterior shear forces created by the hamstrings. Patients also perform "ankle-pumping" exercises to minimize venous stasis in the lower leg. All patients are advised to avoid resting positions that place varus or valgus forces on the knee.

14. Postoperative Rehabilitation

Table 14.1. Multiple ligament reconstruction rehabilitation

Phase I: 0 to 6 weeks
  Goals
    Maximum protection of grafts
    Maintain patella mobility
    Maintain quadriceps tone
    Maintain full passive extension
    Control pain and swelling
  Program
    Non-weight-bearing ambulation with crutches
    Brace locked in extension 24 h/day
    Cryotherapy
    Quadriceps sets: enhance with low intensity electrical stimulation or biofeedback
    Patella mobilization
    Ankle pumps: ROM
    Stretching exercises: gastrocnemius–soleus and gentle hamstrings
Phase II: 6 to 12 weeks
  Goals
    Initiate weight bearing for articular cartilage nourishment
    Increase knee flexion
    Maintain quadriceps tone
    Improve proprioception
    Avoid isolated quadriceps and hamstring contraction
  Program
    Begin partial weight bearing gait of 25% BW and increase by 25% over next 4 weeks
    Open brace to full flexion: with PLC, continue to wear at night
    Prone hangs
    Passive flexion exercises: consider continuous passive motion if no involvement of PLC
    Patella mobilization
    High intensity electric stimulation at 60° of knee flexion
    Initiate closed chain strengthening once full weight bearing has been achieved and quadriceps strength is $3^+/5$ or more
    Stationary bicycle for ROM assist
    Proprioception and weight shift: (KAT) or biomechanical ankle platform system (BAPS) board
    Hip strengthening: no adduction if PLC is involved
    Discontinue brace at end of postoperative week 12
Phase III: 4 to 6 months
  Goals
    Increase knee flexion
    Maintain full passive extension
    Improve quadriceps and hamstring strength
    Improve proprioception
    Improve functional skills
    Increase cardiovascular endurance
  Program
    4 Months
      Closed chain progressive resistance exercises (PREs): avoid flexion beyond 70°
      Isolated quadriceps and hamstring exercises: no resistance
      Single-leg proprioception exercises (KAT, BAPS, mini-trampoline)
      Closed chain conditioning exercises: stair climber, skiing machine, rower, etc.
      Aggressive flexion ROM: consider manipulation if ROM < 90° by end of month 4
      Hip PREs
      Straight-line jogging at end of postoperative month 4
    5 Months
      Initiate resisted quadriceps and hamstring exercises
      Progress closed chain strengthening and conditioning exercises
      Initiate low intensity plyometrics
      Progress jogging and begin sprints
      Advance proprioception training
      Fit for ACL/PCL functional brace
    6 Months
      Progression of all strengthening exercises and plyometrics
      Begin agility drills in brace: carioca, figure 8s, zigzag, slalom running, etc.
      Sport-specific drills
      Isokinetic testing at end of postoperative month 6
Phase IV: 7 to 12 months
  Program: Assess functional strength via single-leg hop for distance, timed hop test, shuttle run, etc. Return to sports if the following criteria are met:
    Minimal or no pain or swelling
    Isokinetic *and* functional tests within 10 to 15% of the uninvolved side
    Successful completion of sport-specific drills
    ACL/PCL functional brace

Weeks 7 to 12

At the end of the sixth postoperative week, the brace is unlocked to allow full flexion and may be removed at night. The patient begins weight bearing of 25% body weight and continues to increase by 25% body weight per week in a progressive fashion, until full weight bearing is attained at the end of postoperative week 10 (Table 14.2). Within this time frame, passive ROM is also increased, guardedly, since flexion greater than 90° places high forces on PCL grafts.[36] To begin flexion exercises with minimal hamstring activity and varus/valgus forces on the knee, the patient is advised to obtain a chair with wheels and to block the involved extremity against a solid object. While maintaining the knee in a straight line, the patient rolls toward the stabilizing object, producing flexion of the knee. Although ROM goals

Table 14.2. Rehabilitation summary following multiple ligament reconstruction

	Postoperative weeks					Postoperative months			
	1–2	3–4	5–6	7–8	9–12	4	5	6	7–12
Long-leg brace at 0° of flexion	×	×	×						
Long-leg brace at 0 to 135° of flexion				×	×				
Functional brace						×	×	×	×
Weight bearing									
Non–weight bearing	×	×	×						
25% BW				×					
50% BW				× wk 8					
75% BW					×				
Fully weight bearing					× wk 10				
ROM goals									
0–70°				×					
0–90°				× wk 10					
0–110°					×				
0–120°						×			
0–130°							×		
Procedures									
Electric stimulation	×	×	×						
Patella mobility	×	×	×						
Exercises									
Stretching									
Hamstring-gastrocnemius	×	×	×						
Prone hangs			×	×	×	×	×		
Strengthening									
Quadriceps sets: straight-leg raise	×	×	×						
Knee extension						×	×	×	×
Short arc					×	×	×	×	×
Resisted						×	×	×	×
Hamstring curls						×	×	×	×
Resisted hamstring curls							×	×	×
Resisted knee extension							×	×	×
Proprioception									
KAT or BAPS					×	×	×	×	×
Plyometrics							×	×	×
Conditioning/Aerobic									
Upper body exercises		×	×						
Stationary bicycle				×	×	×	×	×	×
Walking						×	×	×	×
Stair climber						×	×	×	×
Ski machine						×	×	×	×
Jogging							×	×	×
Sport specific									
Cutting								×	×
Return to sports									×

of 90° by postoperative week 8 and 120° by week 10 are imposed, the patient is cautioned about aggressively forcing motion. Conversely, the patient is also advised that motion gains may be gradual, to avoid discouragement when progress is slow. We have found that patients who achieve the ROM goals gradually have the most favorable functional outcomes and static stability. To facilitate motion, a stationary bicycle may be employed once the patient has achieved flexion beyond 90°. Although flexion ROM is emphasized, the patient also performs prone hangs to assure that full extension is attained and to avoid flexion contractures.

Once the patient is fully weight bearing, closed chain exercises are instituted. As stated earlier, cocontraction occurs during these exercises to minimize anterior and posterior tibial translation. These exercises are restricted to a range of 60 to 0° to contain tibiofemoral shearing and patellofemoral compressive forces. As the patient's tolerance to closed chain exercises improves, progressive, resistive exercises are incorporated. These can be in the form of short-arc squats or by utilizing a leg press machine. Balance and proprioception training activities are initiated as an adjunct to the closed chain exercises. There are several commercial devices available for training proprioception, and the patient may also practice at home in front of a mirror. Isolated, open chain flexion and extension exercises are avoided during this phase of rehabilitation.

Months 4 to 6

Between postoperative weeks 10 and 12, the hinged brace is discontinued. The patient is often fitted with a combined instability functional brace at this time to provide medial and lateral support. Range of motion is expected to approach 120° of knee flexion at this time, and the patient must have full extension. Flexion limitations of 10 to 15° are not uncommon but may resolve over time. Residual flexion deficits of 10° or less can persist; however, this rarely results in any functional limitation and may result in less stress on the graft, since the PCL fibers are most taut at end-range flexion.[34] If active flexion of 90° has not been achieved by the end of postoperative week 12, manipulation under anesthesia and/or arthroscopic debridement may be considered.

Closed chain strengthening exercises are advanced at this time, as well as aerobic conditioning exercises incorporating such devices as a stair climber, rowing machine, and stationary bicycle. Open chain knee extension and flexion are initiated at the end of postoperative month 4, but no resistance is applied. The patient also begins straight-line jogging, assuming that he or she can demonstrate functional strength that is at least 70% of the uninvolved extremity. This is assessed through a single-leg hop test. The patient assumes a single-leg stance beginning with the uninvolved extremity and jumps forward as far as possible, landing on the same extremity. The patient performs 3 trials, and the average distance is calculated. The procedure is then repeated for the involved extremity. When running is permitted, the patient is advised to begin with a fast walk that is gradually progressed to a mild jog. As tolerance improves, the patient advances to a more consistent jogging pace. Aquatic running can be a useful adjunct at this time to provide light resistance and to diminish the impact loading forces on the knee. Resistive exercises begin at the end of postoperative month 5 and gradually progress as tolerated. Toward the end of postoperative month 6, an isokinetic assessment is obtained. Higher velocities are used to minimize shear forces.[37] Quadriceps and hamstring deficits of 20% or less are desired before the patient is allowed to begin sport-specific activities. These are performed with the combined instability brace, and the patient is carefully monitored for signs of pain, swelling, or increased laxity.

Months 7 to 12

At the beginning of postoperative month 7, the patient is allowed to return to sports or heavy labor assuming that several criteria are met. These include the following:

1. No swelling and minimal to no pain
2. Strength (isokinetic) and functional tests within 90% of the contralateral side
3. Grade I laxity with standard physical examination, arthrometric testing, and/or stress radiography
4. Properly fitted combined instability brace

At 1 year following the initial postoperative date, the patient is asked to return for a full reassessment including stress radiography, arthrometric testing, physical examination, and completion of ligament rating forms. The brace is continued for an additional 6 months for sports or rigorous activity; then the patient is given the option to discontinue it. Subsequent appointments are scheduled annually so that long-term effectiveness as well as patient satisfaction can be assessed.

Conclusions

Complete knee dislocation is a serious injury and results in complete disruption of the major stabilizing ligaments of the knee. Following reconstruction, the rehabilitation specialist must consider all patient activities and prescribed exercises on the implanted grafts. The regimen outlined in this chapter is based on current scientific findings and our experience with this patient population over the past 10 years. Attempts to accelerate this process have resulted in less than optimal results.

References

1. Bach BR, Tradonsky S, Bojchuk J, Levy ME, Bush-Joseph CA, Kahn NH. Arthroscopically assisted anterior cruciate ligament reconstruction using patellar tendon autograft. Five- to nine-year follow-up evaluation. Am J Sports Med 1998; 26:20–29.
2. Beynnon BD, Johnson RJ. Anterior cruciate ligament injury rehabilitation in athletes. Biomechanical considerations. Sports Med 1996; 22:54–64.
3. Bynum BD, et al. Open versus closed chain kinetic exercises after anterior cruciate ligament reconstruction. A prospective randomized study. Am J Sports Med 1997; 25:823–829.
4. Fitzgerald GK. Open versus closed kinetic chain exercise: issues in rehabilitation after anterior cruciate ligament reconstructive surgery. Phys Ther 1997; 77: 1747–1754.
5. Frndak PA, Berasi CC. Rehabilitation concerns following anterior cruciate ligament reconstruction. Sports Med 1991; 12:338–346.
6. Hooper DM, Morissey MC, Dreschler W, Morissey D, King J. Open and closed kinetic chain exercises in the early period after anterior cruciate ligament reconstruction. Am J Sports Med 2001; 29:167–174.
7. Noyes FR, Barber-Westin SD. Reconstruction of the anterior cruciate ligament with human allograft. Comparison of early and late results. J Bone Joint Surg Am 1996; 78:524–537.
8. Parker MG. Biomechanical and histological concepts in the rehabilitation of patients with anterior cruciate ligament reconstruction. J Orthop Sports Phys Ther 1994; 20:44–50.

9. Shelbourne KD, Klootwyk TE, Wilkens JH, Carlos MS. Ligament stability two to six years after anterior cruciate ligament reconstruction with autogenous patellar tendon graft and participation in an accelerated rehabilitation program. Am J Sports Med 1995; 23:575–579.
10. Steindler A. Kinesiology of the Human Body Under Normal and Pathological Conditions. Springfield, IL: Charles C Thomas; 1970.
11. Irrgang JJ. Rehabilitation for non-operative and operative management of knee injuries. In: Fu FA, Harner CD, Vince KD, eds. Knee Surgery. Baltimore, MD: Williams & Wilkins; 1994:485–502.
12. Lutz GE, Palmitier RA, An KN, Chao YS. Comparison of tibiofemoral joint forces during open-kinetic-chain and closed-kinetic-chain exercises. J Bone Joint Surg Am 1993; 75:732–739.
13. Wilk KE, Escamilla RF, Fleisig GS, Barrentine SW, Andrews JR, Boyd ML. A comparison of tibiofemoral joint forces and electromyographic activity during open and closed kinetic chain exercises. Am J Sports Med 1996; 24:518–527.
14. Snyder-Mackler L. Scientific rationale and physiological basis for the use of closed kinetic chain exercises in the lower extremity. J Sports Rehabil 1996; 5:2–12.
15. Arms SW, Pope MH, Johnson RJ, Fisher RA, Arvidsson I, Eriksson E. The biomechanics of anterior cruciate ligament rehabilitation and reconstruction. Am J Sports Med 1984; 12:8–18.
16. Grood ES, Suntay WJ, Noyes FR, Butler DL. Biomechanics of the knee-extension exercise: effect of cutting the anterior cruciate ligament. J Bone Joint Surg Am 1984; 66:725–734.
17. Renstrom P, Arms SW, Stanwyck TS, Johnson RJ, Pope MH. Strain within the anterior cruciate ligament during hamstring and quadriceps activity. Am J Sports Med 1986; 14:83–87.
18. Daniel DM, Stone ML, Barrett P, Sachs R. Use of the quadriceps active test to diagnose posterior cruciate ligament disruption and measure posterior laxity of the knee. J Bone Joint Surg Am 1988; 70:387–391.
19. Hungerford DS, Barry M. Biomechanics of the patellofemoral joint. Clin Orthop 1979; 144:9–15.
20. Cohen ZA, Roglic H, Grelsamer RP, Henry JH, Levine WN, Mow VC, Ateshian GA. Patellofemoral stresses during open and closed kinetic chain exercises: an analysis using computer simulation. Am J Sports Med 2001; 29:480–487.
21. Ohkoshi Y, Yasuda K, Kaneda K, Wada T, Yamanaka M. Biomechanical analysis of rehabilitation in the standing position. Am J Sports Med 1991; 19: 605–611.
22. Dahlkuits NJ, Mago P, Seedholm BB. Forces during squatting and rising from a deep squat. Eng Med 1982; 11:69–76.
23. Wilk KE. Rehabilitation of isolated and combined posterior cruciate ligament injuries. Clin Sports Med 1994; 13:649–677.
24. Kvist J, Gillquist J. Sagittal plane knee translation and electromyographic activity during closed and open kinetic chain exercises in anterior cruciate ligament-deficient patients and control subjects. Am J Sports Med 2001; 29:72–82.
25. Ericson MO, Nisell R. Tibiofemoral joint forces during ergometer cycling. Am J Sports Med 1986; 14:285–290.
26. Morrison JB. The biomechanics of the knee joint in relation to normal walking. J Biomech 1970; 3:51–60.
27. Morrison JB. Function of the knee joint in various activities. Biomech Eng 1969; 4:573–580.
28. Smidt GL. Biomechanical analysis of knee extension and flexion. J Biomech 1973; 6:79–92.
29. Beynnon BD, Fleming BC, Johnson RJ. The strain behavior of the anterior cruciate ligament during squatting and active flexion–extension exercise. A comparison of an open and closed kinetic chain exercise. Am J Sports Med 1997; 25:823–829.
30. Lysholm M, Messner K. Sagittal plane translation of the tibia in anterior cruciate ligament-deficient knees during commonly used rehabilitation exercises. Scand J Med Sci Sports 1995; 5:49–56.
31. Vergis A, Hindriks M, Gillquist J. Sagittal plane translations of the knee in anterior cruciate deficient subjects and controls. Med Sci Sports Exerc 1994; 29: 1561–1566.

32. Fanelli GC, Giannotti BF, Edson CJ. Arthroscopically assisted combined posterior cruciate ligament/posterior lateral complex reconstruction. Arthroscopy 1996; 12:521–530.
33. Fanelli GC, Giannotti BF, Edson CJ. Arthroscopically assisted combined anterior and posterior cruciate ligament reconstruction. Arthroscopy 1996; 12:5–14.
34. Noyes FR, Barber-Westin SD. Reconstruction of the anterior and posterior cruciate ligaments after knee dislocation: use of early protected postoperative motion to decrease arthrofibrosis. Am J Sports Med 1997; 25:769–778.
35. Shapiro MS, Freedman EL. Allograft reconstruction of the anterior and posterior cruciate ligaments after traumatic knee dislocation. Am J Sports Med 1995; 23:580–587.
36. Ogata K, McCarthy JA. Measurements of length and tension patterns during reconstruction of the posterior cruciate ligament. Am J Sports Med 1992; 20:351–355.
37. Kaufman KR, An K-N, Litchey WJ, Morrey BF, Chao EYS. Dynamic joint forces during knee isokinetic exercise. Am J Sports Med 1991; 19:305–315.

Chapter Fifteen

Complications Associated with Treatment

John C. Richmond

This chapter reviews the complications that may result from treatment of the multiple ligament injured/dislocated knee, rather than those directly resulting from the injury. The treatment of these complex and potentially devastating injuries presents the possibility of certain complications that are not typically encountered when one is treating injury to the individual ligaments. The timing of treatment may be a major determinant of the risk of these various complications. It is important to identify the specific complications engendered by the acute treatment of a multiligament injured/dislocated knee, as well as those that may be faced in a more chronic situation. Early recognition of the extent of injury is crucial for early identification of certain injuries, particularly vascular injuries. One should always approach a multiple ligament injured knee with the caution employed in the management of the dislocated knee.[1,2] Failure to recognize the extent of all the ligaments involved may result in an inadequate treatment plan. Magnetic resonance imaging (MRI) is a valuable diagnostic tool to identify the injured structures and to define an appropriate treatment schema.[3] In a study of the multiligament injured/dislocated knee, Twaddle et al.[4] revealed that clinical examination alone had significant inaccuracies (53–82% correct) while MRI scan was more accurate (85–100% correct). We routinely obtain an MRI scan early on in all our patients with acute polyligament knee injuries, (Figure 15.1) to most accurately identify all injured structures. Planning for the treatment program is then based on the combination of clinical examination and MRI findings.

In the management of any of these injuries, careful neurovascular assessment supersedes the ligament exam. Failure to recognize damage to the popliteal artery and/or vein may result in an amputation. Vascular injury has been relatively infrequent from low velocity knee dislocations sustained in the athletic venue, 4.8% in a report from Shelbourne et al.[1] Higher velocity injuries, as occur with motor vehicle trauma, have higher rates of vascular injury, typically noted in the 30% range.[5] Knee dislocation following trivial trauma has been described in patients with morbid obesity.[6] There is substantially increased risk for vascular catastrophe in the special case of the morbidly obese.[7] In an ongoing series of this population from the Campbell Clinic Foundation (personal communication: Azar FM, Brandt JC, Phillips BB, Miller RH III, 2001), 41% sustained vascular injury. Focusing on the potential limb-threatening vascular injuries remains the first step. Careful coordination of the treatment plan with the vascular surgeon is paramount, for the goals are to prevent any unnecessary delay in the vascular repair and to protect that repair through the immediate postoperative period and any late reconstruction.

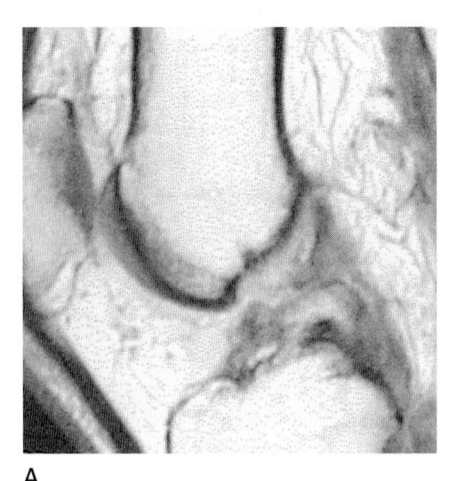

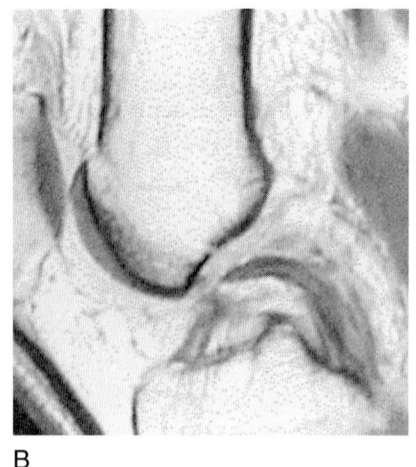

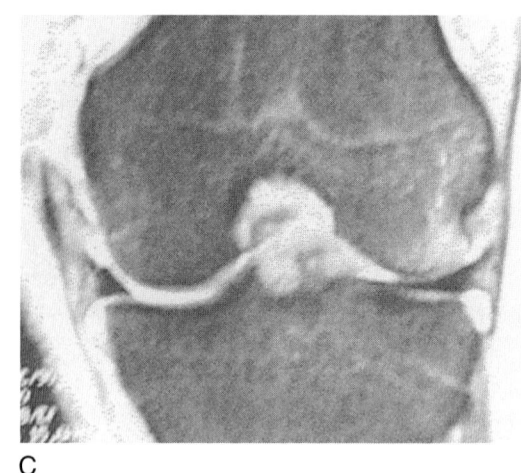

Fig. 15.1. MRI views of a multiple ligament injured knee reveal (A) complete ACL tear, (B) complete PCL tear, and (C) complete MCL tear.

The neurologic injury most commonly encountered is damage to the peroneal nerve from stretching as a result of bicruciate injuries with lateral blowout.[8–10] Initial assessment should identify any sensory or motor deficit, for documentation purposes. Further injury to the nerve has also been identified as a potential complication of the surgical reconstruction[11]; one must be vigilant to avoid excessive manipulation of the knee during surgical treatment.

The ligament injuries associated with the multiligament injured/dislocated knee fall into common patterns that we will discuss individually. Although knee dislocation without posterior cruciate ligament (PCL) tear[12] has been reported, this injury is rare; and bicruciate ligament tears are the norm.[13–16] The most common patterns are (1) bicruciate injuries [to the anterior cruciate ligament (ACL) and PCL], (2) bicruciate with medial side injuries [to the ACL, PCL, and medial collateral ligament (MCL)], and (3) bicruciate injuries (ACL, PCL) with lateral and posterolateral corner injuries (LCL, PLC).

General Complications

The potential of a compromised soft tissue envelope presents a major challenge in the treatment of the multiligament injured/dislocated knee. This heightens the risk of any major surgical procedure. Vascular injury, neurologic injury, compartment syndrome, fluid extravasation, and wound problems are included among the specific perioperative complications that need to be considered.

Iatrogenic Vascular Injury

In treating the polyligament injured knee with associated vascular injury, vascular repair needs to be among the first treatments rendered. The presence of a previous vascular repair must heighten the caution of the orthopaedic surgeon in dealing with these polyligament injuries. A vascular anastomosis could potentially be threatened by excessive manipulation of the knee. The vascular surgeon who performed the repair should be in the operating room or readily available at the time of ligament reconstruction, to provide the best opportunity for avoiding injury to a preexisting anastomosis.[17]

Since posterior cruciate reconstruction will often be a component of the surgeries performed in the treatment of the multiligament injured/dislocated knee, the popliteal vessels and tibial nerve need to be a focus of attention to avoid injury to these structures. Careful protection of these structures, as described by Fanelli et al.[18,19] in their technique, or by Miller and Gordon[20] in their technique, are among the several means that can be utilized to reduce the risk of injury. When performing a delayed PCL reconstruction with an arthroscopically assisted technique, we currently rely on a shielded drill guide for passage of the guide wire through the tibia. Passage of the guide wire through the tibia should be visualized directly, with the arthroscope in the posteromedial portal, or with a C-arm in the lateral view, to reduce the risk of inadvertent penetration of the popliteal space. Care must also be maintained when drilling over the guide wire; hand-drilling through the posterior tibial cortex is a strategy that may reduce the risk of penetration into the neurovascular structures.

Occlusion of the popliteal artery that is identified immediately following ligament reconstruction may, however, be due to an unrecognized subintimal tear that occurred at the time of the injury and did not result from injury at the time of surgery. Preoperative angiography may be of value in identifying such subintimal disruptions, which are potentially treated with either observation or surgical repair.[11,14,15]

Neurologic Injury

Several neurologic structures are put at risk by the extent of open incisions that may be required to repair polyligament injuries. Most frequently injured is the infrapatellar branch of the saphenous nerve, which rarely presents major problems but may cause a symptomatic neuroma or become the focus of sympathetically mediated pain.[17] The major neurologic structures around the knee, including the peroneal nerve at the posterolateral corner, the tibial nerve in close proximity to the popliteal artery and vein, and the saphenous nerve on the medial side, must be carefully preserved.

Lateral side disruptions of the knee not uncommonly result in injury to the peroneal nerve, and it is paramount to prevent further nerve damage during reconstruction of the posterolateral corner. The nerve should be identified and protected throughout surgery. Care to prevent further traction to the nerve by overaggressive manipulation of the joint has been noted and stressed by Shapiro and Freedman[11] Utilization of the biceps tendon in any part of the ligament reconstruction puts the nerve at further risk, and the fascial bands that encompass the peroneal nerve and biceps must be released.

Protection of the tibial nerve is accomplished through similar maneuvers as protection of the popliteal artery and vein. Since the tibial nerve is more superficial than the vascular structures and therefore farther away from penetrating transosseous instrumentation, it is less commonly injured at the time of surgery,

Somewhat variable in its location, the saphenous nerve typically penetrates the sartorius fascia just proximal to the knee joint. Careful retraction of the pes anserine tendons, as well as utilization of the flexed knee position during surgical exposure on the medial side of the knee, can protect this nerve in major open medial reconstructions.

Compartment Syndromes and Fluid Extravasation

Compartment syndrome of the leg is not only a major threat following revascularization of an ischemic limb but also a potential catastrophic event resulting from fluid extravasation during arthroscopy when there is a capsular disruption. Compartment syndrome has been identified in a number of situations characterized by potential for fluid escape from the joint, and extreme care needs to be maintained when the arthroscope is used in this situation.[21-25] Delaying for several weeks from initial injury to surgery may facilitate arthroscopic treatment of these injuries and thus reduce the risk of fluid-related compartment syndromes. Avoiding high pump pressures or utilizing relatively low height gravity flow may decrease the extent of fluid leakage.

Wound Problems

Avoiding narrow skin bridges by careful planning of skin incisions is crucial. High energy dislocations as well as open dislocations are major predispositions for problems in wound healing. Undue tension should be avoided during closure of the incisions. Delaying surgery for 10 days or more, as is now common prior to these major multiple ligament reconstructions, may reduce the perioperative swelling and the potential for wound breakdown.[17]

Knee-Specific Complications

Current consensus is that the nonoperative treatment of the dislocated knee leads to a less satisfactory outcome than surgical repair and/or reconstruction, particularly in the athletic population.[13-15,26-34] Nonoperative treatment leads, in the long term, to both a higher risk of laxity and decreased function. Myers and Harvey[26] have reported 81% good to excellent results in patients who had early repair of all ligamentous structures, while fewer than 10% of their patients treated without surgery had satisfactory results. Roman et al.[13] reported dramatically better results in their operatively treated group.

The major potential complication that may result from surgical repair/reconstruction of the multiple ligament injured knee is stiffness. This may range from mild limitation of motion to severe arthrofibrosis.[11,13-15,29-35] The few series that have compared operative and nonoperative treatments have strongly recommended surgical repair/reconstruction in spite of this potentially devastating complication.[2,12,28,30,35] To reduce the risk of arthrofibrosis, current research efforts in treatment of the polyligament injured knee are focused on identifying the specific injuries that can be treated with delayed surgery. Following the lead of Shelbourne[36] and Mohtadi[37] and their colleagues in the treatment of ACL injuries, some authors have suggested a short delay between the injury and reconstruction of the polyligament injured knee. Three weeks has been suggested as a time frame that will allow the early posttraumatic inflammatory process to subside prior to the second insult of major ligament reconstruction.[14,15,17,31,32] This delay may also allow adequate capsular healing, such that the arthroscope can be safely utilized in reconstruction of the cruciate ligaments. Owing to the complexity of the posterolateral corner, however, most authors recommend early direct repair with augmentation of the posterolateral structures.[17,31,32] The window of opportunity for doing this is probably 10 to 14 days, after which time secondary scarring eliminates the option of repair at the posterolateral corner. Early posterior cruciate reconstruction with no attention paid to the ACL at the time of injury is another means proposed to reduce the risk of arthrofibrosis.[16]

It has been suggested that the complex of ACL, PCL, and MCL tears may be treated with immobilization to allow the MCL to heal prior to bicruciate reconstruction, similar to the treatment schema that has been recommended for the ACL/MCL injury.[2,16] When this pattern of injury is present (ACL, PCL, MCL), the medial tibia may undergo posterior subluxation when placed in a brace. This will lead to inadequate healing of the MCL. If one is to consider nonoperative treatment of the MCL injury, to be followed by cruciate reconstruction, one must demonstrate that the tibia remains located while in the brace. A true lateral radiograph of the knee obtained within the brace can be used to assess position of the tibia in reference to the femur. If this radiograph in the brace demonstrates any rotatory subluxation of the medial tibia, or posterior subluxation of the entire tibia in the sagittal plane, brace treatment is not appropriate, and early surgical reconstruction/repair is indicated.

Arthrofibrosis

If stiffness is encountered as a complication of treatment, the likely cause is excessive scarring as a result of the injury, surgery, or immobilization. An additional etiology that must be considered is inappropriately positioned or tensioned ligament grafts. Graft location can usually be identified on true anteroposterior and lateral radiographs. If routine radiographs are inadequate to visualize tunnel or hardware placement, then MRI or computed tomography scans are reasonable choices to assess graft position. MRI has the added benefit of visualization of the soft tissues, which may also result in the identification of allowing impingement of the grafts against bony structures.

A major potential determinant for both the risks of arthrofibrosis and recurrent laxity is the timing of surgery following injury. In a number of series reporting aggressive surgical treatment (repair of all capsular structures with bicruciate reconstruction), the incidence of arthrofibrosis requiring manipulation and/or arthroscopy averaged 39% (range 29–57%); unfortunately, early-protected motion during the postoperative period in this population was not successful in reducing the risk of motion-related complications.[11,29,32,35]

Although limitation of motion may occur secondary to timing, mechanical, or rehabilitative issues with treatment, this symptom may portend the onset of primary arthrofibrosis, which can be particularly bothersome to treat. Infrapatellar contracture syndrome (IPCS) may develop in this situation.[38–40] Often IPCS presents early on, with warmth and swelling in the region of the patella tendon and fat pad. Limitation of patella mobility, especially superior glide, is the hallmark of IPCS and is also a frequent early finding. Early recognition of the peripatellar inflammation, which will often precede the development of IPCS, will allow the surgeon to develop a prompt treatment plan. A short course of high dose oral corticosteroids offers a good chance of successfully treating this early inflammatory phase and of reducing or preventing the major problems associated with a full-blown IPCS.[41,42] Nonsteroidal anti-inflammatory drugs have also been recommended.[43,44] It is the author's personal experience that corticosteroids do work better. In this early inflammatory phase, aggressive stretching, through physiotherapy or manipulation under anesthesia, seems to exacerbate the inflammation in many patients and is often counterproductive.[38,40] A paradoxical increase in scar formation can occur when abnormal fibroblasts are stretched. This may be the case in this inflammatory phase of IPCS, where aggressive stretching often aggravates the problem.[45–47] At this time the best rehabilitation program is gentle, nonforceful mobilization performed actively by the patient, with little, if any manipulation by a physiotherapist. This seems to allow a number of patients to at least stabilize, if not improve, early in the course of IPCS.

Although most of the motion restrictions that occur following surgical treatment of the dislocated knee have limitations of both flexion and extension, these are not true IPCS. Within the first 3 months after surgery, lesser restrictions of motion may be treated with manipulation alone. If 4 or more months have elapsed from the initial surgery, I favor surgical treatment, performed arthroscopically. Manipulation is not encouraged without the release of the intra-articular scar, since there is a risk of articular cartilage injury when potential adhesions to the articular surface have matured past 4 months. The surgical treatment should include scar removal, release of the fat pad from the anterior tibia and notch, freeing the quadriceps from the anterior femur, and lateral (and occasionally medial retinacular) release when patella mobility is limited.[39]

Stiffness is not limited to patients who have been treated surgically. This was also one of the problems noted by the early proponents of the nonoperative treatment, when excessive periods of immobilization resulted in major restriction of motion.[26-28] While nonoperative treatment remains an option for low demand patients, prolonged immobilization should be avoided. The older studies of nonoperative treatment suggested that less than 6 weeks of immobilization may be appropriate, because motion limitation frequently followed longer periods of cast treatment. When nonoperative treatment is selected, the availability of easily fitted braces, with adjustable motion stops, speaks for a lesser period of immobilization, with prolonged protection through limited ranges of motion.

Recurrent or Persistent Ligamentous Laxity

As early surgical treatment of the multiligament injured knee has become more frequent, persistent laxity has become less common but remains an issue.[12-14,26,28-34] The difficulty of obtaining stability of the posterior cruciate due to its complex anatomy or posterior sag as a direct result of the weight of the tibia against the graft is frequently cited as contributing to persistent laxity. An additional source of residual laxity is failure to recognize or address the collateral ligament and corner injuries. As noted earlier, the nonoperative treatment is more likely to result in inadequate stability. This may require complex late polyligament reconstruction, which has proven far less satisfactory in dealing with the posterolateral complex and medial collateral ligament than for the cruciates. A prolonged delay from injury to reconstruction, with the increased translation associated with the excess laxity, also increases the risk of injury to the articular surfaces and menisci. In Noyes and Barber-Westin's series,[35] though 75% of those being treated in the chronic situation had significant articular damage and required meniscectomy, there was no meniscal or articular cartilage damage noted in the joints treated with early surgery.

Conclusions

The treatment of the multiligament injured/dislocated knee presents the orthopaedic surgeon with the potential for many complications. The extent of the injury to the surrounding soft tissue and neurovascular structures, as well as to the ligamentous support of the knee, can lead to debilitating long-term outcomes. Attention to detail, with strict protection of the neurovascular structures, will minimize the potential risk of devastating neurovascular complications. Magnetic resonance imaging improves the identification of injured structures and should be utilized as an important diagnostic adjunct for the careful planning of surgical treatment and the timing of surgical repair/reconstruction. Stiffness remains a major potential threat with early surgical treatment of all involved ligaments.

Consideration may be given to limited early (during the first 2 weeks from injury) repairs to injuries that involve the lateral and posterolateral corners. On the medial side, one option is to allow the MCL to heal through bracing and then deal with the bicruciate injury arthroscopically. Early recognition of developing limitations of motion depends on heightened suspicion and allows appropriate treatment. Nonoperative treatment is currently reserved for special situations, such as low demand individuals or cases in which associated injuries prevent early surgical treatment. Prolonged immobilization can also result in significant restriction of motion and should be avoided.

The treatment of the multiple ligament injured knee initially depends on early recognition and treatment of all potential neurovascular complications. Complete diagnosis of all injured structures needs to be followed by careful planning of the extent and timing of surgeries. Meticulous surgery is needed to protect the neurovascular structures. Postoperative and nonoperative treatments must include carefully planned rehabilitation programs. Limitation of motion remains a complex issue that should be addressed promptly for optimal results.

References

1. Shelbourne KD, Porter DA, Clingman JA, et al. Low velocity knee dislocation. Orthop Rev 1991; 20:995–1004.
2. Cole BJ, Harner CD. The multiple ligament injured knee. Clin Sports Med 1999; 18:241–262.
3. Lonner JH, Dupuy DE, Siliski JM. Comparison of magnetic resonance imaging with operative findings in acute dislocations of the adult knee. J Orthop Trauma 2000; 14(3):183–186.
4. Twaddle BC, Hunter JC, Chapman JR, et al. MRI in acute knee dislocation: a prospective study of clinical, MRI and surgical findings. J Bone Joint Surg Br 1996; 78b:573–579.
5. Armstrong PJ, Franklin DP. Management of arterial and venous injuries in the dislocated knee. Sports Med Arthrosc Rev 2001; 9:219–226.
6. Marin EL, Bifulco SS, Fast A. Obesity: a risk factor for knee dislocation. Am J Phys Med Rehabil 1990; 69:132–134.
7. Hagino RT, DeCaprio JD, Valentine RJ, et al. Spontaneous popliteal vascular injury in the morbidly obese. J Vasc Surg 1998; 28:458–462.
8. White J. The results of traction injuries to the common peroneal nerve. J Bone Joint Surg Br 1968; 50:346–350.
9. Rorabeck CH, Kennedy JC. Tourniquet induced nerve ischemia complicating knee ligament surgery. Am J Sports Med 1980; 8:98–102.
10. Tomaino M, Day C, Papageorgiou C, et al. Peroneal nerve palsy following knee dislocation: pathoanatomy and implications for treatment. Knee Surg Sports Traumatol Arthrosc 2000; 8:163–165.
11. Shapiro MS, Freedman EL. Allograft reconstruction of the anterior and posterior cruciate ligaments after traumatic knee dislocation. Am J Sports Med 1995; 23:580–587.
12. Toritsuka Y, Horibe S, Hiro-oka A. Knee dislocation following anterior cruciate ligament disruption without any other ligament tears. Arthroscopy 1999; 15:522–526.
13. Roman PD, Hopson CN, Zenni EJ. Traumatic dislocation of the knee: a report of thirty cases and literature review. Orthop Rev 1987; 16:917–924.

14. Good L, Johnson RJ. The dislocated knee. J Am Aced Orthop Surg 1995; 3: 284–292.
15. Schenck RC, Jr. et al. Knee dislocations. Instructional Course Lect 1999; 48:515–522.
16. Shelbourne KD, Klootwyk TE. Low-velocity knee dislocations with sports injuries: treatment principles. Clin Sports Med 2000; 19:443–456.
17. Hegyes MS, Richardson MW, Miller MD. Knee dislocation: complications of nonoperative and operative management. Clin Sports Med 2000; 19:519–543.
18. Fanelli GC, Giannotti BF, Edson CJ. Arthroscopically assisted combined anterior and posterior cruciate ligament reconstruction. Arthroscopy 1996; 12:5–14.
19. Fanelli GC, Giannotti BF, Edson CJ. Arthroscopically assisted combined posterior cruciate ligament/posterior lateral complex reconstruction. Arthroscopy 1996; 12:521–530.
20. Miller MD, Gordon WT. Posterior cruciate ligament reconstruction: tibial inlay technique—principles and procedure. Oper Techniques Sports Med 1999; 7: 127–133.
21. Noyes FR, Spievack ES. Extraarticular fluid dissection in tissues during arthroscopy: a report of clinical cases and a study of intraarticular thigh pressure in cadavers. Am J Sports Med 1982; 12:1006–1011.
22. Bomberg BC, Hurley PE, Clark CA, McLaughlin CS. Complications associated with the use of an infusion pump during knee arthroscopy. Arthroscopy 1992; 8:224–228.
23. Elkman EF, Poehling GG. An experimental assessment of the risk of compartment syndrome during knee arthroscopy. Arthroscopy 1996; 12:193–199.
24. Amendola A, Faber K, Willits K, Miniaci A, Labib S, Fowler P. Compartment pressure monitoring during anterior cruciate ligament reconstruction. Arthroscopy 1999; 15:607–612.
25. Marti CB, Jakob RP. Case report: accumulation of irrigation fluid in the calf as a complication during high tibial osteotomy combined with simultaneous arthroscopic anterior cruciate ligament reconstruction. Arthroscopy 1999; 15: 864–866.
26. Myers MH, Harvey JP Jr. Traumatic dislocation of the knee joint: a study of eighteen cases. J Bone Joint Surg Am 1971; 53:16–29.
27. Taylor AR, Arden GP, Rainey HA. Traumatic dislocation of the knee: a report of forty-three cases with special reference to conservative treatment. J Bone Joint Surg Br 1972; 54:96–102.
28. Myers MH, Moore TM, Harvey JP Jr. Follow-up notes on articles previously published in the Journal: traumatic dislocation of the knee joint. J Bone Joint Surg Am 1975; 57:430–433.
29. Sisto DJ, Warren RF. Complete knee dislocation: a follow-up study of operative treatment. Orthop Clin North Am 1985; 198:94–101.
30. Montgomery TJ, Savoie FH, White JL, et al. Orthopedic management of knee dislocations. Comparison of surgical reconstruction and immobilization. Am J Knee Surg 1995; 8:97–103.
31. Wascher DC, Dvirnak PC, DeCoster TA. Knee dislocation: initial assessment and implications for treatment. J Orthop Trauma 1997; 11:525–529.
32. Wascher DC, Becker JR, Dexter JG, et al. Reconstruction of the anterior and posterior cruciate ligaments after knee dislocation. Am J Sports Med 1999; 27: 189–196.
33. Ibrahim SA. Primary repair of the cruciate and collateral ligaments after traumatic dislocation of the knee. J Bone Joint Surg Br 1999; 81:987–990.
34. Dedmond BT, Almekinders LC. Operative versus nonoperative treatment of knee dislocations: a meta-analysis. Am J Knee Surg 2001; 14:33–38.
35. Noyes FR, Barber-Westin SD. Reconstruction of the anterior and posterior ligaments after knee dislocation: use of early protected postoperative motion to decrease arthrofibrosis. Am J Sports Med 1997; 25:769–778.
36. Shelbourne KD, Wilckens JH, Mollabashy A, et al. Arthrofibrosis in acute anterior cruciate ligament reconstruction. The effect of timing of reconstruction and rehabilitation. Am J Sports Med 1991; 19:332–336.
37. Mohtadi NGH, Webster-Bogaert S, Fowler PJ. Limitation of motion following anterior cruciate ligament reconstruction. A case-control study. Am J Sports Med 1991; 19:620–625.

38. Paulos LE, Rosenberg TD, Drawbert J, et al. Infrapatellar contracture syndrome. An unrecognized cause of knee stiffness with patella entrapment and patella infera. Am J Sports Med 1987; 15:331–341.
39. Richmond JC, Assal MA. Arthroscopic management of arthrofibrosis of the knee, including infrapatellar contraction syndrome. Arthroscopy 1991; 7: 144–147.
40. Paulos LE, Wnorowski DC, Greenwald AE. Infrapatellar contracture syndrome diagnosis, treatment, and long-term follow-up. Am J Sports Med 1994; 22: 440–449.
41. Vargas JH, Ross DG. Corticosteroids and anterior cruciate ligament repair. Am J Sports Med 1989; 17:532–534.
42. Highgenboten CL, Jackson AW, Meske NB. Arthroscopy of the knee. Ten-day pain profiles and corticosteroids. Am J Sports Med 1993; 21:503–506.
43. Nelson WE, Henderson RC, Almekinders LC, et al. An evaluation of pre- and postoperative nonsteroidal anti-inflammatory drugs in patients undergoing knee arthroscopy. A prospective, randomized, double-blind study. Am J Sports Med 1993; 21:510–516.
44. Rasmussen S, Thomsen S, Madsen SN, et al. The clinical effect of naproxen sodium after arthroscopy of the knee. A randomized, double-blind, prospective study. Arthroscopy 1993; 9:375–380.
45. Alman BA, Nabor SP, Terek RM, et al. Platelet-derived growth factor in fibrous musculoskeletal disorders: a study of pathologic tissue sections and primary cell cultures. J Orthop Res 1995; 13:66–77.
46. Richmond JC, Alman BA, Pojerski M. Growth factor expression in arthrofibrosis. Arthroscopy 1996; 12:352–353.
47. von Deck MD, Richmond JC, Alman BA. Arthrofibrosis: a potential treatment based on growth factor manipulation. Arthroscopy 1997; 13:393–394.

Chapter Sixteen

Revision Surgery

Gregory C. Fanelli

Revision surgery in the multiple ligament injured knee is a complex procedure, and to the best of our knowledge, at the time of writing, there is nothing published on this topic, although several authors have presented their work at various meetings.[1-3] Principles for revision surgery in the multiple ligament injured knee are extrapolated from the literature on anterior cruciate ligament (ACL) reconstruction revision surgery and posterior cruciate ligament (PCL) reconstruction surgery.[4-12] This chapter presents our methods for evaluation and treatment of failed surgery in the multiple ligament injured knee.

Surgery in the multiple ligament injured knee may be labeled "unsuccessful" because of motion loss, extensor mechanism dysfunction, posttraumatic arthrosis, recurrent patholaxity, or any combination of these. Causes of failed multiple ligament knee surgery include technical errors, iatrogenic factors, biomechanical factors, associated structural injuries, postsurgical reinjury, and infection.

Causes of Failed Surgery

Technical Errors

Inadequate notchplasty may lead to graft impingement of the anterior cruciate ligament reconstruction with attenuation and subsequent graft failure. Improper tunnel placement can lead to excessive graft forces, graft impingement, and loss of motion, resulting in a captured knee that adversely affects the outcome of cruciate and collateral ligament reconstructions. Improper graft tensioning, whether too tight or too loose, can also lead to failure of both cruciate and collateral ligament surgeries.

Inadequate graft fixation will allow the position of the graft to change prior to biologic incorporation, resulting in patholaxity. Improper (i.e., too vigorous) postoperative rehabilitation can lead to overstressing the surgical procedure and subsequent reinjury, while inadequate rehabilitation can lead to loss-of-motion problems.

Biomechanical Factors

Biomechanical characteristics of the graft material will affect the outcome in multiple ligament knee reconstructive surgery. Graft strength is proportional to the cross-sectional area of the graft, so a larger graft will be stronger. Irradiation of allograft tissue may affect allograft strength, depending on the radiation dose, and can ultimately affect the surgical outcome. Synthetic graft material may have a place in reconstruction of the multiple ligament injured knee; however, the success of the operation is highly dependent on the synthetic material and the surgical technique.[13]

Associated Structural Injuries

Failure to recognize and treat associated structural injuries has been identified as a cause of failure in ACL reconstructions, PCL reconstructions, and reconstructions in the multiple ligament injured knee.[6–12] Associated structural injuries that if left untreated will compromise surgical results include the following:

1. Varus or valgus knee with a lateral or medial thrusting gait, respectively
2. Unrecognized and untreated medial side, and/or posterolateral–lateral side injuries
3. Severe meniscus pathology
4. Articular cartilage injury
5. Unstable patellofemoral joint or compromised extensor mechanism

Postreconstruction Trauma

Postreconstruction trauma can cause failure of surgical reconstruction in the multiple ligament injured knee. Overaggressive rehabilitation that stresses the fixation of grafts beyond the capabilities of the initial mechanical fixation and before biologic incorporation has occurred can cause surgical reconstruction failure. A high force reinjury in the postoperative period (early or late) may cause graft failure. Chronic repetitive microtrauma occurring in the ACL and PCL grafts owing to failure to recognize and treat associated ligament instability will lead to excess forces in the grafts and cause graft attentuation and the development of progressive laxity over time.

Infection

Infection can occur as a superficial or deep infection. This includes cellulitis, septic arthritis, localized infection around hardware external to the joint, and osteomyelitis. All these processes may cause graft failure directly by destroying the graft material, or they may necessitate graft removal to treat the infection. Sterile abscess formation may occur in response to allograft tissue, synthetic graft material, or various fixation devices that have adversely affected the surgical outcome.

Revision Surgery

Surgical Indications

The main reason patients present to our clinic for revision multiple ligament knee surgery is functional instability of the involved knee in sports, work, and the activities of daily living. These knees have increased anterior and/or posterior laxity on physical examination, arthrometer testing, and stress radiography. A patient's chief complaint may be instability, pain, or both.

Preoperative Evaluation

Preoperative evaluation of the multiple ligament injured knee requiring revision surgery includes history and physical examination, imaging studies, and instrumented measurement. It is important to determine the patient's chief complaint, which may be instability, pain, or both. Assessment of the previous surgical procedure is essential with respect to graft source, surgical technique, and associated pathology. Did the previous surgical procedure use autograft, allograft, or synthetic material as the graft source? What was the associated pathology at the time of the original procedure, and how was the associated pathology addressed? Were the menisci intact, repaired, or resected? What was the condition of the articular cartilage, and how was any damage to this tissue addressed? What is the condition of the extensor mechanism? The patellofemoral joint? Is there patellofemoral joint instability, anterior knee pain, or both? Assessment of range of motion and strength is important, as well as gait analysis to evaluate for varus or valgus thrust during ambulation.

Radiographic evaluation includes 30° anterior–posterior axial x-ray of the patellofemoral joint to assess for alignment, subluxation, and arthrosis. Standing anterior–posterior tibiofemoral radiographs are used to assess lower extremity alignment and tibiofemoral arthrosis, and 45° posterior–anterior flexed tibiofemoral radiographs of both knees are used to evaluate for occult tibiofemoral degenerative joint disease. Lateral and intercondylar notch radiographs are used to complement the other x-ray views in the evaluation of tunnel position and size, the degree of arthrosis, and hardware position, type, and size.

Specialized studies that may be used include stress radiography to evaluate displacement, magnetic resonance imaging (MRI) for bone bruises and meniscus pathology, bone scan to detect early arthrosis, and computer tomography for the evaluation of tunnel expansion, synovial fluid analysis, and strength evaluation.

Technical Considerations

The goal of revision surgery in the multiple ligament injured knee is restoration of functional stability for the patient's desired level of activity. These complex revision surgical procedures may be accomplished as a single-stage operation or as staged surgical procedures depending on the complexity of the individual case. Staged surgical procedures may be considered when range-of-motion restoration is required, in the presence of bone grafting for bony deficiency, when tibial or femoral osteotomies are needed, and for meniscus transplantation and articular surface grafting procedures.

Graft Sources

Graft materials used for revision surgery in the multiple ligament injured knee include autograft, allograft, and synthetic materials. The ideal graft material is strong, available, and easy to pass and secure with the appropriate fixation devices; it has little or no donor site morbidity. Our preferred graft materials for revision surgery in the multiple ligament injured knee are as follows: allograft tissue for the cruciate ligaments, allograft or autograft tissue for the lateral and medial side reconstructions, and combinations of autograft and allograft tissue as required for individual patients. The graft material used in the preceding surgical reconstruction affects the type of graft material employed in the revision surgery (Figure 16.1).

Fig. 16.1. Our preferred graft material for revision surgery in the multiple ligament injured knee is allograft tissue. The Achilles tendon allograft is particularly useful because the material is strong, easy to pass, and easy to fix, and the calcaneal bone plug can be used to graft bony defects.

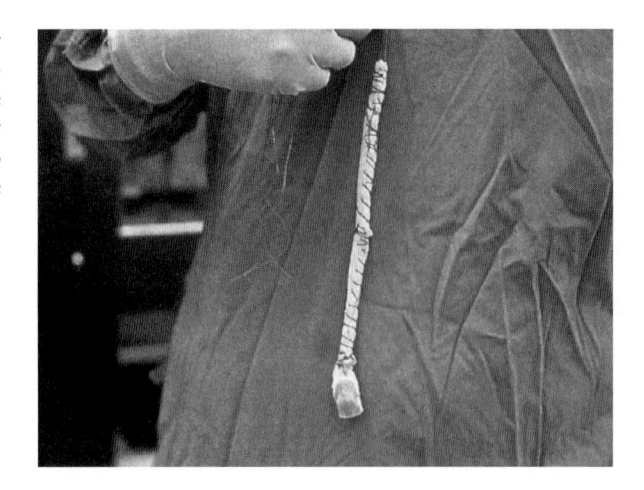

Hardware Removal

Hardware removal during revision surgery of the multiple ligament injured knee can be very difficult. The primary strategy is maximum preservation of bone stock, and a staged procedure with hardware removal and bone grafting, followed by revision reconstructive surgery at a later time, is sometimes necessary. The old hardware may be left in place when it does not interfere with the revision reconstructive procedure (Figure 16.2). Special equipment is needed for the removal of metal implant (Figure 16.3). Bioabsorbable fixation devices are technically easier to remove or drill through; if however, osteolysis has occurred, staged bone grafting procedures will be required. Prosthetic ligament removal may be difficult and will often require staged procedures that include prosthetic ligament removal, arthroscopic synovectomy and joint debridement, and bone grafting, followed at a later date by multiple ligament reconstruction (Figure 16.4).

Fig. 16.2. Metallic hardware (A, B) may be difficult to remove from a failed synthetic reconstruction of a multiple ligament injured knee, and special equipment may be necessary. Preservation of maximum bone stock is essential in these complex cases. (X-ray films courtesy of Don Johnson, MD, Ottawa, Ontario, Canada.)

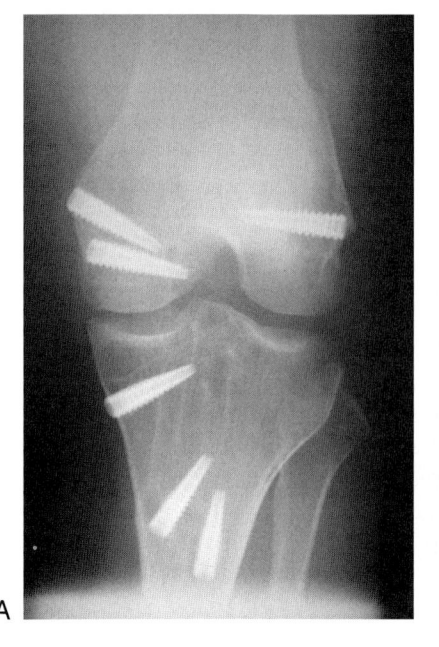

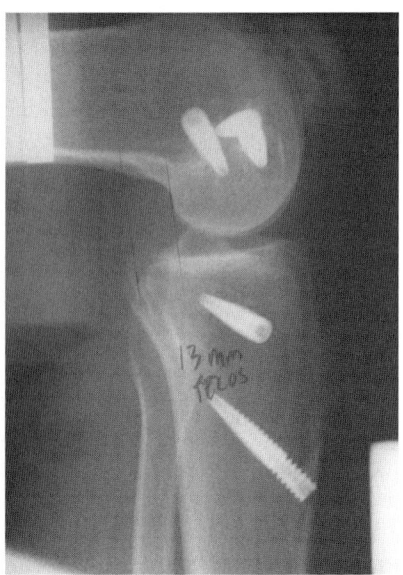

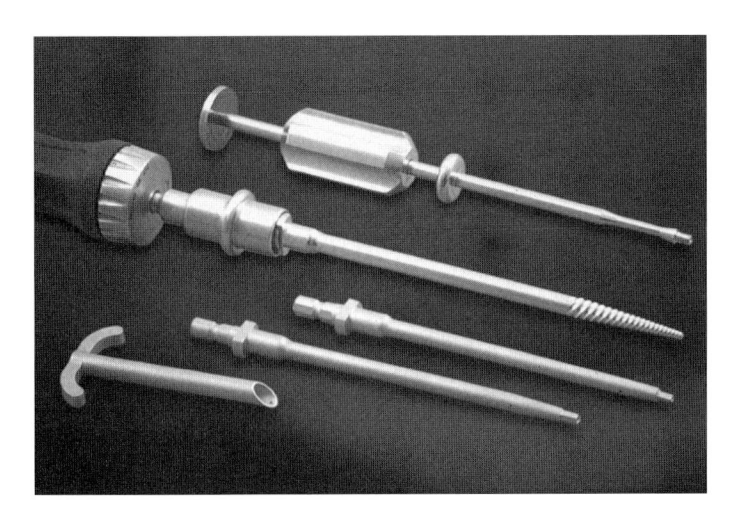

Fig. 16.3. Arthrotek revision PCL-ACL instruments. Multiple hexagonal driver sizes, an "easy out," a slap hammer, and a cannulated delivery system facilitate hardware removal. (Photograph courtesy of Arthrotek, Inc., Warsaw, IN, used with permission.)

Operative Technique

Revision multiple knee ligament surgery includes the following steps, which may be done in a single stage, or in two staged procedures, depending on the individual:

Clearly defining the pathology
Preoperative planning
Hardware removal
Bone grafting if necessary
Osteotomy if necessary
Meniscus surgery
Notchplasty
Tunnel creation
Graft passage
Graft tensioning
Graft fixation
Associated ligament surgery
Associated articular surface surgery

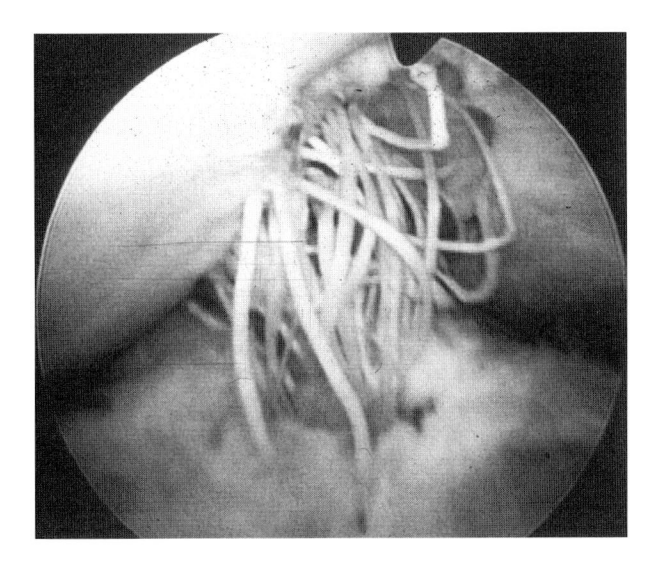

Fig. 16.4. Failed synthetic ligament used for the ACL reconstruction in a multiple ligament injured knee. Osteolysis required bone grafting of the defects after extensive debridement of the synthetic material.

Defining the pathology calls for history, physical examination, imaging studies, arthrometer measurements, stress radiographs, gait analysis, and possibly diagnostic arthroscopy. This preoperative evaluation enables the creation of the surgical plan. Skin condition is assessed for the position of previous incisions, taking care to leave adequate skin bridges between old and new incisions. If indicated, hardware removal, bone grafting, osteotomy, and meniscus transplant surgery may be performed at this time as part of a staged procedure.

The ideal graft material is strong, and provides secure fixation; it is easy to pass, readily available, and has low donor site morbidity. The available options in the United States are autograft and allograft sources. Our preferred graft for posterior cruciate ligament revision reconstruction is the Achilles tendon allograft because of its large cross-sectional area and strength, absence of donor site morbidity, and easy passage with secure fixation (Figure 16.1). We also prefer Achilles tendon allograft for revision ACL reconstruction. The preferred graft material for the revision posterolateral corner reconstruction is a split or complete biceps tendon transfer, or free autograft or allograft tissue combined with posterolateral capsular shift, depending on how the primary posterolateral repair or reconstruction was performed. Revision medial side reconstruction is performed with Achilles tendon or other allograft tissue, capsular shift procedures, or a combination of both procedures depending on the surgical technique used for the primary repair or reconstruction.

Notchplasty is performed to prevent graft impingement and to allow good visualization of the over-the-top position for anterior cruciate ligament femoral tunnel placement, as well as for posterior capsular elevation in preparation for posterior cruciate ligament surgery.

Bone tunnels are created around existing bone tunnels, if possible, but are bone-grafted if necessary because of potential tunnel overlap. This may require a staged surgical procedure. Alternate techniques for tunnel creation (e.g., over-the-top positioning of the ACL graft during revision of the ACL; the tibial inlay technique for revision PCL reconstruction following failure of a transtibial tunnel technique) may need to be used, depending on the index procedure.

Associated ligament reconstructions are performed after revision of the ACL and PCL reconstructions. The collateral ligament surgeries may address previously untreated collateral ligament injuries, failed collateral ligament reconstructions, or failed primary repair. Careful physical examination is required for clear delineation of the type and degree of the collateral ligament instability present.

Revision ACL-PCL Reconstruction

This section describes our technique for reconstruction of the multiple ligament injured knee and our utilization of that technique in revision ACL-PCL reconstruction.[14-20]

Operative Technique

The patient is positioned supine on the operating room table. The surgical leg hangs over the side of the operating table, and the well leg is supported by the fully extended table. A lateral post is used for control of the surgical leg (Figure 16.5). We do not use a leg holder. The surgery may be done

16. Revision Surgery

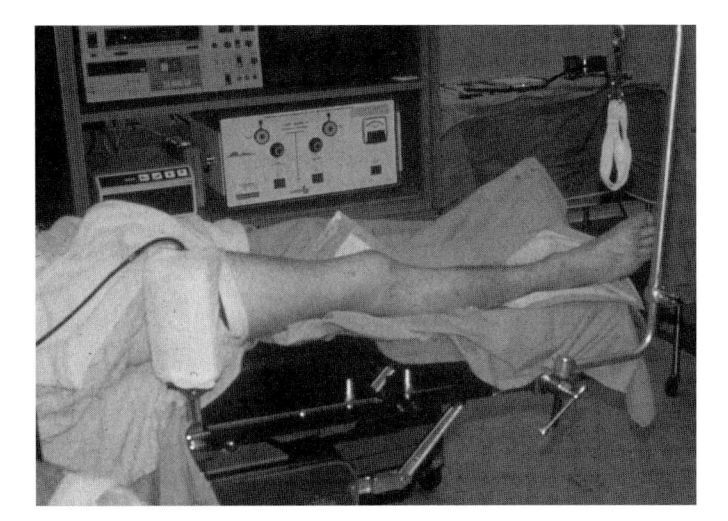

Fig. 16.5. Patient is positioned supine on the operating table with the non-surgical leg resting on the fully extended operating table. A lateral post is used for control of the surgical lower extremity.

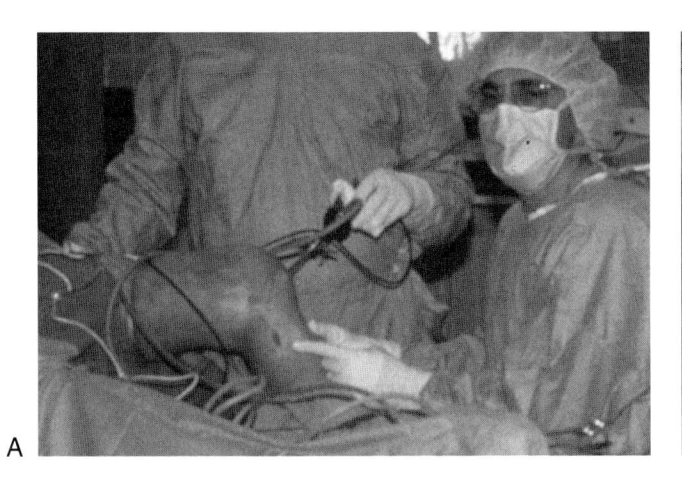

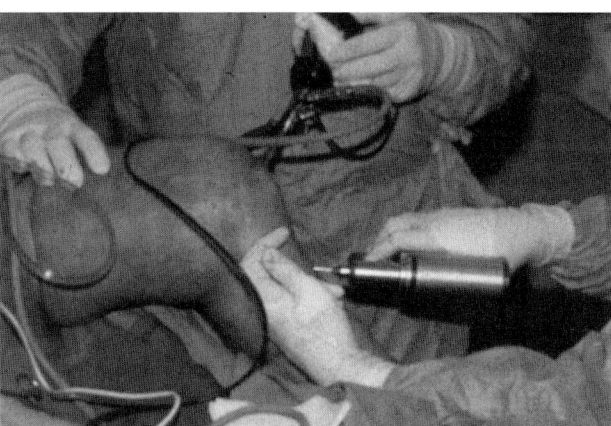

Fig. 16.6. A 1 to 2 cm extracapsular extra-articular posterior medial safety incision allows the surgeon's fingers to protect the neurovascular structures (B) and to confirm the position of instruments on the posterior aspect of the proximal tibia (A).

under tourniquet control, and fluid inflow is by gravity. We do not routinely use an arthroscopic fluid pump.

Arthroscopic instruments are placed with the inflow in the superior lateral patellar portal, arthroscope in the inferior lateral patellar portal, and instruments in the inferior medial patellar portal. Instruments are interchanged between portals as necessary. An accessory extracapsular extra-articular posteromedial safety incision is used to protect the neurovascular structures and to confirm the accuracy of tibial tunnel placement (Figure 16.6).

The notchplasty is performed first and consists of ACL and PCL failed graft debridement, bone removal, and contouring of the medial wall of the lateral femoral condyle and the intercondylar roof. This allows visualization of the over-the-top position and prevents ACL graft impingement throughout the full range of motion. Specially curved PCL instruments (Arthrotek) are used to elevate the capsule from the posterior aspect of the tibia (Figure 16.7).

The PCL tibial and femoral tunnels are created with the help of the Fanelli PCL/ACL drill guide (Arthrotek) (Figure 16.8). Two techniques are currently available to create the point of insertion of the posterior cruciate ligament graft on the tibia: the transtibial tunnel technique and the tibial inlay technique. The technique employed depends on the technique that was used in

Fig. 16.7. Specially curved PCL reconstruction instruments used to elevate the capsule from the posterior aspect of the tibial ridge during PCL reconstruction. Posterior capsular elevation is critical in transtibial PCL reconstruction because it facilitates accurate PCL tibial tunnel placement and subsequent graft passage. (Photograph courtesy of Arthrotek, Inc., Warsaw, IN, used with permission.)

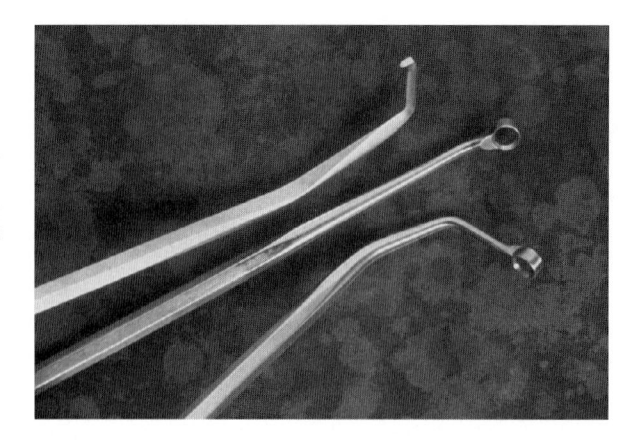

the primary reconstruction, the position of the existing tunnels, and the condition of the proximal tibial bone stock. Large amounts of osteolysis and bone resorption require a staged procedure of bone grafting followed later with PCL reconstruction. Correctly placed tibial tunnels with good bone stock can use the same tunnel for revision surgery, provided metallic hardware can be easily removed. Poorly placed tibial tunnels that are far from the PCL anatomic insertion sites may be treated by drilling new tunnels in the appropriate place. Poorly placed tibial tunnels not far from the correct placement, or well-placed tunnels with questionable bone stock, are best treated by using the tibial inlay method of PCL reconstruction.[21]

The transtibial PCL tunnel is drilled from the anteromedial aspect of the proximal tibia 1 cm below the tibial tubercle to exit in the inferior lateral aspect of the PCL anatomic insertion site. This provides a relatively vertically oriented PCL tunnel and minimizes acute angle graft bending around the back of the proximal tunnel, eliminating the killer turn. The extracapsular extra-articular posteromedial safety incision protects the neurovascular structures.[14–17,22–24]

When it is not possible to use the transtibial tunnel technique, the tibial inlay technique is employed.[21] The patient is positioned in the lateral position with the surgical extremity draped free. A posterior medial surgical approach is used, proceeding in the interval between the medial hamstring and medial head of the gastrocnemius muscles. The medial head of the gas-

Fig. 16.8. The PCL/ACL drill guide system is used to precisely create both the PCL femoral and tibial tunnels and the ACL tunnels made by the single- and double-incision techniques. To use the system, the drill guide is positioned for the PCL tibial tunnel so that a guide wire enters the anteromedial aspect of the proximal tibia approximately 1 cm below the tibial tubercle, at a point midway between the posteromedial border of the tibia and the tibial crest anteriorly. The guide wire exits in the inferior lateral aspect of the PCL tibial anatomic insertion site. The guide is positioned for the PCL femoral tunnel so the guide wire enters the medial aspect of the medial femoral condyle midway between the medial femoral condyle articular margin and the medial epicondyle, 2 cm proximal to the medial femoral condyle distal articular surface (joint line). The guide wire exits through the center of the stump of the anterolateral bundle of the posterior cruciate ligament. The drill guide is positioned for the single-incision endoscopic ACL technique so that the guide wire enters the anteromedial surface of the proximal tibia approximately 1 cm proximal to the tibial tubercle at a point midway between the posteromedial border of the tibia and the tibial crest anteriorly. The guide wire exits through the center of the stump of the tibial ACL insertion. (Photograph courtesy of Arthrotek, Inc., Warsaw, IN, used with permission.)

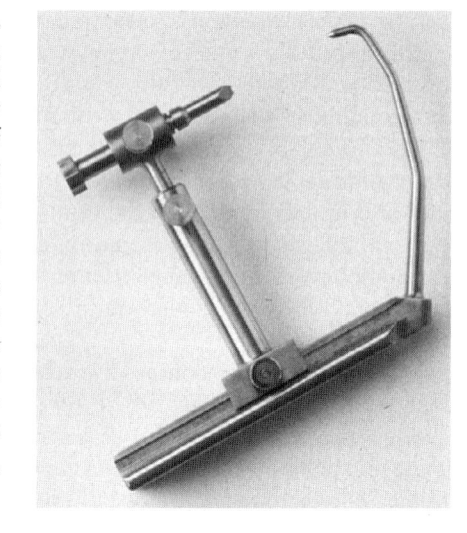

trocnemius muscle is retracted medially, exposing the posterior proximal tibia and protecting the neurovascular structures. A posterior capsulotomy is made for graft passage, and a trough is made in the posterior aspect of the proximal tibia to inlay and secure the PCL graft with screw-and-washer technique.[21]

Options available for revision of the PCL femoral tunnel include using staged bone grafting for large cavitating osteolytic lesions and for tunnels that just miss being well placed, followed by PCL reconstruction; reusing a well-placed existing femoral tunnel; and drilling a new femoral tunnel around a very poorly placed femoral tunnel. The femoral tunnel may be drilled from outside in, or from inside out, which may slightly alter the tunnel angle in the medial femoral condyle and route the tunnel to avoid poor quality distal femoral bone stock.

The outside-in PCL femoral tunnel originates externally between the medial femoral epicondyle and the medial femoral condylar articular surface approximately 2 cm proximal to the distal medial femoral condyle articular surface, emerging through the center of the stump of the anterolateral bundle of the posterior cruciate ligament. This external position of the femoral tunnel minimizes the chance of avascular necrosis or subchondral fracture of the medial femoral condyle.[7,9–12] The inside-out femoral tunnel is created through a low anterolateral patellar arthroscopic portal by drilling a guide wire through the center of the anatomic insertion of the anterolateral bundle of the posterior cruciate ligament. An endoscopic reamer is used to create the femoral tunnel. Either method, or a combination of both, may be utilized for both single- and double-bundle techniques.

The same principles of staged bone grafting of large osteolytic lesions of the ACL tibial and femoral tunnels, almost well-placed tunnels, and very poorly placed tunnels apply to revision ACL reconstruction. The ACL tunnels are created using the single-incision technique.[18–20] The tibial tunnel begins externally at a point 1 cm proximal to the tibial tubercle on the anteromedial surface of the proximal tibia to emerge through the center of the stump of the ACL tibial footprint. The femoral tunnel is positioned next to the over-the-top position on the medial wall of the lateral femoral condyle near the ACL anatomic insertion site. The tunnel is created to leave a 1 to 2 mm posterior cortical wall, which will permit interference fixation.

Revision ACL-PCL Reconstruction Graft Fixation

Graft fixation is enhanced by using primary and backup fixation. Our methods of fixation are primary aperture opening fixation with bioabsorbable interference screws and backup fixation that consists of screw and spiked ligament washer, post and washer, or ligament fixation buttons (Figure 16.9). It is essential in revision ACL-PCL reconstruction surgery to ensure secure fixation of each graft that may involve several different methods not routinely used by the surgeon for primary reconstructions. Poor bone quality and decreased biologic healing capabilities may necessitate creative graft fixation methods.

Revision Posterolateral Reconstruction Operative Technique

For posterolateral reconstruction, we use the split and full biceps tendon transfer to the lateral femoral epicondyle and the allograft or autograft figure-of-eight techniques.[25–28] The requirements for the biceps tendon procedures include an intact proximal tibiofibular joint, intact posterolateral capsular attachments to the common biceps tendon, and intact biceps femoris tendon insertion into the fibular head. These techniques reproduce the function of the popliteofibular and lateral collateral ligaments, tighten the posterolateral capsule, and provide a post of strong autogenous tissue to reinforce the posterolateral corner.

A lateral hockey stick incision is made.[25,27,29] The peroneal nerve is dissected free and protected throughout the procedure. The long head and the common biceps femoris tendon are isolated, and the anterior two-thirds is separated from the short head muscle. The tendon is detached proximal and left attached distally to its anatomic insertion site on the fibular head. The strip of biceps tendon is approximately 12 to 14 cm long. The iliotibial band is incised in line with its fibers, and the fibular collateral ligament and popliteus tendon are exposed. A drill hole is made 1 cm anterior to the fibular collateral ligament femoral insertion. A longitudinal incision is made in the lateral capsule just posterior to the fibular collateral ligament. The split biceps tendon is passed medial to the iliotibial band and secured to the lateral femoral epicondylar region with a screw and spiked ligament washer at the above-mentioned point. The residual tail of the transferred split biceps tendon is passed medial to the iliotibial band and secured to the fibular head. The posterolateral capsule that had been incised earlier is then shifted and sewn into the strut of transferred biceps tendon to eliminate posterolateral capsular redundancy. If the proximal tibiofibular joint has been disrupted, a two-tailed allograft reconstruction is utilized to control the tibia and fibula independently.[30]

Posterolateral reconstruction with the free graft figure-of-eight technique utilizes semitendinosus autograft or allograft, Achilles tendon allograft, or other soft tissue allograft or autograft material. A curvilinear incision is made in the lateral aspect of the knee extending from the lateral femoral epicondyle to the interval between Gerdy's tubercle and the fibular head. The fibular head is exposed, and a tunnel is created in an anterior-to-posterior direction at the area of maximal fibular diameter. The tunnel is created by passing a guide pin followed by a cannulated drill, usually 7 mm in diameter. The peroneal nerve is protected during tunnel creation and

Fig. 16.9. (A) Anteroposterior and (B) lateral radiographs status after revision ACL-PCL-posterolateral reconstruction. Primary aperture opening fixation is achieved with bioabsorbable interference screws, and backup fixation is achieved with ligament fixation buttons, and/or screw and washer devices.

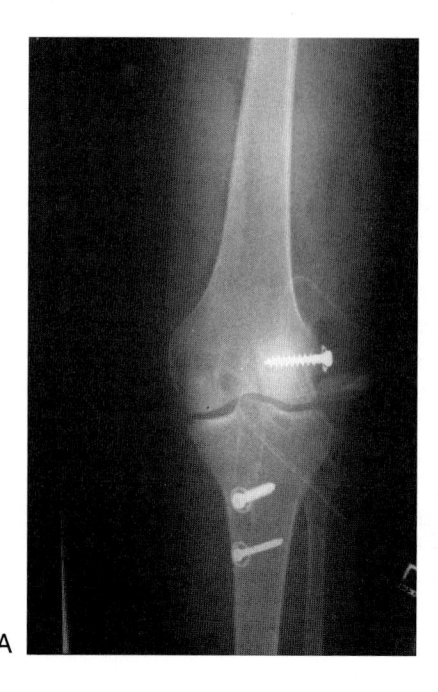

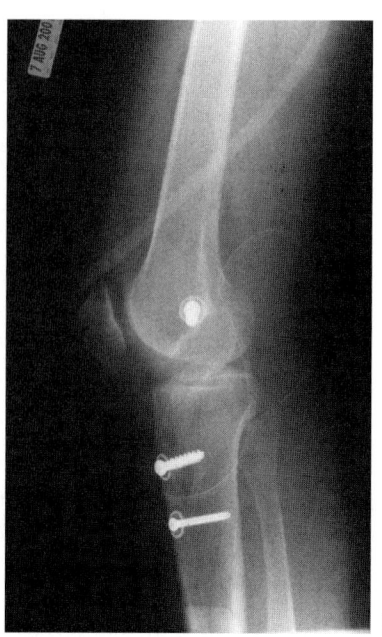

16. Revision Surgery

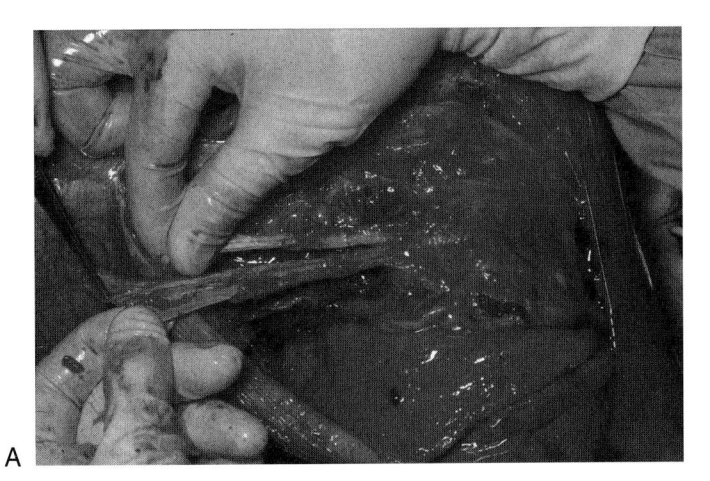

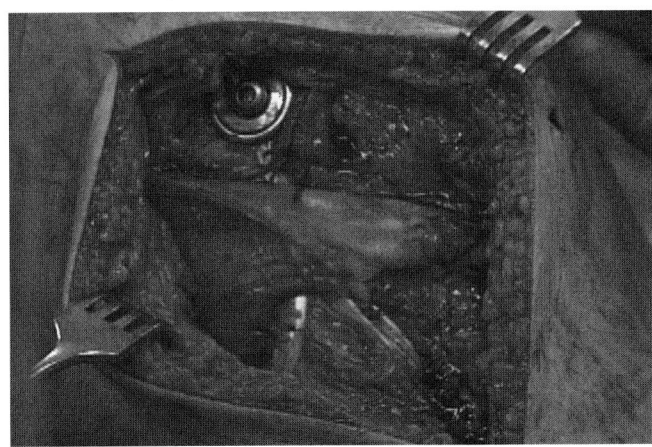

Fig. 16.10 A and B. Our preferred surgical technique for posterolateral and lateral reconstruction is the split biceps tendon transfer (A) or the allograft or autograft figure-of-eight reconstruction (B) combined with posterolateral capsular shift and primary repair of injured structures as indicated. These complex surgical procedures reproduce the function of the popliteofibular ligament and the lateral collateral ligament and eliminate posterolateral capsular redundancy. The split biceps tendon transfer utilizes anatomic insertion sites and preserves the dynamic function of the long head and common biceps femoris tendon.

throughout the procedure. The free tendon graft is then passed through the fibular head drill hole. An incision is then made in the iliotibial band in line with the fibers directly overlying the lateral femoral epicondyle. The graft material is passed medial to the iliotibial band, and the limbs of the graft are crossed to form a figure-of-eight. A drill hole is made 1 cm anterior to the fibular collateral ligament femoral insertion. A longitudinal incision is made in the lateral capsule just posterior to the fibular collateral ligament. The graft material is passed medial to the iliotibial band and secured to the lateral femoral epicondylar region with a screw and spiked ligament washer at the above-mentioned point. The posterolateral capsule that had been incised is then shifted and sewn into the strut of figure-of-eight graft tissue material to eliminate posterolateral capsular redundancy. The anterior and posterior limbs of the figure-of-eight graft material are sewn to each other to reinforce and tighten the construct (Figure 16.10; see color plate). The iliotibial band incision is closed. The procedures described are intended to eliminate posterolateral and varus rotational instability.

The particular surgical technique utilized for revision posterolateral reconstruction depends on the surgical procedure employed for the primary repair or reconstruction, on bone quality, and on available local autogenous soft tissue. Methods of fixation may vary depending on bone quality, and a combination of fixation methods may be necessary. It is our opinion that all lateral and posterolateral revision reconstruction requires allograft or autograft augmentation and not just primary repair.

Revision Medial Reconstruction Operative Technique

Posteromedial and medial reconstructions are performed through a medial hockey stick incision. Care is taken to maintain adequate skin bridges between incisions. The superficial medial collateral ligament (MCL) is exposed, and a longitudinal incision is made just posterior to the posterior border of the MCL. Care is taken not to damage the medial meniscus during the capsular incision. The interval between the posteromedial capsule and the medial meniscus is developed. The posteromedial capsule is shifted anterosuperiorly. The medial meniscus is repaired to the new capsular position, and the shifted capsule is sewn into the medial collateral ligament. Superficial MCL reconstruction is performed with allograft or autograft tissue. This graft material is attached at the anatomic insertion sites of the superficial medial collateral ligament on the femur and tibia. The posteromedial capsular advancement is performed and sewn into the newly reconstructed MCL (Figure 16.11; see color plate).

The particular surgical technique utilized for revision medial side reconstruction depends on the surgical procedure employed for the primary repair or reconstruction, bone quality, and available local autogenous soft tissue. Methods of fixation may vary depending on bone quality, and a combination of fixation methods may be necessary.

Graft Tensioning and Fixation

The PCL is reconstructed first, followed by the ACL, followed by the posterolateral complex and the medial ligament complex. Tension is placed on the PCL graft distally using the Arthrotek knee ligament tensioning device (Figure 16.12; see color plate). This restores the anatomic tibial step-off. The knee is cycled through a full range of motion 25 times to allow pretensioning and settling of the graft. After the knee has been placed in 0 or 70° of flexion, fixation is achieved on the tibial side of the PCL graft with a bioabsorable interference screw, and backup fixation is ensured with a screw and spiked ligament washer. The Arthrotek knee ligament tensioning device is applied to the ACL graft. The knee is placed in 0 or 70° of flexion (the same position the PCL graft was tensioned in), and final fixation of the ACL graft is achieved with a bioabsorbable interference screw, and spiked ligament washer or button backup fixation. The knee is then placed in 30° of flexion, the tibial internally rotated; slight valgus force applied to the knee, and final tensioning and fixation of the posterolateral corner is achieved. The MCL reconstruction is tensioned with the knee in 30° of flexion with the leg in a figure-four position. Full range of motion is confirmed on the operating table to ensure that the knee has not been "captured" by the reconstruction.

Technical Hints for Operative Technique

The posteromedial safety incision protects the neurovascular structures, confirms accurate tibial tunnel placement, and allows the surgery to proceed at an accelerated pace. The single-incision ACL reconstruction technique prevents lateral cortex crowding and eliminates multiple through-and-through drill holes in the distal femur, reducing stress riser effect. It is important to be aware of the two tibial tunnel directions and to have a 1 cm bone

Fig. 16.11. The Achilles tendon allograft's broad anatomy can anatomically reconstruct the superficial medial collateral ligament. Screws and spiked ligament washers are used to secure the Achilles tendon allograft to the anatomic insertion sites of the superficial MCL. The posteromedial capsule can then be secured to the Achilles tendon allograft to eliminate posteromedial capsular laxity. This technique will address all components of the medial side instability. (See color plate.)

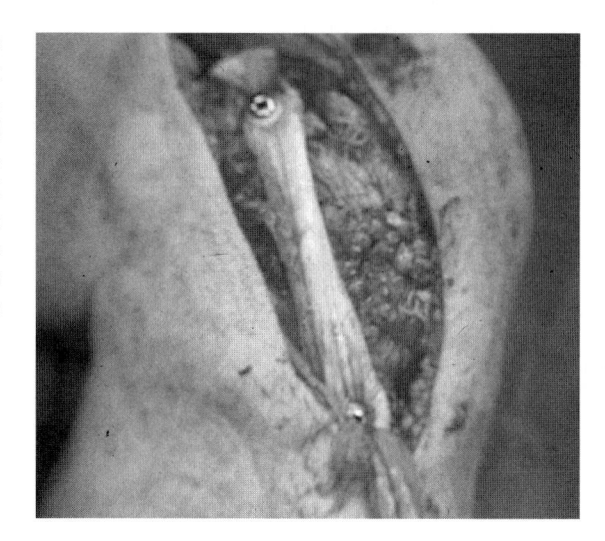

16. Revision Surgery

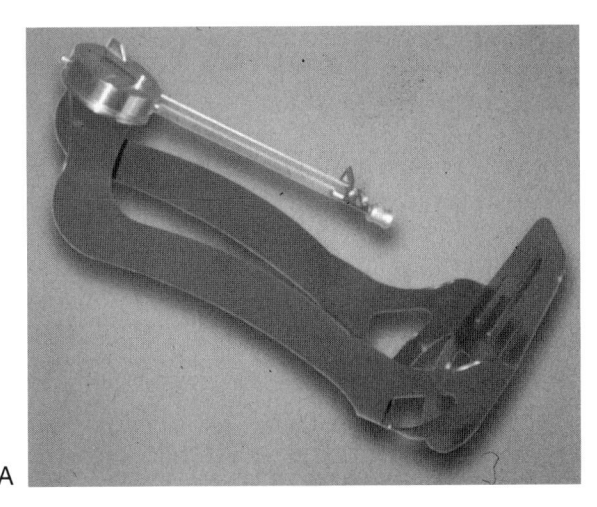

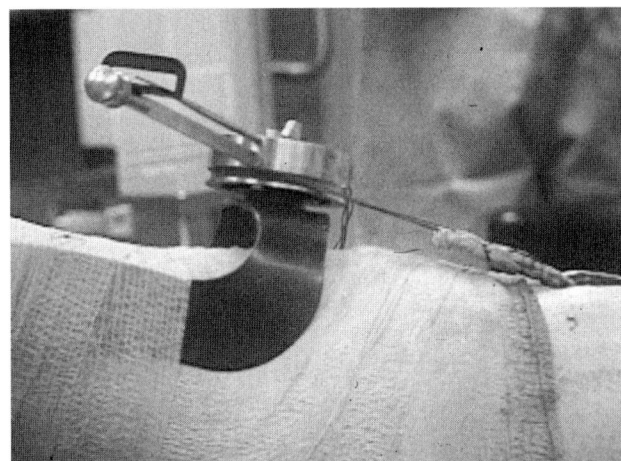

bridge between the PCL and ACL tibial tunnels. This will reduce the possibility of fracture. We have found it useful to use primary and backup fixation. Primary fixation is anchored with bioabsorbable interference screws, and backup fixation is performed with a screw and spiked ligament washer. Secure fixation is critical to the success of this surgical procedure.

Certain chronic multiple ligament injured knees may present with varus deformity combined with a lateral thrust. This may result from the ligament injury alone, or a combination of the ligament injury and a malunited tibial plateau fracture. These injuries require a high tibial osteotomy to correct bony malalignment prior to ligament reconstruction. The correction of the bony malalignment will eliminate the varus thrust and improve the chance of successful ligament surgical reconstruction (Figure 16.13). At times revision multiple knee ligament reconstruction may require meniscus transplant surgery and/or osteochondral grafting procedures as outlined earlier.

Postoperative Rehabilitation

Rehabilitation following multiple ligament reconstruction is an evolving process, with principles based on existing knowledge and scientific rationale.[17] Rehabilitation guidelines consider operative technique and the natural alignment of the lower extremity. Postoperative weeks 1 to 6 comprise the maximum protection phase. During this period, the patient is non–weight bearing, and the surgical extremity is braced in full extension. During postoperative weeks 4 to 6, range of motion is progressed. In postoperative weeks 7 to 10, the rehabilitation brace is unlocked, and during this period progressive weight bearing is progressed at 25% of body weight per week. The patient is fully weight bearing with crutches at the end of postoperative week 10. Varus and/or valgus forces are avoided during range-of-motion exercises to protect the collateral ligaments that have been reconstructed. The long-leg rehabilitation brace is discontinued at the end of postoperative week 10, and an ACL-PCL functional brace is used for activities of daily living for continued protection. Range-of-motion exercises are progressed using stationary bicycle, and closed chain exercises are performed with stair stepping machines, rowing machines, leg press, and elliptical trainers. Proprioceptive skill training is advanced. Straight-line jogging is initiated between postoperative months 4 and 5 depending on the patient's strength and proprioceptive skill level.

Fig. 16.12. The mechanical graft knee ligament tensioning device (A) is used as in (B) to precisely tension PCL and ACL grafts. During PCL reconstruction, the tensioning device is attached to the tibial end of the graft and the torque wrench ratchet is set to 20 lb to restore the anatomic tibial step-off. The knee is cycled through 25 full flexion–extension cycles, and with the knee at 70° of flexion, final PCL tibial fixation is achieved with a Lactosorb resorbable interference screw; backup fixation is provided by screw and spiked ligament washer. The tensioning device is applied to the ACL graft, and set to 20 lb, whereupon the graft is tensioned with the knee in 70° of flexion. Final ACL fixation is achieved with Lactosorb bioabsorbable interference screws and spiked ligament washer back-up fixation. The mechanical tensioning device ensures consistent graft tensioning and eliminates graft advancement during interference screw insertion. It also restores the anatomic tibial step-off during PCL graft tensioning and applies a posterior drawer force during ACL graft tensioning. (See color plate.) (Photograph 16.12A courtesy of Arthrotek, Inc., Warsaw, IN, used with permission.)

Fig. 16.13. Opening wedge high tibial osteotomy in a patient with a multiple ligament injured knee. This patient had a malunited tibial plateau fracture in addition to cruciate ligament and lateral side injuries, resulting in a lateral thrusting gait during ambulation. Opening wedge high tibial osteotomy was performed below the level of the tibial tubercle to avoid interference with cruciate ligament reconstruction tunnels. The realignment of the lower extremity after the osteotomy eliminated the varus thrusting gait even before ligament reconstruction was performed. This is critically important in primary and revision reconstructions.

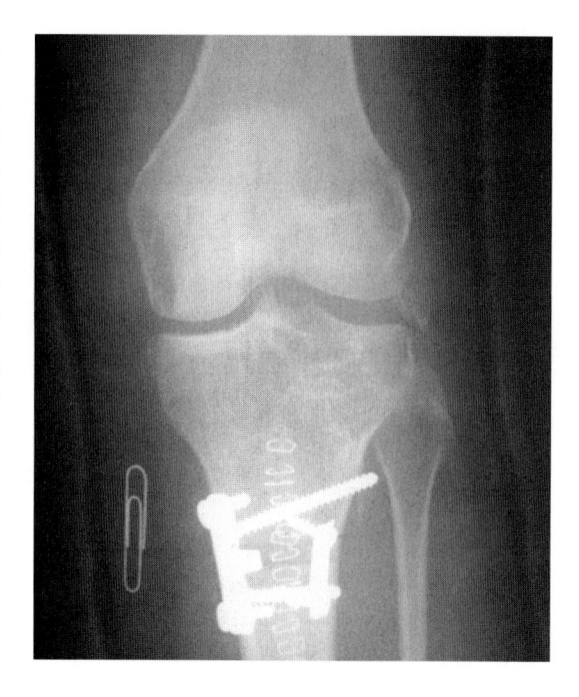

Sport-specific exercises and training begin between postoperative months 4 and 5, with return to sports at the end of postoperative month 6 to 9 if the following criteria are met: quadriceps and hamstring strength is 90% or greater than the uninvolved extremity; patient can perform all necessary skills without pain or restriction; and a functional brace (combined instability brace) is obtained. It should be noted that a loss of 10 to 15° of terminal flexion can be expected in these complex knee ligament reconstructions. This does not cause a functional problem for these patients and is not a cause for alarm.

Results

There is little published material that addresses the results of revision surgery in the multiple ligament injured knee.[2,3,31] The trends in revision combined ACL-PCL reconstruction indicate that these knees are improved subjectively and objectively from their preoperative status; however, the results are not as good as primary multiple ligament knee injury reconstructions. Results depend not only on achieving functional stability but also on the condition of the articular cartilage, and the meniscus, and other structural injuries.

Conclusions

Unsuccessful multiple ligament knee surgery may result from motion loss, extensor mechanism dysfunction, arthrosis, and recurrent patholaxity. Recurrent patholaxity is the most common indication for revision ACL/PCL/collateral ligament revision reconstruction. Technical errors such as inaccurate tunnel placement and failure to address associated ligament instability are the most frequent causes of recurrent patholaxity.

Regardless of the specific surgical techniques employed, the revision multiple ligament injured knee surgery must address all components of the instability. Preoperative planning must be meticulous to ensure detection of all components of the combined instability, anticipation of the technical difficulties, and choice of the appropriate surgical strategy. The surgeon should be aware of several potential pitfalls, including varus alignment, reversed tibial slope, and the existence of a fixed posterior drawer.[2] These complex surgical procedures require preoperative planning, possible staged procedures, an individualized rehabilitation program, and realistic goals and expectations.

References

1. Fanelli GC. ACL and PCL complications and revisions. Paper presented at: International Congress of Arthroscopy and Related Sciences; May 23–26, 2002; Buenos Aires, Argentina.
2. Christel P. Basic principles for posterior cruciate ligament revision surgery. Paper presented at: meeting of the PCL Study Group; July 14–17, 2002; Millennium Hotel, Anchorage, AK.
3. Cooper D. Reconstruction of the posterior cruciate ligament using the tibial inlay fixation technique: minimum two year follow-up. Paper presented at: meeting of the PCL Study Group; July 14–17, 2002; Millennium Hotel, Anchorage, AK.
4. Giffin JR, Harner CD. Failed anterior cruciate ligament surgery. Overview of the problem. Am J Knee Surg 2001; 14(3):185–192.
5. Tredinnick TJ, Friedman MJ. Revision anterior cruciate ligament reconstruction. Technical considerations. Am J Knee Surg 2001; 14(3):193–200.
6. Fanelli GC, Edson CJ, Maish DR. Revision anterior cruciate ligament reconstruction. Associated patholaxity, tibiofemoral malalignment, rehabilitation, and results. Am J Knee Surg 2001; 14(3):201–204.
7. Fanelli GC. Complications of multiple ligamentous injuries of the knee. In: Schenck RC Jr, ed. Multiple Ligamentous Injuries of the Knee in the Athlete. Rosemont, IL: American Academy of Orthopaedic Surgeons; 2002:101–107.
8. Hegyes MS, Richardson MW, Miller MD. Knee dislocation: complications of nonoperative and operative management. Clin Sports Med 2000; 19:519–543.
9. Fanelli GC, Monahan TJ. Complications of posterior cruciate ligament reconstruction. Sports Med Arthrosc Rev 1999; 7(4):296–302.
10. Fanelli GC, Monahan TJ. Complications in posterior cruciate ligament and posterolateral complex surgery. Oper Techniques Sports Med 2001; 9(2):96–99.
11. Fanelli GC. Complications and pitfalls in posterior cruciate ligament reconstruction. In: Monahan TJ, ed; Malek MM, ed in chief; Fanelli, GC, Johnson J, Johnson D, section eds. Knee Surgery: Complications, Pitfalls, and Salvage. New York: Springer-Verlag; 2001:121–128.
12. Fanelli GC. Complications in PCL surgery. In: Fanelli GC, ed. Posterior Cruciate Ligament Injuries. A Practical Guide to Management. New York: Springer-Verlag; 2001:291–302.
13. Johnson DJ, Laboureau JP. Cruciate ligament reconstruction with synthetics. Complications in PCL surgery. In: Fanelli, GC, ed. Posterior Cruciate Ligament Injuries. A Practical Guide to Management. New York: Springer-Verlag; 2001: 189–214.
14. Fanelli GC, Giannotti BF, Edson CJ. Current concepts review. The posterior cruciate ligament arthroscopic evaluation and treatment. Arthroscopy 1994; 10; 6:673–688.
15. Fanelli GC, Giannotti BF, Edson CJ. Arthroscopically assisted combined posterior cruciate ligament/posterior lateral complex reconstruction. Arthroscopy 1996; 12(5):521–530.
16. Fanelli GC, Giannotti BF, Edson CJ. Arthroscopically assisted combined anterior and posterior cruciate ligament reconstruction. Arthroscopy 1996; 12(1): 5–14.
17. Fanelli GC, Edson CJ. Arthroscopically assisted combined ACL/PCL reconstruction. 2–10 year follow-up. Arthroscopy 2002; 18(7):703–714.

18. Malek MM, Fanelli GC, DeLuca JV. Intraarticular and extraarticular anterior cruciate ligament reconstruction. In: Scott WN, ed. The Knee. St Louis, MO: CV Mosby; 1994:791–812.
19. Malek MM, Fanelli GC, Golden MD. Combined intraarticular and extraarticular anterior cruciate ligament reconstruction. In: Scott WN, ed. Ligament and Extensor Mechanism Injuries of the Knee. St Louis, MO: CV Mosby; 1991: 267–284.
20. Fanelli GC, Desai BM, Cummings PD, Hanks GA, Kalenak A. Divergent alignment of the femoral interference screw in single incision endoscopic reconstruction of the anterior cruciate ligament. Contemp Orthop 1994; 28;1:21–25.
21. Berg EE. Posterior cruciate ligament tibial inlay reconstruction. Arthroscopy 1995; 11(1):69–76.
22. Fanelli, GC. Arthroscopic posterior cruciate ligament reconstruction: transtibial tunnel technique. Surgical technique and 2–10 year results. Arthroscopy 2002; 18(9; December, suppl 2):44–49.
23. Fanelli GC. Arthroscopic PCL reconstruction: transtibial technique. In: Fanelli GC, ed. Posterior Cruciate Ligament Injuries. A Practical Guide to Management. New York: Springer-Verlag; 2001:141–156.
24. Fanelli GC. Arthroscopic combined ACL/PCL reconstruction. In: Fanelli GC, ed. Posterior Cruciate Ligament Injuries. A Practical Guide to Management. New York: Springer-Verlag; 2001:215–236.
25. Fanelli GC, Feldmann DD. The dislocated/multiple ligament injured knee. Oper Techniques Orthop 1999; 9(4):298–308.
26. Clancy WG. Repair and reconstruction of the posterior cruciate ligament. In: Chapman M, ed. Operative Orthopaedics. Philadelphia: JB Lippincott; 1988: 1651–1665.
27. Fanelli GC, Larson RV. Practical management of posterolateral instability of the knee. Arthroscopy 2002; 18(2; February, suppl 1):1–8.
28. Wascher DC, Grauer JD, Markoff KL. Biceps tendon tenodesis for posterolateral instability of the knee. An in vitro study. Am J Sports Med 1993; 21;3: 400–406.
29. Fanelli GC, Feldmann DD. Management of combined ACL/PCL/posterolateral complex injuries of the knee. Oper Techniques Sports Med 1999; 7(3):143–149.
30. Muller W. The Knee: Form, Function, and Ligamentous Reconstruction. New York: Springer-Verlag; 1983.
31. Cooper D. Revision posterior cruciate ligament reconstruction using the tibial inlay technique. Arthroscopy 1999; 15(7, suppl 1):S45.

Chapter Seventeen

Brace Treatment

H. Jurgen Eichhorn and Daniel Pflaster

Knee braces play a significant role in the treatment of the multiple ligament injured knee. Used in conjunction with both operative or nonoperative treatment programs, a variety of knee braces exist to allow healing of the soft tissue structures in a protected environment. In its 1984 Knee Braces Seminar Report, the American Academy of Orthopaedic Surgeons (AAOS) classified knee braces into three groups:

Prophylactic knee braces, designed to prevent or reduce the severity of knee injuries
Rehabilitative knee braces, designed to allow protected motion of injured knees or knees that have been treated operatively
Functional knee braces, designed to provide stability for the unstable knee

The AAOS position statement on knee braces, published on their Web site (www.AAOSoorg) states:

AAOS believes that rehabilitative knee braces and functional knee braces can be effective in many treatment programs, and that this efficacy has been demonstrated by long-term scientifically conducted studies.
Rehabilitative knee braces have been designed to provide a compromise between protection and motion. That is, they allow the knee to move, but within specific limits, which has been shown to be beneficial to the injured knee. Rehabilitative knee braces generally are more effective in protecting against excessive flexion and extension than in protecting against anterior and posterior motion.
Functional knee braces aid in the control of unstable knees. Studies have shown that some of the currently available braces are very effective in controlling abnormal motions under low load conditions but not under high loading conditions that occur during many athletic activities. Most studies designed to test whether functional knee braces protect against the knee "giving way" have demonstrated some beneficial effect of the brace. However, the patient and the physician must guard against a false sense of security evoked by the use of such a brace; bio-mechanical studies show that functional knee braces do not restore normal knee stability under high forces related to certain activities. However, when it is properly fitted, used in conjunction with a knee rehabilitation program, and the patient modifies his or her activities appropriately, a functional knee brace can provide an important adjunct in the treatment of knee instability.

In the AAOS classification, modern postoperative braces fall into the rehabilitative brace category. Anterior cruciate ligament (ACL), or "derotation," braces fall into the functional brace category. This chapter reviews rehabilitative and functional knee braces and their practical use in managing the multiple ligament injured patient.

Postoperative Braces

After any neurovascular injuries in the multiple ligament injured knee have been evaluated and managed, long-leg postoperative braces are used to immobilize the limb. The brace can be locked at the desired flexion angle or unlocked with range-of-motion (ROM) stops set to limit the flexion and extension extremes. An example of a postoperative brace with telescoping uprights to improve patient fit is shown in Figure 17.1.

Although most clinicians will recommend operative treatment for patients with multiple ligament injuries, nonoperative treatment is indicated for some older and more sedentary patients, as well as those who are stable following reduction. If nonoperative treatment is chosen, a postoperative brace can be used to stabilize the knee during early range-of-motion exercises and activities of daily living.

Routine surgical repair of the disrupted ligaments in the multiple ligament injured knee started in the 1970s and continues to be the preferred treatment for most of these patients. After surgical repair of the soft tissue structures, postoperative braces are used to protect the multiple reconstructions. Postoperative braces are also used in nonsurgical treatment of acute ligament injuries [e.g., to medial collateral ligaments (MCLs) and posterior cruciate ligaments (PCLs)] to reduce loads in structures that can heal without surgery. Postoperative braces can also be fitted with pneumatic condyle pads or formed to apply varus or valgus loading after medial or lateral side injuries and to effect repairs aimed at reducing loads in the healing structure. For example, a pneumatic pad has been used to apply a varus moment to the knee after microperforation of the MCL to inducing a healing response in a chronic grade III MCL injury.[1] In another variation, postoperative braces designed with a posterior tibial support (PTS) to counter gravity and reduce a fixed posterior tibial subluxation of the tibia have been shown to be effective in treating acute and chronic injuries involving the PCL.[2] Current postoperative braces are compatible with cryotherapy systems used for control of pain and edema after surgery.

Postoperative brace features must accommodate the various protocols used immediately after surgery, when maximal protection is needed. The patient should be able to lock and unlock the brace easily to allow passive and active exercises during this period. A number of researchers have demonstrated increased ACL loading at the limits of extension and flexion.[3-5] ROM stops can be used to limit the knee flexion and extension during exercise to protect against high strains seen in the ACL at the limits of extension and flexion. These stops should be easy to use so the patient can adjust them in relation to activity level and postoperative progression.

Range-of-motion and muscle-strengthening exercises in the early phase of rehabilitation can be assisted with the use of an instrumented postoperative brace such as the DonJoy Vista. The Vista system provides patients with feedback on their efforts, quantifying the progression. The handheld unit also records a patient's performance and generates a report that can be uploaded to the clinician's computer. The Vista System, including a handheld unit, is shown in Figure 17.2.

Functional Braces

Functional braces have been shown to reduce anterior tibial translation 70 to 85% in ACL-deficient knees.[6] Use of a knee brace during nonoperative treatment of the ACL-deficient knee may help protect meniscus, cartilage,

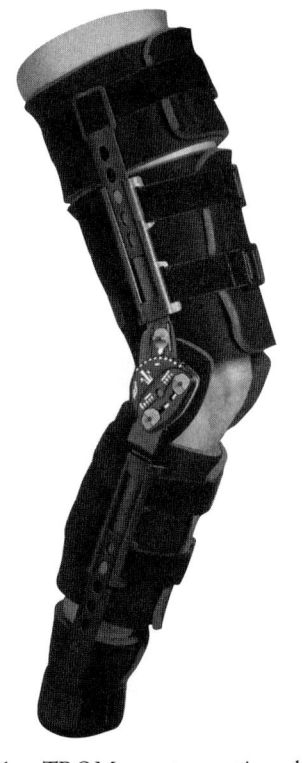

Fig. 17.1. TROM postoperative brace. (Courtesy of dj Orthopedics, Vista, CA.)

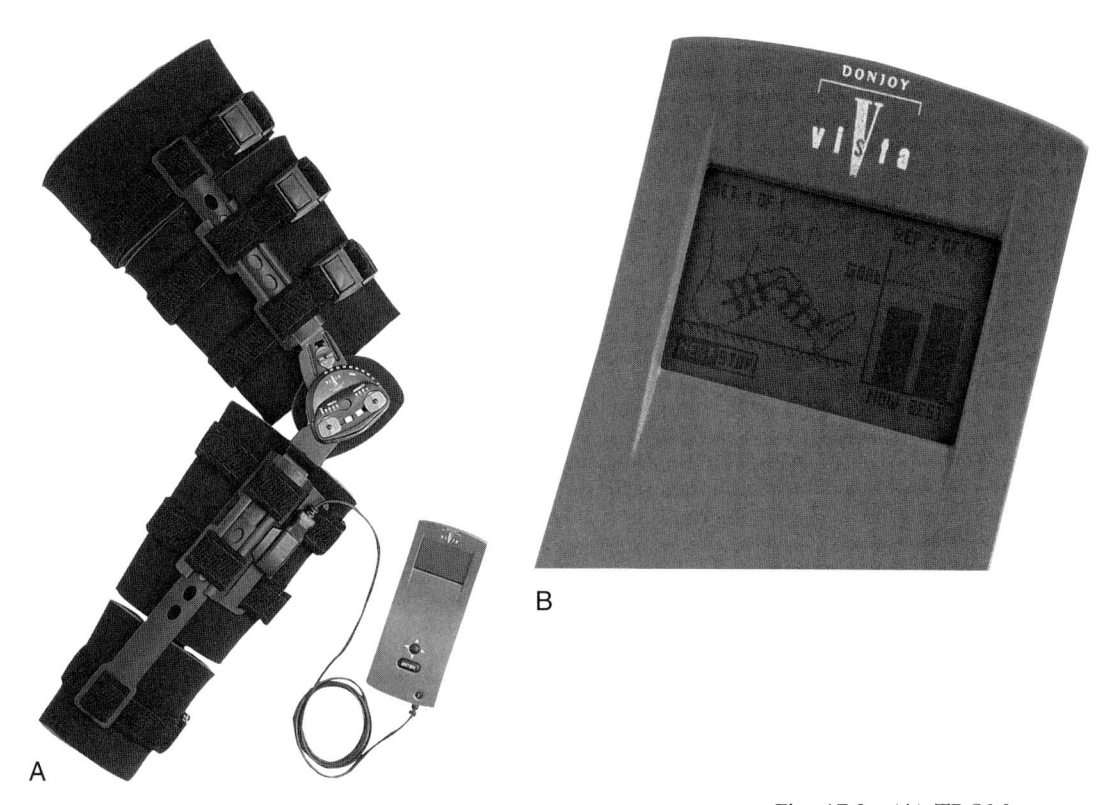

Fig. 17.2. (A) TROM postoperative brace and (B) Vista handheld unit. (Courtesy of dj Orthopedics, Vista, CA.)

and secondary restraints by limiting the amount of pathologic motion in the knee. Functional braces are also used during activity after surgical repair of soft tissue structures in the knee. Dynamic braces uniquely designed to apply a posterior preload to the tibia have been shown to reduce strain in an ACL graft in vivo.[7] These dynamic braces use four points of leverage (4-point ACL) to apply the dynamic posterior preload. Conversely, PCL versions of this dynamic brace design (4-point PCL) are applied to the knee to effect an anterior preload to the tibia, reducing the load in the PCL or its graft. Finally, combined instability (CI) braces are designed without any preload for combined ACL and PCL injuries.

Healing of autogenous ACL grafts follows a predictable healing curve: graft strength initially decreases, followed by an increase in graft strength with new collagen formation and tissue ligamentization.[8] Actual ACL graft strength is difficult to measure in vivo, but graft strength is thought to be impaired up to a year after surgery. In fact, it is unknown whether the graft ever regains 100% of its strength. Functional braces are commonly used during the first postoperative year to protect the graft material during ligamentization. Multiple ligament injured patients who have surgical repair of the soft tissue structures in the knee would similarly benefit from use of a functional brace during activity. A commercially available 4-point ACL brace is shown in Figure 17.3.

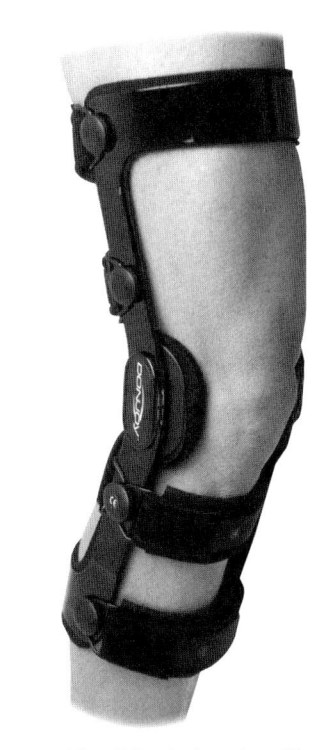

Load-Shifting Braces

Braces designed to shift the compressive knee loads in the frontal plane have been used successfully for patients with unicompartmental knee osteoarthritis. A number of approaches to brace design have been used to accomplish a redistribution of the compressive loads away from the affected compart-

Fig. 17.3. The 4Titude functional knee brace. (Courtesy of dj Orthopedics, Vista, CA.)

Fig. 17.4. (A) Montana single upright load-shifting brace and (B) OAdjuster double upright load-shifting brace. (Courtesy of dj Orthopedics, Vista, CA.)

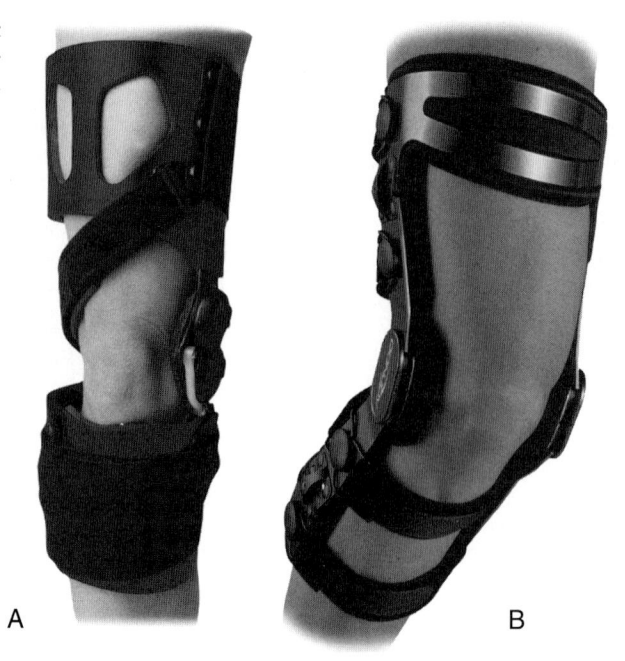

ment. Both single- and double-hinge designs attempt to accomplish the load shift by a three point loading system as shown in Figure 17.4. Single upright braces are effective in shifting the load in the frontal plane but not in the sagittal plane. Double upright braces are designed to apply a moment in the frontal plane and also preload in the sagittal plane. Double upright load-shifting braces can therefore be used where both anterior/posterior and medial/lateral injuries are present. These braces are available in 4-point ACL, 4-point PCL, and CI versions.

Fig. 17.5. Reduction of COP shift with flexion increasing angle for eight different load-shifting brace designs.

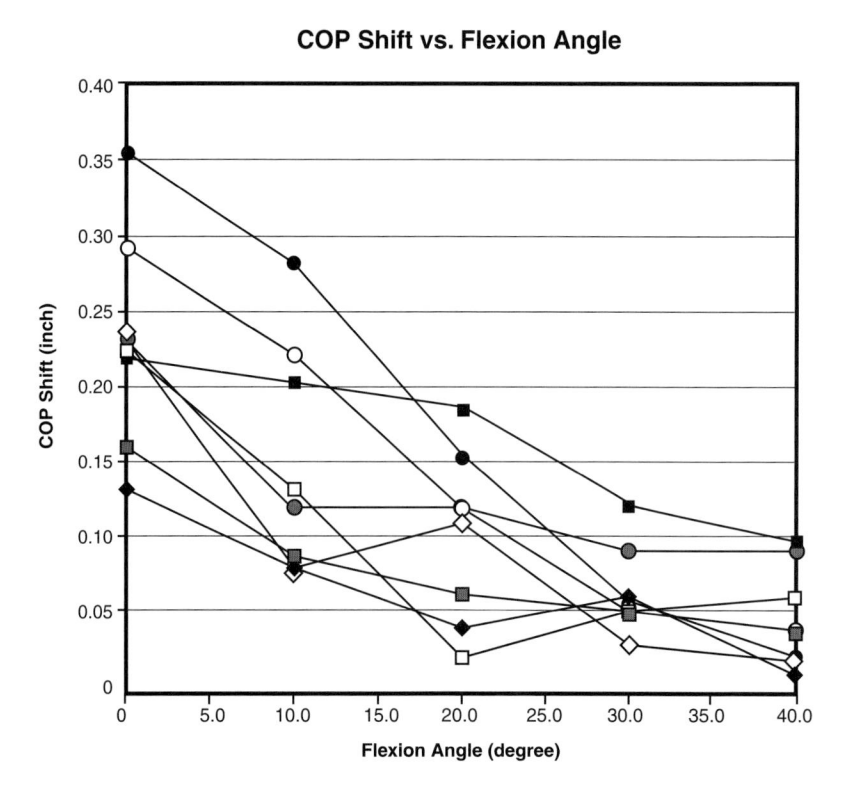

17. Brace Treatment

The load-shifting capacity of these braces has been demonstrated on a mechanical knee surrogate. The surrogate has load sensors in the medial and lateral compartments to measure the changes and compressive force and resulting shift in center of pressure (COP) due to application of a load-shifting brace. Data from eight different brace designs are shown in Figure 17.5. All brace designs show a reduction of COP shift with increasing flexion angle, with maximum load shifting at full extension. Since the knee is near full extension during maximum joint loading, which occurs at heel strike, the maximum brace effectiveness coincides with maximal joint loading. Additional load-shifting and functional improvements may be attained by maintaining load shift through a range of motion. To provide load shifting through an increased range of motion, current braces are designed to reduce the effect of knee flexion on COP shift (curve indicated by solid diamonds in Figure 17.5 represents data from the OAdjuster from dj Orthopedics).

Table 17.1. Brace indications for specific ligament injuries

Ligament injury	Treatment	Indicated brace[a]		
		Postoperative	Functional	Load shifter
Acute partial tear of ACL	Nonsurgical		4-Point ACL	
	Surgical		4-Point ACL	
Complete tear of ACL	Nonsurgical		4-Point ACL	
	Surgical		4-Point ACL	
Acute MCL grade I and II	Nonsurgical	With varus moment	Soft brace	
Acute MCL grade III	Nonsurgical	With varus moment	Soft brace	
	Surgical	With varus moment	Soft brace	
Acute ACL + MCL	Nonsurgical	With varus moment	4-Point ACL	
	Surgical	ACL reconstruction after MCL heals, with varus moment if residual laxity treated (e.g., microperforation)	4-Point ACL	
Chronic ACL + MCL	Nonsurgical			4-Point ACL with varus moment
	Surgical	With varus moment if MCL treated		4-Point ACL with varus moment
Chronic ACL + lateral side	Nonsurgical			4-Point ACL with valgus moment
	Surgical	With valgus moment		4-Point ACL with valgus moment
Acute PCL	Nonsurgical	Standard or PTS	4-Point PCL	
Chronic PCL	Nonsurgical		4-Point PCL	
	Surgical	Standard or PTS	4-Point PCL	
Acute PCL + lateral side	Nonsurgical	Standard or PTS	4-Point PCL	
	Surgical	Standard or PTS		4-Point PCL with valgus moment
Chronic PCL + lateral side	Nonsurgical			4-Point PCL with valgus moment
Acute ACL + PCL	Nonsurgical	Standard or PTS	CI	
Chronic ACL + PCL	Nonsurgical		CI	
	Surgical	Standard or PTS	CI	
Acute ACL + PCL + lateral side	Nonsurgical	Standard or PTS		CI with valgus moment
	Surgical	Standard or PTS		CI with valgus moment
ACL + PCL + medial and lateral side	Nonsurgical	Standard or PTS	CI	
	Surgical	Standard or PTS	CI	

Load-shifting braces are also being used after surgical repair of lateral or medial soft tissue structures. The frontal plane load generated by the brace will reduce loads on the healing structures during weight-bearing and non-weight-bearing activities. A balance is necessary between range-of-motion exercises to avoid a stiff knee and protection of the surgical repair to allow complete incorporation of the graft into the bone tunnels and remodeling of the graft in its new loading environment. In comparison to long-leg postoperative braces, load-shifting braces allow patients to perform more normal range-of-motion exercises and activities of daily living, while providing protection of lateral or medial structure repairs.

Conclusions

Knee bracing plays a significant role in the operative and nonoperative treatment of the multiple ligament injured knee. The various combinations of ligament injury are best treated using specific brace designs depending on the type of injury. Differences in patient requirements and treatment protocols in this population need to be evaluated to ensure that the correct brace is chosen for the specific application. The various combinations of ligament injuries in the knee are as varied as the protocols used to treat them. It is important to choose a brace that is compatible with the protocol best suited to address the unique requirements seen in the multiple ligament injured knee. Table 17.1 summarizes brace indications for various ligament injuries.

References

1. Rosenberg TD. Microperforation for chronic ACL/MCL laxity: results in a rabbit animal model and human experience. Paper presented at: meeting of the ACL Study Group; July 14–17, 2002; Millennium Hotel; Anchorage, AK.
2. Strobel MJ, Weiler A, Schulz MS, Russe K, Eichhorn HJ. Fixed posterior subluxation in posterior cruciate ligament deficient knees: diagnosis and treatment of a new clinical sign. Am J Sports Med 2002; 30(1):32–38.
3. Beynnon BD, Fleming BC. Anterior cruciate ligament strain in-vivo: a review of previous work. J Biomech 1998; 31(6):519–525.
4. Wallace MP, Howell SM, Hull ML. In vivo tensile behavior of a four-bundle hamstring graft as a replacement for the anterior cruciate ligament. J Orthop Res 1997; 15(4):539–545.
5. Markoff KL, Burchfield DM, Shapiro MM, Cha CW, Finerman GAM, Slauterbeck JL. Biomechanical consequences of replacement of the anterior cruciate ligament with a patellar ligament allograft. J Bone Joint Surg Am 1996; 78: 1728–1734.
6. Wojtys EM, Kothari SU, Huston LJ. Anterior cruciate ligament functional brace use in sports. Am J Sports Med 1996; 24(4):539–546.
7. Fleming BC, Renstrom PA, Beynnon BD, Engstrom B, Peura G. The influence of functional knee bracing on the anterior cruciate ligament strain biomechanics in weightbearing and nonweightbearing knees. Am J Sports Med 2000; 28(6): 815–824.
8. Amiel D, Kleiner JB, Roux RD, Harwood FL, Akeson WH. The phenomena of "ligamentization": anterior cruciate ligament reconstruction with autogenous patellar tendon. J Orthop Res 1986; 4(2):162–172.

Chapter Eighteen

Selected Case Studies

Gregory C. Fanelli

This chapter presents selected cases in treatment of the multiple ligament injured knee that are representative of my practice. I have written the chapter in the first person to provide a more personal approach. These selected cases represent real-life management examples in the treatment of difficult knee ligament instability problems.

Details of the surgical technique and postoperative rehabilitation are not presented in this chapter because the surgery and postoperative rehabilitation were performed as described in Chapter 8. The purpose of this case study section is to afford the reader insight into management and treatment strategies in complex knee ligament injuries.

Case Study 1: Acute ACL-PCL-High Grade Medial Side Injury

A 24-year-old male professional bicycle motocross trick rider sustained a fall of approximately 12 feet during a failed bicycle trick. The patient landed on his right foot, and forced valgus, external rotation, and flexion forces were applied to the knee, resulting in a tibiofemoral dislocation. The patient was transported from the scene of the accident to the hospital, where closed reduction of the dislocated knee was performed. An arteriogram showed the arterial vascular status of the lower extremity to be intact. There was no clinical evidence of venous insufficiency. The sensory and motor functions of the nerves of the lower extremity were intact.

Physical examination of the knee revealed grade III+ anterior–posterior laxity of the knee at 25 and 90° of knee flexion. The tibial step-off was negative. There was grade III+ laxity of the knee to valgus stress at 0 and 30° of knee flexion and a palpable defect in the medial retinaculum; the patella could be easily dislocated laterally. The lateral and posterolateral ligament complex were stable to examination with varus stress at 30 and 0° of knee flexion, and the posterior lateral drawer test was negative.

Magnetic resonance imaging study revealed complete disruption of the ACL, PCL, and medial collateral ligament–medial retinacular complex. There was also peripheral detachment of the medial meniscus and lateral patellar tilting.

The assessment of this patient revealed a knee with complete disruption of the ACL and PCL with high grade medial side injury, medial meniscus tear, and laterally dislocating patella. Dislocated knees with high grade medial side injuries seem to be associated with a higher risk of stiffness and heterotopic ossification. My treatment strategy was to try to reduce the risk of these two complications by doing a staged surgical procedure.

The patient was taken to surgery 3 days after the injury, and open medial collateral ligament primary repair augmented with an Achilles tendon allograft, medial meniscus repair, and extensor mechanism repair–realignment were performed as the first stage of a two-stage procedure. Postoperatively, the knee was first protected in an immobilizer in full extension. Range of motion was progressed; the patient was non–weight bearing the entire time. The second-stage surgical procedure was performed approximately 4 weeks after the first and consisted of an arthroscopically assisted combined ACL-PCL reconstruction using Achilles tendon allograft tissue for the anterior and posterior cruciate ligament reconstructions.

The postoperative rehabilitation program was as follows. During weeks 1 to 6 following the second-stage surgical procedure, the patient was non–weight bearing, and the surgical extremity was braced in full extension. During postoperative weeks 4 to 6, range of motion was progressed. During postoperative weeks 7 to 10, the rehabilitation brace was unlocked, and weight bearing was progressed at 25% of body weight per week over those 4 weeks. The patient was fully weight bearing and using crutches at the end of postoperative week 10. Varus and/or valgus forces were avoided during range-of-motion exercises to protect the collateral ligaments that had been reconstructed. The long-leg rehabilitation brace was discontinued at the end of postoperative week 10, and an ACL-PCL functional brace was used for activities of daily living for continued protection. Range-of-motion exercises were progressed using a stationary bicycle, and closed chain exercises were performed with stair-stepping machines, rowing machines, leg press, and elliptical trainers. Proprioceptive skill training was advanced. Straight-line jogging was initiated between postoperative months 4 and 5, since this patient had excellent strength and proprioceptive skills. The patient returned to competitive bicycle motocross trick riding approximately 6 months postreconstruction.

This patient's Tegner, Lysholm, and Hospital for Special Surgery knee ligament rating scale scores 14 months postreconstruction were 7, 95, and 94, respectively. The KT1000 arthrometer side-to-side difference values for the PCL screen, corrected posterior, and corrected anterior measurements were −8.0, −8.5, and 0.5 mm, respectively. The Telos stress radiographic side-to-side difference measurement at 90° of knee flexion with a 32 lb posteriorly directed force applied to the tibial tubercle area to assess PCL reconstruction stability was −7.0 mm. The patient had an isolated PCL tear on his nonsurgical knee; these results indicate that the surgical knee is tighter than the nonsurgical knee. The following additional results were obtained: Lachman test normal, pivot shift negative, tibial step-off normal, posterior drawer negative, valgus stress test symmetric to the nonsurgical knee, and range of motion 0 to 120° of knee flexion (nonsurgical side range of motion, 0–130°), with a stable extensor mechanism. Follow-up radiographs show no indication of heterotopic ossification.

Case Study 2: Acute ACL-PCL-MCL Injury

A 23-year-old unrestrained male driver was involved in a motor vehicle accident. The patient was transported to the hospital via the trauma system. The patient had cuts and abrasions on both legs, and both knees were painful. Physical examination of the right knee revealed a positive Lachman test, positive pivot shift, and grade III varus laxity at 30° of knee flexion. The right knee PCL, lateral and posterolateral structures, and extensor mechanism were stable. Physical examination of the left knee revealed grade III+ anterior–posterior laxity of the knee at 25 and 90° of knee flexion. The tibial step-off was negative. There was grade III+ laxity of the knee to valgus stress at 0 and 30° of knee flexion; there was no palpable defect in the medial retinaculum, and the extensor mechanism was stable. The lateral and posterolateral ligament complex were stable to examination with varus stress at 30 and 0° of knee flexion, and the posterior lateral drawer test was negative.

Arteriography of the left lower extremity revealed the arterial vascular status of the left lower extremity to be intact. There was no clinical evidence of venous insufficiency. Sensory and motor functions of the nerves of both the right and the left lower extremities were intact. The patient had no other orthopaedic or systemic injuries.

Plain radiographs of the right knee demonstrated avulsion of the fibular head. There were no other fractures or ligament bony avulsions. The tibiofemoral and patellofemoral joints were normally aligned. Plain radiographs of the left knee demonstrated no fractures or evidence of ligament bony avulsions. The tibiofemoral joint and extensor mechanism were aligned normally. Magnetic resonance imaging (MRI) examination of the right knee demonstrated complete disruption of the ACL, avulsion of the fibular head, and tearing of the lateral and posterolateral structures from their tibial insertions. MRI examination of the left knee revealed complete disruption of the ACL, PCL, and MCL with the medial collateral ligament torn from its femoral insertion site. There were no meniscus tears or articular surface injuries in either knee.

A summary of the patient's orthopaedic injuries included a right knee anterior cruciate ligament tear combined with a fibular head avulsion and lateral and posterolateral corner tears. The patient also had a left knee injury consisting of anterior and posterior cruciate ligament tears, and a grade III complete medial collateral ligament tear located at the femoral insertion of the medial collateral ligament.

The treatment of the right knee consisted of early primary repair of the fibular head avulsion and the lateral and posterolateral capsular and ligament tears. This was followed by arthroscopic ACL reconstruction using autogenous bone–patellar tendon–bone graft as a second-stage procedure done approximately 4 weeks after the lateral side repair. The left knee had a medial side injury at a lower level than the knee of the patient discussed in case study 1, and the treatment plan was to treat the MCL tear with bracing for approximately 4 to 6 weeks, followed by arthroscopic ACL-PCL reconstruction using autogenous bone–patellar tendon–bone graft for the ACL and Achilles tendon allograft for the PCL reconstruction.

This treatment strategy could be employed for the left knee for several reasons. The tibiofemoral joints were well aligned on both the AP and lateral x-rays and stayed that way during brace treatment of the medial collateral ligament as documented with serial radiographs. This particular medial side injury, though a complete MCL tear, was a relatively low level injury in that the medial retinaculum was intact, the extensor mechanism was stable, and the medial meniscus was intact and stable. These factors enabled nonsurgical treatment of the medial collateral ligament, which also seemed to decrease the risk of stiffness and heterotopic ossification.

The postoperative rehabilitation program consisted of non–weight bearing for both the right and left lower extremities until healing had occurred both for the right knee, which had had the lateral side surgery, and for the left knee medial collateral ligament, which had been braced. Progressive range of motion was initiated for both knees, and both knees had near full range of motion restored prior to their respective second-stage procedures. Postoperative rehabilitation following the second-stage surgical procedures consisted of progressive range of motion and progressive protected weight bearing with return to strenuous activities at 6 to 9 months after the surgical reconstructions.

This patient's postoperative Tegner, Lysholm, and Hospital for Special Surgery knee ligament rating scale scores 24 months postreconstruction were 7, 100, and 96, respectively. The KT1000 side-to-side difference values for the PCL screen, corrected posterior, and corrected anterior measurements were 1.0, 0.0, and 1.5 mm, respectively. The left knee Lachman test was normal, pivot shift was negative, tibial step-off was normal, posterior drawer was negative, and valgus stress test was symmetric to the nonsurgical knee. Knee range of motion was 0 to 140°, with a stable extensor mechanism. Follow-up radiographs showed no indication of heterotopic ossification. The right knee Lachman test, pivot shift, and varus stress test at 30° of knee flexion were normal, with range of motion 0 to 140°. The patient had returned to full unrestricted work as heavy laborer and roofer.

Case Study 3: Acute ACL-PCL-Posterolateral Type B Injury

A 19-year-old male jumped across a puddle of water, slipped upon landing, and sustained a complete anterior tibiofemoral right knee dislocation. The patient was evaluated in the emergency room, where the knee dislocation was reduced. Physical examination of the injured knee in comparison to the normal knee revealed grade III+ anterior–posterior laxity of the right knee at 25 and 90° of knee flexion. The tibial step-off was negative. There was grade II+ laxity of the knee to varus stress at 0 and 30° of knee flexion with a firm end point. The external rotation thigh–foot angle test (dial test) was positive at 30 and 90° of flexion with the right foot externally rotating 15° greater than the left foot. The posterolateral drawer test was positive. The medial collateral ligament complex was stable to examination with valgus stress at 30 and 0° of knee flexion, and the posterior medial drawer test was negative.

Arteriography of the right lower extremity revealed the arterial vascular status of the right lower extremity to be intact. The sensory and motor function of the nerves of both the right and the left lower extremities were intact. The patient had no other orthopaedic or systemic injuries. The patient did develop calf pain and swelling. Venography revealed a 2.5 cm posttraumatic deep venous thrombosis in the popliteal vein.

Plain radiographs of the right knee demonstrated anterior dislocation of the tibiofemoral joint. There were no other fractures or ligament bony avulsions. Postreduction x-ray films revealed that the tibiofemoral and patellofemoral joints were normally aligned. MRI examination of the right knee revealed complete disruption of the ACL, PCL, and femoral insertion site injuries to the fibular collateral ligament and the popliteus tendon. There were no meniscus tears or articular surface injuries in the injured knee.

In summary, this patient's right knee injury was a complete tibiofemoral dislocation with complete disruption of the anterior and posterior cruciate ligament and posterolateral instability type B. Posterolateral instability includes at least 10° of increased tibial external rotation in comparison to the normal knee at 30 and 90° of knee flexion (positive dial test, and external rotation thigh–foot angle test), and variable degrees of varus instability depending on the injured anatomic structures. Posterolateral instability (PLI) type A has increased external rotation only, corresponding to injury to the popliteofibular ligament, and popliteus tendon only. PLI type B presents with increased external rotation and mild varus of approximately 5 mm increased lateral joint line opening to varus stress at 30° knee flexion.

18. Selected Case Studies

This occurs with damage to the popliteofibular ligament and popliteus tendon, as well as attenuation of the fibular collateral ligament. PLI type C presents with increased tibial external rotation and varus instability of 10 mm greater than the normal knee tested at 30° of knee flexion with varus stress. This occurs with injury to the popliteofibular ligament, popliteus tendon, fibular collateral ligament, and lateral capsular avulsion, in addition to cruciate ligament disruption. The intact medial collateral ligament, tested with valgus stress at 30° of knee flexion, is the stable hinge in the ACL/PCL/PLC injured knee.

Surgical timing was affected by the presence of the deep venous thrombosis of the surgical lower extremity. The patient was treated with heparin initially and then switched to Coumadin under the direction of the anticoagulation medicine specialists. The knee was immobilized in a long-leg brace locked in full extension. Serial weekly anteroposterior and lateral radiographs were obtained to make sure that the tibiofemoral joint was reduced and that there was no posterior tibial subluxation. The patient's surgical reconstruction was performed between 2 and 3 weeks after the injury.

Surgical treatment of this patient's right knee consisted of a single-stage combined arthroscopically assisted ACL-PCL reconstruction and open lateral–posterolateral primary repair-reconstruction. The PCL reconstruction was an arthroscopically assisted single-bundle single-femoral transtibial technique using a fresh-frozen Achilles tendon allograft. The ACL reconstruction performed was an arthroscopically assisted single-incision technique using a fresh-frozen bone–patellar tendon–bone allograft. Lateral and posterolateral instability was surgically corrected using a combined procedure: primary repair of the fibular collateral ligament and popliteus tendon femoral insertions, and reconstruction using a split biceps tendon tenodesis and posterolateral capsular shift procedures.

The postoperative rehabilitation program was as follows. During weeks 1 to 6, the patient was non–weight bearing, and the surgical extremity was braced in full extension. During postoperative weeks 4 to 6, range of motion was progressed. Postoperative weeks 7 to 10, the rehabilitation brace was unlocked, and progressive weight bearing progressed at 25% of body weight per week over those weeks. The patient was fully weight bearing using crutches at the end of postoperative week 10. Varus forces were avoided during range-of-motion exercises to protect the lateral and posterolateral structures that had been reconstructed. The long-leg rehabilitation brace was discontinued at the end of postoperative week 10, and an ACL-PCL functional brace was used for activities of daily living for continued protection. Range-of-motion exercises were progressed using a stationary bicycle, and closed chain exercises were performed with stair-stepping machines, rowing machines, leg press, and elliptical trainers. Proprioceptive skill training was advanced. Straight-line jogging was initiated between postoperative months 4 and 5, and activity level progressed as strength and proprioceptive skills improved.

This patient's Tegner, Lysholm, and Hospital for Special Surgery knee ligament rating scale scores 24 months postreconstruction were 7, 91, 90, respectively. The KT1000 arthrometer side-to-side difference values for the PCL screen, corrected posterior, and corrected anterior measurements were 3.0, 0.5, and 0.0 mm, respectively. The Telos stress radiographic side-to-side difference measurement at 90° of knee flexion with a 32 lb posteriorly directed force applied to the tibial tubercle area to assess PCL stability was 5.0 mm. Other results were as follows: Lachman test normal, pivot shift negative, tibial step-off normal, posterior drawer negative, varus stress test symmetric to the nonsurgical knee, dial test less than (tighter than) the normal knee at 30 and 90° of knee flexion, and range of motion 0 to 130° (normal side, 0–135°).

Case Study 4: Chronic ACL-PCL-Posterolateral Type B Injury

A 32-year-old male presented to my sports injury clinic 10 years after having sustained a left knee injury while skiing. The patient's chief complaint was functional instability of his left knee with activities of daily living as well as with pivoting and twisting in recreational sports. Physical examination of the injured knee in comparison to the normal knee revealed grade III+ anterior–posterior laxity of the left knee at 25 and 90° of knee flexion. The tibial step-off was negative. There was grade II+ laxity of the knee to varus stress at 0 and 30° of knee flexion with a firm end point. The external rotation thigh–foot angle test (dial test) was positive at 30 and 90° of flexion with the left foot externally rotating 20° greater than the right foot. The posterolateral drawer test was positive. The medial collateral ligament complex was stable to examination with valgus stress at 30 and 0° of knee flexion, and the posterior medial drawer test was negative. The patient's left and right lower extremity mechanical axes were symmetric, and his gait was normal with no lateral thrust.

Preoperative KT1000 arthrometer measurements demonstrated side-to-side difference values on the PCL screen, corrected posterior, and corrected anterior measurements of 10.5, 12.5, and 2.0 mm, respectively. A preoperative Telos stress radiographic side-to-side difference measurement at 90° of knee flexion with a 32 lb posteriorly directed force applied to the tibial tubercle area to assess PCL stability was 17.0 mm.

Plain radiographs of the left knee demonstrated normally aligned tibiofemoral and patellofemoral joints with no evidence of degenerative joint disease. MRI examination of the left knee revealed complete disruption of the ACL and PCL, as well as attenuation of the fibular collateral ligament and the popliteus tendon. The lateral meniscus was torn, the medial meniscus intact. There was no osteonecrosis and no MRI-diagnosed articular surface injuries in the knee.

In summary, this patient's chronic left knee injury was a complete disruption of the anterior and posterior cruciate ligaments, combined with posterolateral instability type B. The patient had a normal gait with no varus thrust and no radiographic evidence of degenerative joint disease. As outlined earlier, posterolateral instability includes at least 10° of increased tibial external rotation compared with the normal knee at 30 and 90° of knee flexion (positive dial test, and external rotation thigh–foot angle test), and variable degrees of varus instability depending upon the injured anatomic structures. Posterolateral instability type A has increased external rotation only, corresponding to injury to the popliteofibular ligament and popliteus tendon only. PLI type B presents with increased external rotation and mild varus of approximately 5 mm increased lateral joint line opening to varus stress at 30° knee flexion. This occurs with damage to the popliteofibular ligament and popliteus tendon, as well as attenuation of the fibular collateral ligament. PLI type C presents with increased tibial external rotation and varus instability of 10 mm greater than the normal knee tested at 30° of knee flexion with varus stress. This occurs with injury to the popliteofibular ligament, popliteus tendon, fibular collateral ligament, and lateral capsular avulsion, in addition to cruciate ligament disruption.

Since this patient presented to my clinic with chronic functional instability 10 years after his injury, any reconstructive procedure was purely elective, and surgical timing was determined by patient convenience. Surgical treatment of this patient's left knee consisted of a single-stage combined arthroscopically assisted ACL-PCL reconstruction and open lateral–posterolateral reconstruction. The PCL reconstruction was an arthroscopically assisted single-bundle single-femoral transtibial technique using a fresh-frozen Achilles tendon allograft. The ACL reconstruction performed was an arthroscopically assisted single-incision technique using a fresh-frozen Achilles tendon allograft. Lateral and posterolateral instability was surgically corrected using a combined reconstruction using a split biceps tendon tenodesis and posterolateral capsular shift procedure. Since the patient had normal lower extremity alignment and no lateral thrusting gait, high tibial osteotomy was not indicated.

The postoperative rehabilitation program during weeks 1 to 6 had the patient non–weight bearing and the surgical extremity braced in full extension. During postoperative weeks 4 to 6, range of motion was progressed. During postoperative weeks 7 to 10, the rehabilitation brace was unlocked, and weight bearing progressed at 25% of body weight per week over those weeks. The patient was fully weight bearing using crutches at the end of postoperative week 10. Varus forces were avoided during range of motion exercises to protect the lateral and posterolateral structures that had been reconstructed. The long-leg rehabilitation brace was discontinued at the end of postoperative week 10, and an ACL-PCL functional brace was used for activities of daily living for continued protection. Range-of-motion exercises were progressed using a stationary bicycle. Strength and proprioceptive skill training were progressed using stair-stepping machines, rowing machines, leg press, elliptical trainers, and balance devices. Straight-line jogging was initiated between postoperative months 4 and 5, and activity level progressed as strength and proprioceptive skills improved.

This patient's Tegner, Lysholm, and Hospital for Special Surgery knee ligament rating scale scores 36 months postreconstruction were 4, 90, and 87, respectively. The KT1000 arthrometer side-to-side difference values for the PCL screen, corrected posterior, and corrected anterior measurements were 3.5, 5.5, and 1.5 mm, respectively. The Telos stress radiographic side-to-side difference measurement at 90° of knee flexion with a 32 lb posteriorly directed force applied to the tibial tubercle area to assess PCL stability was 7.0 mm. Other test results were as follows: Lachman test normal, pivot shift negative, tibial step-off decreased 5 mm, posterior drawer grade I, varus stress test symmetric to the nonsurgical knee, dial test equal to the normal knee at 30 and 90° of knee flexion, and range of motion 0 to 125° compared with the normal knee of 0 to 135°. The patient has returned to his desired level of activity.

Case Study 5: Open Knee Dislocation

A 25-year-old male was injured at a building site when a large piece of construction equipment struck him on the anterior medial aspect of the left knee. The patient was transported to the hospital through the emergency trauma system. Physical examination of the injured lower extremity revealed deformity of the lower extremity and a 25 cm open wound on the lateral aspect of the knee, with gross contamination from dirt and clothing fabric. There were no pulses in the involved lower extremity, and the patient was able to plantar flex his toes but not dorsiflex them. Radiographs revealed an anterior tibiofemoral dislocation with no fractures. Immediate reduction was performed in the emergency department; however, there was no return of pulses to the lower extremity.

Vascular surgery consultation was obtained, and the patient was immediately taken to the operating room for arteriography, irrigation and debridement, and repair of the popliteal artery disruption with a vein bypass graft. Compartment pressures were monitored, and no fasciotomies were required. The surgical lower extremity was placed in a knee immobilizer. The patient was taken back to the operating room 2 days later for repeat irrigation and debridement, examination under anesthesia, and primary repair of the injured lateral side structures.

Physical examination of the injured knee compared with the normal knee revealed grade III+ anterior–posterior laxity of the left knee at 25 and 90° of knee flexion. The tibial step-off was negative. There was grade III+ laxity of the knee to varus stress at 0 and 30° of knee flexion with no firm end point. The external rotation thigh–foot angle test (dial test) was positive at 30 and 90° of flexion with the left foot externally rotating 20° greater than the right foot. The posterolateral drawer test was positive. The medial collateral ligament complex was stable to examination with valgus stress at 30 and 0° of knee flexion, and the posterior medial drawer test was negative. There was no damage to the extensor mechanism.

The lateral side injury included avulsion of the common biceps tendon, fibular collateral ligament, and popliteofibular ligament from the fibular head. The lateral and posterolateral capsules were avulsed from the proximal tibia, and the iliotibial band had been avulsed from Gerdy's tubercle. The lateral meniscus was peripherally detached but was not displaced. There was complete midsubstance disruption of the anterior and posterior cruciate ligaments. The medial meniscus and the articular surfaces were intact, as was the medial collateral ligament. The peroneal nerve had been avulsed from its muscular insertion into the lateral compartment muscles, with substance loss in the nerve.

In summary, this patient's acute left knee injury was a complete disruption of the anterior and posterior cruciate ligaments, combined with lateral and posterolateral instability type C with peroneal nerve avulsion and popliteal artery disruptions. As outlined earlier, posterolateral instability includes at least 10° of increased tibial external rotation compared to the normal knee at 30 and 90° of knee flexion (positive dial test and external rotation thigh–foot angle test), and variable degrees of varus instability depending on the injured anatomic structures. Posterolateral instability type A has increased external rotation only, corresponding to injury to the popliteofibular ligament and popliteus tendon only. PLI type B presents with increased external rotation and mild varus of approximately 5 mm increased lateral joint line opening to varus stress at 30° knee flexion. This occurs with damage to the popliteofibular ligament and the popliteus tendon, as well as attenuation of the fibular collateral ligament. PLI type C presents with increased tibial external rotation and varus instability of 10 mm greater than the normal knee tested at 30° of knee flexion with varus stress. This occurs with injury to the popliteofibular ligament, popliteus tendon, fibular collateral ligament, and lateral capsular avulsion, in addition to cruciate ligament disruption.

Surgical timing was influenced by the popliteal artery repair and the open lateral wound. The popliteal artery repair was performed emergently along with initial wound debridement. Two days after the initial surgery, repeat irrigation and debridement, primary repair of the injured lateral and posterolateral structures, lateral meniscus repair, and wound closures were performed. The proximal end of the peroneal nerve was identified and tagged with appropriate suture material. The primary repair of these structures was very stable, and I chose not to use allograft augmentation because of the open wound and increased risk of infection. The knee was immobilized in full extension, and serial radiographs were taken to ensure that tibiofemoral alignment and a good reduction were maintained.

Stage 2 of the patient's surgical treatment consisted of a combined arthroscopically assisted ACL-PCL reconstruction. The PCL reconstruction was an arthroscopically assisted single-bundle single-femoral transtibial technique using a fresh-frozen Achilles tendon allograft. The ACL reconstruction performed was an arthroscopically assisted single-incision technique using a fresh-frozen bone–patellar tendon–bone allograft. The lateral and posterolateral instability and lateral meniscus were surgically corrected as outlined earlier, had healed very well, and were very stable at the time of the second stage of reconstruction.

The postoperative rehabilitation program was as follows. During weeks 1 to 6 following the second-stage surgical procedure, the patient was non–weight bearing, and the surgical extremity was braced in full extension. During postoperative weeks 4 to 6, range of motion was progressed. Postoperative weeks 7 to 10, the rehabilitation brace was unlocked, and weight bearing was progressed at 25% of body weight per week over those weeks. The patient was fully weight bearing using crutches at the end of postoperative week 10. Varus forces were avoided during range-of-motion exercises to protect the lateral and posterolateral structures that had been repaired. The long-leg rehabilitation brace was discontinued at the end of postoperative week 10, and an ACL-PCL functional brace was used for activities of daily living for continued protection. Range-of-motion exercises were progressed using a stationary bicycle, while strength and proprioceptive skill training were progressed using stair-stepping machines, rowing machines, leg press, elliptical trainers, and balance devices. Straight-line jogging was initiated between postoperative months 4 and 5, and activity level progressed as strength and proprioceptive skills improved. An ankle–foot orthosis was used for treatment of the footdrop resulting from the peroneal nerve injury.

This patient's Tegner, Lysholm, and Hospital for Special Surgery knee ligament rating scale scores 60 months postreconstruction were 6, 90, and 89, respectively. The KT1000 arthrometer side-to-side difference values for the PCL screen, corrected posterior, and corrected anterior measurements were 0.5, 0.5, and 0.0 mm, respectively. The Telos stress radiographic side-to-side difference measurement at 90° of knee flexion with a 32 lb posteriorly directed force applied to the tibial tubercle area to assess PCL stability was 4.0 mm. Other results were as follows: Lachman test normal, pivot shift negative, tibial step-off normal, posterior drawer negative, varus stress test symmetric to the nonsurgical knee, dial test less than (surgical side tighter than) the normal knee at 30 and 90° of knee flexion, and range of motion 0 to 130° on the surgical knee and 0 to 140° on the nonsurgical knee. The patient has returned to his desired level of activity.

Case 6: Revision Multiple Ligament Reconstruction

A 40-year-old woman injured her left knee in an equestrian accident. The patient apparently sustained a left tibial shaft fracture combined with a multiple ligament injured left knee. Another orthopaedic surgeon had treated the tibial fracture with casting. When the tibial fracture was healed, the patient had had combined ACL and PCL reconstruction performed as a staged procedure with allograft tissue. The anterior cruciate ligament reconstruction was done first, followed by the PCL reconstruction approximately 6 months later. The patient continued to have pain and instability following the reconstructive surgical procedure, and the operating orthopaedic surgeon then performed an arthroscopic debridement procedure, combined with removal of the fixation hardware. The patient continued to have pain and instability with her activities of daily living and was referred to me for evaluation and treatment.

Physical examination of the injured knee compared with the normal knee revealed grade III+ anterior–posterior laxity of the left knee at 25 and 90° of knee flexion. The tibial step-off was negative. There was grade II+ laxity of the knee to varus stress at 0 and 30° of knee flexion with a firm end point. The external rotation thigh–foot angle test (dial test) was positive at 30 and 90° of flexion with the left foot externally rotating 20° greater than the right foot. The posterolateral drawer test was positive. The medial collateral ligament complex was stable to examination with valgus stress at 30 and 0° of knee flexion, and the posterior medial drawer test was negative. The patient's left and right lower extremity mechanical axes were symmetric, and her gait was normal with no lateral thrust. Quadriceps strength was symmetric.

Plain radiographs of the left knee demonstrated normally aligned tibiofemoral and patellofemoral joints with no evidence of degenerative joint disease, and well-positioned ACL and PCL tibial and femoral tunnels. MRI examination of the left knee revealed attenuation of the ACL and PCL grafts with well-positioned ACL and PCL femoral and tibial tunnels. The menisci were intact; there was no osteonecrosis, and MRI examination did not reveal any articular surface injuries in the knee. Telos stress radiographic measurements comparing the injured knee and the normal knee, measuring posterior tibial displacement in millimeters with a 32 lb posteriorly directed force applied to the tibial tubercle to assess PCL stability, revealed a 13 mm side-to-side difference. The KT1000 arthrometer side-to-side difference values for the PCL screen, corrected posterior, and corrected anterior measurements were 7.0, 7.0, and 3.0 mm, respectively.

Analysis of this patient's problem revealed that her anterior and posterior cruciate ligament reconstructions had failed for several reasons. The patient's initial operating surgeon did not recognize the associated posterolateral instability. As outlined earlier, posterolateral instability includes at least 10° of increased tibial external rotation compared with the normal knee at 30 and 90° of knee flexion (positive dial test, and external rotation thigh–foot angle test), and variable degrees of varus instability depending on the injured anatomic structures. Posterolateral instability type A has increased external rotation only, corresponding to injury to the popliteofibular ligament, and popliteus tendon only. PLI type B presents with increased external rotation, and mild varus of approximately 5 mm increased lateral joint line opening to varus stress at 30° knee flexion. This occurs with damage to the popliteofibular ligament and popliteus tendon, as well as attenuation of the fibular collateral ligament. PLI type C presents with increased tibial external rotation and varus instability of 10 mm greater than the normal knee tested at 30° of knee flexion with varus stress. This occurs with injury to the popliteofibular ligament, popliteus tendon, fibular collateral ligament, and lateral capsular avulsion, in addition to cruciate ligament disruption.

Since the patient had a type B posterolateral instability, her central pivot reconstruction had chronic repetitive varus and axial rotation forces applied to the ACL/PCL reconstruction, resulting in attenuation, graft failure, and subsequent anterior–posterior and posterolateral laxity. Another contribution to failure may have been the order in which the patient's original operating surgeon performed the ACL and PCL reconstructions. The ACL reconstruction was done first, the PCL reconstruction 6 months later. This order of reconstruction probably displaced the proximal posteriorly, creating a situation of chronic posterior tibial subluxation and compromising the

ACL reconstruction. There may have also been inadequate reduction at the time of the second-stage PCL reconstruction, resulting in a reconstructed knee in which the tibiofemoral joint was never reduced and centered. This condition, combined with the continued posterolateral instability led to the reconstruction failure.

The patient had chronic functional instability with activities of daily living in the setting of a failed ACL-PCL reconstruction. Any reconstructive procedure was purely elective, and surgical timing was determined by patient convenience. Surgical treatment of this patient's left knee consisted of revision single-stage combined arthroscopically assisted ACL-PCL reconstruction and open lateral–posterolateral reconstruction. Since the ACL and PCL tunnels were well positioned, the same tunnels were used. Care was taken to ensure that the tibiofemoral joint was easily reduced and radiographically documented preoperatively, and that there was no fixed posterior tibial subluxation. The PCL reconstruction was an arthroscopically assisted single-bundle single-femoral transtibial technique using a fresh-frozen Achilles tendon allograft. The ACL reconstruction performed was an arthroscopically assisted single-incision technique using a fresh-frozen Achilles tendon allograft. Lateral and posterolateral instability was surgically corrected by a combined reconstruction using a split biceps tendon tenodesis and posterolateral capsular shift procedure. Because the patient had normal lower extremity alignment and no lateral thrusting gait, high tibial osteotomy was not indicated.

During weeks 1 to 6 of the postoperative rehabilitation program the patient was non–weight bearing, and the surgical extremity was braced in full extension. During postoperative weeks 4 to 6, range of motion was progressed. During postoperative weeks 7 to 10, the rehabilitation brace was unlocked, and weight bearing was progressed at 25% of body weight per week over those weeks. The patient was fully weight bearing using crutches at the end of postoperative week 10. Varus forces were avoided during range-of-motion exercises to protect the lateral and posterolateral structures that had been reconstructed. The long-leg rehabilitation brace was discontinued at the end of postoperative week 10, and an ACL-PCL functional brace was used for activities of daily living for continued protection. Range-of-motion exercises were progressed using a stationary bicycle, while strength and proprioceptive skill training were progressed using stair-stepping machines, rowing machines, leg press, elliptical trainers, and balance devices. Straight-line jogging was initiated between postoperative months 4 and 5, and activity level progressed as strength and proprioceptive skills improved.

This patient's Tegner, Lysholm, and Hospital for Special Surgery knee ligament rating scale scores 24 months postreconstruction were 4, 83, 77, respectively. The KT1000 side-to-side difference values for the PCL screen, corrected posterior, and corrected anterior measurements were 4.0, 5.0, and 2.5 mm, respectively. Telos stress radiographic measurements comparing the injured knee and the normal knee, measuring posterior tibial displacement in millimeters with a 32 lb posteriorly directed force applied to the tibial tubercle to assess PCL stability, revealed a 4.0 mm side-to-side difference. Other test results were as follows: Lachman test normal, pivot shift negative, tibial step-off decreased 5 mm, posterior drawer grade I laxity, varus stress test symmetric to the nonsurgical knee, dial test equal to the normal knee at 30 and 90° of knee flexion, and range of motion 0 to 128° on the surgical knee compared with 0 to 142° on the nonsurgical knee. The patient has returned to her desired level of activity.

Index

A

Achilles' tendon, contractures of, 178
Achilles' tendon allografts, 60, 60*f*
   for anterior cruciate ligament/posterior cruciate ligament reconstruction, 118f
   for anterior cruciate ligament reconstruction, 115
   for medial collateral ligament reconstruction, 120f
   for medial side injury reconstruction, 115
   for posterior cruciate ligament reconstruction, 79, 79t, 80, 82, 83f
   for posterolateral reconstruction, 101, 118
   for revision surgery, 230f, 232
   for superficial medial collateral ligament reconstruction, 238
ACL. *See* Anterior cruciate ligament(s)
Allografts, 58, 60–61. *See also* specific types of allografts
   for revision surgery, 229, 230f, 232
American Academy of Orthopedic Surgeons, knee brace classification system of, 243
Amputations
   effect of delayed arterial injury repair on, 23–24, 66
   knee dislocation-related, 52, 161
   popliteal artery injury-related, 151, 152t, 160, 162, 217
   popliteal vein injury-related, 217
Anesthesia, knee examination under, 45, 46, 47, 76–77
Angiography
   versus ankle-brachial index, 134
   of knee dislocations, 157
   of popliteal artery injuries, 155f
Ankle-brachial index (ABI), 65, 97, 134, 157, 158
Anterior cruciate ligament(s)
   anatomy of, 1–2, 3f, 22

   anteromedial band, 21
   posterolateral band, 21
   biomechanics of, 10
   effect of open- and closed-chain knee exercises on, 209
   functions of, 10
   interaction with posterior cruciate ligaments, 11f
   physical examination of
      in acute knee injuries, 25–27, 26f
      in chronic knee injuries, 28
   strain rate in, 40–41, 42, 42f
   tensile strength of, 15
Anterior cruciate ligament injuries, 38–39
   anterior knee dislocation-associated, 63
   avulsion-type, 40
   hyperextension-related, 40
   magnetic resonance imaging of, 30
   mechanism of injury in, 40, 134
   tears
      complete, 218f
      low-velocity knee dislocation-related, 70
      tibial side avulsion injury-related, 72
Anterior cruciate ligament/posterior cruciate ligament injuries
   incidence of, 111
   initial evaluation of, 112
Anterior cruciate ligament/posterior cruciate ligament/medial side knee injuries, 134
   initial evaluation of, 113, 134
   surgical repair of, 70–79, 135
      anterior cruciate ligament reconstruction in, 71, 72, 85, 87–88, 87f, 88f
      arthroscopy in, 77, 78f, 79
      examination under anesthesia in, 76–77
      medial side surgery in, 88–93, 89f, 89t, 90f, 91f, 92f

      patient positioning for, 75–76
      posterior cruciate ligament reconstruction in, 71, 72–75, 79–85, 88f
      preoperative preparation for, 75–76
      timing of, 75
      vascular examination in, 77
Anterior cruciate ligament/posterior cruciate ligament/posterolateral knee injuries, 134
   initial evaluation of, 112–113
   mechanisms of injury in, 112
   open surgical reconstruction of, 136–146
      anterior cruciate ligament tunnels in, 140–141, 141f
      autograft harvest and preparation in, 137, 137f, 138f, 139f, 145, 145f, 146f
      autograft passage and fixation in, 140–141, 141f, 142f
      complications of, 147
      medial side injury repair in, 145–146
      notchplasty in, 138, 139f
      posterior cruciate ligament tunnels in, 139–140, 140f
      posterolateral corner injury repair in, 141, 143
   physical examination of, 112–113
   postoperative rehabilitation of, 147
   surgical treatment for, 135
Anterior cruciate ligament/posterior ligament cruciate/medial/lateral knee side injuries, 111–131
   diagnostic imaging of, 113–114
   initial evaluation of, 112–113
   mechanism of injury in, 112
   surgical treatment for, 114–129
      graft selection for, 115
      graft tensioning and fixation of, 119–121
      surgical technique, 115–119
      timing of, 114–115

Anterior cruciate ligament reconstruction
　in combined posterior cruciate ligament/medial knee injuries, 72
　in combined posterior cruciate ligament reconstruction, 85, 87–88, 87f, 88f, 116–117
　　anterior cruciate ligament tunnels in, 117, 118f, 121, 121f
　　drill guide system in, 116–117, 117f
　　Fanelli Sports Injury Clinic results, 123–126
　　posterior cruciate tunnels in, 116–117, 117f, 121, 121f
　with fresh-frozen allografts, 71
　in posterolaterally-injured knees, 102, 102f, 103–104, 103f, 105, 106
　rehabilitation guidelines for, 93
　tibial side fixation in, 87–88
　with valgus osteotomy, 186
Anterior drawer test, 67
　in anesthetized patients, 77
Arterial injuries. *See also* Popliteal artery injuries
　evaluation of, 155–159
　knee dislocation-associated, 23–24, 23t, 45, 151–165
　　incidence of, 112
　multiple ligament injured knee-associated, 33, 134
　signs of, 156, 156t
Arteriography, 33
　diagnostic, 65, 65f, 112, 134
　for high-energy knee dislocation evaluation, 97
　indications for, 23, 113–114, 170–171
　routine, 158–159
Arteriovenous fistulas, 157–158
Arthroscopy
　diagnostic, 114, 134
　dry setting, 77, 78f
　instruments for, 116, 116f
　intraoperative, 77, 79
　of posterolateral knee injuries, 101
Arthrosis, degenerative, 113
Atherosclerosis, of popliteal artery, 154f
Autografts, 58–60
　contralateral, 58
　ipsilateral, 57
　for revision surgery, 229, 232
Avulsion injuries, 40
　to biceps femoris tendon, 98
　to fibular head, 98, 99f
　to fibular styloid process, 170
　to iliotibial band tendon, 98
　magnetic resonance imaging of, 31, 31f
　to posterior cruciate ligaments, 40
　repair of, 84–85, 86f
　posterolateral knee injury-associated, 100, 101
　radiographic evaluation of, 29, 29f

Axonotmesis, 168, 169
　reinnervation in, 172

B
Barr technique, of peroneal nerve palsy treatment, 176, 177, 178
Biceps femoris complex, 21–22
Biceps femoris tendon
　anatomy of, 4, 4f, 5, 96
　avulsion injuries to, 98
Biceps tenodesis, in posterolateral reconstructions, 105
Biomechanics
　definition of, 9
　of the knee, 9–15
Bone bruises, magnetic resonance imaging of, 31, 32
Bone grafts, 230, 231f
Bone-patellar tendon-bone allografts, 106
　for lateral ligament reconstruction, 106
　for posterolateral knee injury repair, 101
Bone-patellar tendon-bone autografts, 58, 59f
Bone scans, 112, 113
Braces, 243–248
　classification of, 243
　functional, 122, 243, 244–245, 245f
　hinged, postoperative use of, 107, 210, 212, 213
　versus internal fixation, 75
　load-shifting, 245–248, 246f
　for multiple ligament injured knees, 115
　for posterolateral knee injuries, 100, 101
　postoperative, 122, 213–214, 244, 244f, 245f
　　hinged, 107, 210, 212, 213
　for specific ligament injuries, 247t

C
Case studies, 249–259
Cast immobilization, of dislocated knees, 70
Closed-chain exercises, postoperative, 122, 209, 213
　versus open-chain knee exercises, 207–208
　for posterolateral knee injury rehabilitation, 107
Collateral ligaments. *See also* Fibular collateral ligament; Lateral collateral ligament; Medial collateral ligament
　functions and biomechanics of, 13
Color flow duplex scans, 157, 158–159

Common peroneal nerve, anatomy of, 6–7, 168, 169f
Common peroneal nerve injuries
　anatomic basis of, 167–169, 169f
　failed repair or regeneration of, 176–178
　follow-up observations of, 173–176
　history of treatment for, 171–172
　incidence of, 167
　initial evaluation of, 169–171
　natural history of, 172–173
　surgical interventions for, 173–176
　traction injuries, 172
Compartment syndrome
　diagnosis of, 67, 156
　as nerve injury cause, 173
　popliteal artery injury-related, 161, 162
　signs of, 156
　treatment for, 67
　treatment-related, 219–220
Complications, treatment-related, 217–225
　general complications, 218–220
　　compartment syndrome, 219–220
　　fluid extravasation, 219–220
　　iatrogenic vascular injuries, 218–219
　　neurologic injuries, 219
　knee-specific complications, 220–222
　　arthrofibrosis, 221–222
　　ligamentous laxity, 222
Computed tomography, of fractures, 32–33
Contractures, of Achilles' tendon, 178
Coronal alignment, measurement of, 188–189, 188f
Cruciate ligaments. *See also* Anterior cruciate ligament(s); Posterior cruciate ligament(s)
　anatomy of, 21
　biomechanics of, 10–13
　four-bar linkage system of, 11, 12f, 42f
　interplay of, 11–13
Crush injuries, 65

D
Deep peroneal nerve, anatomy of, 168, 169f
Dial external rotation test, 77f
Dial sign/spin-out sign, 28
Dimple sign, 24, 33, 113
Dislocations. *See also* Knee dislocations
　undiagnosed, 193–194
Drawer sign, 25. *See also* Anterior drawer sign; Posterior drawer sign

E
Electrical stimulation, effect on nerve regeneration, 179, 180

Index

Electromyography
- follow-up, in nerve injuries, 173
- intraoperative, in peroneal nerve injury repair, 174
- for nerve injury severity evaluation, 169
- serial, 22, 33

Equinovarus deformity, as peroneal nerve palsy cause, 172

Extensor mechanism injuries, 22
- magnetic resonance imaging of, 30

External fixation, of posterolateral knee injuries, 101

External fixators, 100
- hinged, 75, 76f

External rotation recurvatum test, 98

F

Fabellofibular ligament, anatomy of, 95–96, 96f

Falls, as knee dislocation cause, 154, 154t

Fanelli Sports Injury Clinic, multiple ligament-injured knee reconstruction results of
- for combined anterior cruciate ligament/posterior cruciate ligament reconstructions, 123–126
- for combined posterior cruciate ligament/posterolateral reconstructions, 123–126

Fascia lata allografts, 61

Fascia lata autografts, 60

Fasciotomy, 100
- four-compartment, 162

Femoral artery, anatomy of, 151

Femoral condyles
- anatomy of, 1
- lateral, 1, 2
  - biomechanics of, 12–13
- medial, 1, 2

Femoral nerve, muscles innervated by, 5

Femur
- distal, fractures of, 22, 64, 66
- knee dislocation-associated bruising of, 67f

Fibula, knee dislocation-associated fractures of, 22

Fibular collateral ligament
- anatomy of, 21, 95
- complete femoral rupture of, 32f
- functions of, 21

Fibular head
- avulsion injuries to, 98, 99f
- fractures of, 66, 103, 104f

Fibular styloid process, avulsion of, 170

Figure-of-eight technique, 117, 118–119, 119f

Figure-of-four position, 27

Flexion angles, of the knee, 9–10

Fluid extravasation, 219–220

Footdrop
- L4 or L5 radiculopathy-related, 170
- peroneal nerve injury-related, 97, 107
- correction of, 176–178

Four-bar linkage system, of cruciate ligaments, 11, 12f, 42f

Fracture-dislocations, of the knee, 38, 44, 45f, 46t, 104f

Fractures. *See also* specific types of fractures
- computed tomography of, 32–33
- knee dislocation-associated, 22, 38, 66
  - as popliteal artery injury cause, 155, 156f
- open, 114
- radiographic evaluation of, 29
- undiagnosed, 193–194

G

Gerdy's tubercle, avulsion of, 99

Godfrey's sign, 24, 25f, 72, 73f

Grafts, 57–62, 115. *See also* specific types of grafts
- for anterior cruciate ligament reconstruction, 119, 121
- failure of, 227–228
- inadequate fixation of, 227
- for posterior cruciate ligament reconstruction, 119, 120f
- for posterolateral knee injury repair, 101
- for revision surgery, 229, 230f, 232
- strength of, 227–228
- structural properties of, 15

H

Hamstring tendon grafts, 58, 59–60, 59f, 61

Hardware removal
- of painful hardware, 129
- in revision surgery, 230, 230f, 231f

Hinged braces, for posterolateral knee injuries, 107

Hinges, use in chronic fixed posterior tibial subluxation treatment, 199–204
- biomechanics of, 200–203, 200f, 201t, 202f
- clinical results of, 203–204, 203f, 204f
- placement of, 199–200, 199f, 200f

Hyperextension
- as knee dislocation injury mechanism, 40, 41, 42, 42f, 112
- as popliteal artery injury mechanism, 155
- as posterolateral knee injury mechanism, 97

Hyperextension recurvatum test, 41f

I

Iliotibial band
- anatomy of, 4, 4f, 5, 96, 96f
- avulsion injuries to, 98

Imaging studies. *See also* Computed tomography; Magnetic resonance imaging; Radiography
- of acute anterior cruciate ligament/posterior cruciate ligament injuries, 112
- for initial knee injury assessment, 29–33

Infection, as graft failure cause, 228

Innervation, of the knee, 6-7, 7f. *See also* specific nerves

Instruments, arthroscopic, 116, 116f

Internal fixation, *versus* bracing, 75

Intimal injuries
- delayed presentation of, 112
- popliteal, 155, 155f, 158

Ischemia, arterial injury or occlusion-related, 156, 157, 170, 171

J

Jerk test of Hughston, 26

K

Kinetics
- definition of, 9
- of the knee, 9–15

Knee
- anatomy of, 1–7, 38–39
  - cruciate ligaments, 2–3, 3f
  - innervation, 6–7, 7f
  - lateral and posterolateral stabilizers of the knee, 4, 4f
  - medial stabilizers, 3–4, 4f
  - menisci, 5
  - musculature, 5–6
  - osteology, 1–2, 2f
  - vasculature, 6, 7f
- biomechanics and kinetics of, 9–15
- functions of, 9
- passive motion of, 9–10
- posterolateral
  - anatomy of, 95–96, 96f
  - injuries to. *See* Posterolateral knee injuries
- surgical approaches to, 8–9
  - lateral, 8, 9f
  - medial, 8, 8f
  - medial parapatellar, 8

Knee dislocations
- as amputation cause, 52, 161
- anatomic factors in, 38–39
- anterior, 19, 44, 63, 111, 133–134
  - intimal injuries associated with, 155
  - mechanism of, 63
  - vascular injuries associated with, 65
- causes of, 154t

Knee dislocations (*cont.*)
  classification of, 19–20, 20t, 37–38, 42–47, 63, 111, 133–134
    anatomy-based, 46–47, 46t, 95
    position-based, 44–45
  cruciate-intact, 37, 38f
  definition of, 37, 51
  elective reconstruction of, 135
  emergency treatment for, 68–70
    in irreducible dislocations, 69–70
    in open dislocations, 69
    in popliteal artery injuries, 68–69
  evaluation of, 155–156
  high-velocity/energy, 39–40, 112, 133, 134
    initial management of, 99–100
    life-threatening injuries associated with, 155–156
    physical examination of, 97–98
  incidence of, 37, 51
  initial evaluation and management of, 66–68, 66t, 113, 134–135, 155–156
  injuries associated with, 22, 37, 38, 51–54, 64
    ligamentous injuries, 51
    nerve injuries, 51–52, 66
    vascular injuries, 52, 64–66, 133–134
  with intact anterior cruciate ligaments, 43, 43f
  with intact posterior cruciate ligaments, 42–43, 44
  irreducible, surgical treatment for, 69–70, 135
  lateral, 19, 44, 63, 111
  low-velocity/energy, 39–40, 112, 133, 134
    ultra-low velocity, 169
  mechanism of injury in, 39–42, 63, 134
  medial, 19, 44, 63, 64f, 111, 133
  nonoperative treatment for, 51–55
    cast immobilization, 52
    comparison with operative treatment, 52–54
  open, 111–112
    soft-tissue injuries associated with, 19–20
    treatment for, 69, 111–112
  posterior, 19, 44, 63, 64f, 111, 133–134
    mechanism injury in, 63
    vascular injuries associated with, 65, 155
  posterolateral
    irreducible, 24, 33
    open reduction of, 170, 173
  reduction of, 66, 66t
  rotational, 19, 44, 63, 111, 133
    mechanism of injury in, 64
  spontaneous, morbid obesity-related, 20, 154, 217
  spontaneous reduction of, 37, 51, 111, 112, 133, 156
  sports-related, 39–40
  ultra-low velocity, 169
  undiagnosed, 193–194
Knee ligament tensioning device, 119, 120f, 121, 238, 239f
Knee malalignment, osteotomy treatment for, 185–191
Knee recurvatum, 27, 27f, 28
  posterolateral complex injury-associated, 30f
Knee stability testing, for knee dislocation evaluation, 66–67
Knee subluxation, 111

L
Lachman's test, 25, 66, 98, 112–113, 135
Lateral capsular avulsion sign, 29f
Lateral collateral ligament, anatomy and function of, 4, 4f
Lateral collateral ligament reconstruction, in posterolaterally-injured knees, 103, 105–106
Lateral ligament reconstruction, implication of nerve injuries for, 174
Lateral sural cutaneous artery, anatomy of, 7, 7f
Lateral surgical approach, 8, 9f
Ligament(s). *See also* specific ligaments
  anatomy of, 21–22
  examination of, 33, 135
    post-reduction, 25
  knee dislocation-related injuries to, 51
  tensile strength of, 15
Ligament of Humphrey, function of, 5
Ligament of Wrisberg, function of, 5
Ligamentous laxity
  postoperative, 222
  in varus/valgus plane, 66–67
Ligamentous peroneal nerve syndrome, 167, 168f
Ligament reconstruction, biomechanics of, 14–15

M
Magnetic resonance imaging (MRI)
  under anesthesia, 134
  of bone bruises, 32
  of chronic fixed posterior tibial subluxation, 196, 196f
  of cruciate ligament injuries, 30–31, 31f, 33
  of dislocated knees, 32, 67–68, 67f, 68f
    under anesthesia, 46
    preoperative, 46–47
  of fractures, 32–33
  of meniscal injuries, 31–32, 33
  of multiple ligament injured knee, 113, 217, 218f
  of posterior cruciate ligament tears, 72
  of posterolateral knee injuries, 31, 99, 100f, 135
  preoperative, in revision surgery patients, 229
Mannitol, 161
MCL. *See* Medial collateral ligament
Medial capsular ligament, anatomy of, 3–4
Medial collateral ligament
  anatomy of, 3, 4, 21
  deep, 21
  physical examination of, 27, 135
    in acute knee injury, 27
    in chronic knee injury, 28
  role in valgus stability, 13
  tensile strength of, 15
Medial collateral ligament injuries
  with anterior cruciate ligament and posterior ligament injuries, 135–136
  complete tears, 218f
  conservative treatment for, 135
  mechanism of injury in, 134
Medial collateral ligament reconstruction, 119, 120f, 136
  in revision surgery, 237–238, 238f
Medial parapatellar surgical approach, 8
Medial patellofemoral ligament, anatomy and function of, 14, 14f
Medial side knee injuries, 63–94
  high-grade, 113
  nonoperative treatment for, 145
  reconstruction of, 70–79, 88–92, 89f, 89t, 90f, 91f, 92f, 119, 120f
    in chronic medial side laxity, 90–92, 91f, 92f
    grafts for, 115
    open surgical reconstruction, 145–146, 147
  rehabilitation guidelines for, 93
Medial surgical approach, 8, 8f
Meniscus
  anatomy of, 1–2, 10
  biomechanics and kinetics of, 10
  injuries to, magnetic resonance imaging of, 31–32, 33
  lateral
    anatomy of, 5, 5f
    mobility of, 10
  medial
    anatomy of, 5, 5f
    knee dislocation-related extrusion of, 67, 68f
    tears of, in anterior cruciate ligament-deficient knees, 10

Metaphyseal fractures, magnetic resonance imaging of, 32
Motion planes, of the knee, 9
Motor vehicle accidents, as knee injury cause, 20, 39, 63, 154, 154t
Multiple ligament injured knees, 111–131. *See also* specific ligament injuries
  classification of, 19–20, 20t, 111–112
  initial evaluation of, 112–113, 134–135
    diagnostic arthroscopy, 114
    imaging studies, 113–114
  mechanism of injuries in, 112
  postoperative rehabilitation of, 122
  reconstruction of
    anterior cruciate ligament/posterior cruciate ligament reconstruction, 116–117, 117f, 118f
    causes of failure of, 227–229
    complications of, 129
    graft selection for, 115
    indications for, 114
    medial reconstruction, 119, 120f
    posterolateral reconstruction, 117–119, 119f
    results of, 122–129
    surgical techniques, 115–116, 115f, 116f
    timing of, 114–115
  three-ligament injuries, as potential dislocation, 170
Musculature, of the knee, 5–6

N
Nerve grafting, 22
  in peroneal nerve repair, 174, 175
Nerve injuries, 22, 51–52, 66, 167–183
  anatomic basis of, 168–169
  follow-up observations of, 173–176
  history of treatment for, 171–172
  incidence of, 167
  initial evaluation of, 169–171
  mechanisms of, 167–168
  severity classification of, 168–169
  treatment-related, 219
Nerve regeneration
  electrical stimulation-enhanced, 179, 180
  rate of, 172
Neurolysis, 52, 107, 171, 175
Neuromas, medial parapatellar approach-related, 8
Neuropraxia, 168, 169, 170, 175
  reinnervation in, 172
Neurotmesis, 168, 169
  reinnervation in, 172
Notchplasty
  inadequate, 227
  in multiple ligament injured knee reconstruction, 116

O
Ober method, of peroneal nerve palsy treatment, 176, 178
Obesity
  morbid, as knee dislocation cause, 20, 154, 217
  vascular complications of, 217
Open-chain knee exercises, postoperative, 213
  for posterolateral knee injury rehabilitation, 107
Open ligament reconstruction, 133–149
  complications of, 147
  indications for, 135–136
  postoperative rehabilitation in, 147
  surgical technique in, 136–146
Open reduction, of posterolateral knee dislocations, 170, 173
Orthosis, ankle-foot, 107, 173, 176
Osteolysis, as bone grafting indication, 230, 231f
Osteotomy
  high tibial, 190
    in chronic posterolateral instability patients, 104
  opening wedge, 188, 190–191
  opening wedge high tibial, 121–122, 122f, 239, 240f
  in the unstable knee, 185–191
    limb alignment considerations in, 185–187
    operative technique, 188–190
    results of, 190–191
    tibial, indications for, 187–188, 188t
  valgus, 186

P
Patella, anatomy and functions of, 2, 2f
Patellar plexus, anatomy of, 7
Patellar retinaculum, anatomy of, 4, 4f
Patellar tendon allografts, for posterolateral knee injury repair, 101
Patellar tendon autografts, 58
Patellar tendon grafts, tensile strength of, 15
Patellofemoral joint, biomechanics of, 13–14, 14f
Patellofemoral joint forces, during open chain knee exercises, 208
Patellofemoral ligaments, anatomy of, 4, 4f, 14, 14f
PCL. *See* Posterior cruciate ligament(s)
Pellegrini-Stieda sign, 29f
Peripheral nerve stimulators, 179
Peroneal nerve. *See also* Common peroneal nerve; Deep peroneal nerve
  examination of, pre- and postreduction, 97
  location of, 4
Peroneal nerve injuries
  incidence of, 107
  knee dislocation-associated, 22, 66
    classification of, 97
  posterolateral knee injury-associated, 107
  prognosis for, 107
  traction injuries, 174, 176
Peroneal nerve palsy, 172
  fibular styloid process avulsion-related, 170
  as footdrop cause, 97, 107
    correction of, 176–178
  posterolateral knee dislocation-associated, 45
Physical examination, of knee
  of acute knee injuries, 24–28
  under anesthesia, 45, 46, 47, 76–77
  of anterior cruciate ligament injuries, 25–27, 26f
    in acute knee injuries, 25–27, 26f
    in chronic knee injuries, 28
  of anterior cruciate ligament/posterior cruciate ligament/medial side injured knees, 113
  of anterior cruciate ligament/posterior cruciate ligament/posterolateral injured knees, 112–113
  of chronic knee injuries, 27f, 28
  of high-velocity knee dislocations, 97–98
  of ligaments, 135
  of posterolateral knee injuries, 97–98
  for vascular injury detection, 157–159
Pivot shift test, 26, 112–113
  for chronically-injured knee evaluation, 28
  contraindication in acutely-dislocated knees, 67
  false-negative results in, 135
  Slocum variation of, 26–27
Popliteal artery
  anatomy of, 6f, 64–65, 151–152
  atherosclerosis of, 154f
  normal angiogram of, 152, 152f
  occlusion of, 170
  pseudoaneurysms of, 155, 158
  spasms of, 161, 162f
  surgical exposure of, 152–153, 153f
  thrombosis of, 20, 155, 155f, 158
    posterior surgical approach in, 153
Popliteal artery injuries, 64–65
  as amputation cause, 151, 152t, 160, 162, 217
  emergency treatment for, 68–69
  intimal, 155, 155f
  in irreducible dislocations, 69–70

Popliteal artery injuries (cont.)
  limb salvage in, 161, 162
  mechanism of injury in, 52, 154–155, 154t
  nonoperative treatment for, 52, 158
  palpable pulses associated with, 156–157, 157t
  peroneal nerve injury-associated, 22
  prevalence of, 154t
  surgical treatment for, 159–161, 160f
  venous ligation in, 160–161
Popliteal fibular ligament, anatomy and function of, 21
Popliteal fossa, anatomy of, 6
Popliteal nerve injuries, 51–52
  incidence of, 52
  prognosis of, 52
Popliteal vein
  anatomy of, 152
  duplicated, 152
  surgical exposure of, 153, 153f
Popliteofibular ligament
  anatomy and function of, 4
  biomechanics of, 97
  reconstruction of, 105
  surgical access to, 101–102
Popliteus complex
  anatomy and function of, 21
  reconstruction of, 106
Popliteus muscle
  anatomy of, 5, 96, 96f
  functions of, 11
Popliteus tendon
  anatomy of, 4, 4f, 5, 21, 96
  function of, 4
Posterior capsule. See also Posterolateral capsule
  in transtibial posterior cruciate ligament reconstruction, 116
Posterior cruciate ligament(s)
  anatomy of, 2, 3, 22
    anterolateral band/bundle, 21, 74, 74f
    anterolateral bundle, 74, 74f
    meniscofemoral ligaments, 74–75
    posterolateral band/bundle, 21, 74–75, 74f
    secondary restraints, 22
  biomechanics of, 10–11
  effect of open- and closed-chain knee exercises on, 208, 209
  femoral insertion of, 21
  functions of, 10
  interaction with anterior cruciate ligament, 11f
  physical examination of, 27
    in acute knee injury, 27
    in chronic knee injury, 28
  strain rate in, 41, 42, 42f
  tensile strength of, 15

Posterior cruciate ligament-deficient knees, popliteus muscle function in, 11
Posterior cruciate ligament injuries, 38–39
  with anterior cruciate ligament injuries, 14
  anterior knee dislocation-related, 63
  arthroscopic evaluation of, 114
  avulsion injuries, 40
    imaging of, 31, 31f
    magnetic resonance imaging of, 67, 68f
    repair of, 84–85, 86f
  complete tears, 218f
  incidence of, 11
  isolated, 11
    reconstruction of, 14
  magnetic resonance imaging of, 30–31, 31f
  mechanism of injury in, 134
  peel-off, 40, 41, 99
  physical examination of, 135
  with posterolateral corner injuries, 14
  severity grading of, 72–74
Posterior cruciate ligament reconstruction
  allograft use in, 70–71
  with anterior cruciate ligament reconstruction, 71, 72–75, 79–85, 88f, 116–117
    with Achilles tendon allografts, 79, 79t, 80, 82, 83f
    double-bundle technique, 84, 88f
    drill guide system in, 116–117, 117f
    endoscopic technique, 81, 82
    Fanelli Sports Injury Clinic results, 123–126
    graft choice for, 79–80, 79t
    guide pins for, 80–81, 81f, 82f
    guides for, 80f, 81
    outside-in technique, 82, 83f
    posterior cruciate tunnels in, 116–117, 117f, 121, 121f
    posterior tibial inlay technique in, 84, 85f
    transtibial, 79–83, 80f, 81f, 83f
  autograft patellar tendon graft use in, 70, 71
  in combined anterior cruciate ligament/medial side knee injuries, 72–75
  double-bundle technique in, 11
  in posterolaterally-injured knee, 102–104, 102f, 103f, 105, 106, 126–129
  with posterolateral reconstruction, 126–129
  rehabilitation guidelines for, 93

  in revision surgery, 238, 239f
  ruptures of
    isolated, 11
    with posterolateral corner injuries, 11
  transtibial, posterior capsule elevation in, 116, 116f
Posterior drawer test, 26f, 27, 67, 72, 73f, 98
  in anesthetized patients, 77
  in chronically-injured knees, 28
  in posterolateral complex injuries, 28
Posterior tibial tendon transfer, 176–177, 178
Posterolateral capsule
  anatomy of, 95–96
  knee-stabilizing function of, 74
Posterolateral complex
  anatomy of, 95–96, 96f
  biomechanics of, 96–97
  failed reconstruction of, 27f
  physical examination of, 27–28
    in acute knee injury, 27–28
Posterolateral complex injuries, as excessive varus cause, 24, 24f
Posterolateral corner
  knee-stabilizing function of, 74
  physical examination of, in chronic knee injuries, 28
Posterolateral corner injuries
  after posterior cruciate ligament reconstruction, 22
  delayed reconstruction of, 71
  imaging studies of, 31, 32t, 135
  tibial laxity associated with, 25–26
Posterolateral instability, types of, 113
Posterolateral knee injuries, 44–45, 95–110
  dimple sign of, 113
  imaging studies of, 98–99, 99f, 100f
  initial management of, 99–100
  irreducibility of, 44–45
  peroneal nerve injuries associated with, 107
  postoperative rehabilitation of, 107
  surgical treatment/reconstruction of, 100–106, 117–119
    acute repairs/reconstruction, 102–104, 102f, 103f, 104f
    chronic, 104–106
    combined with posterior cruciate ligament reconstruction, 126–129
    timing of, 100–101
Posterolateral sling procedure, 106
Proprioceptive training, postoperative, 122, 213
Pseudoaneurysms, popliteal, 155, 158
Pulse examination
  of dislocated knee, 156–157
  in high-energy knee dislocations, 97

Q
Q angle, 14
Quadriceps active testing, 27, 28
Quadriceps muscle
    anatomy and innervation of, 5
    anterior cruciate ligament rupture-related atrophy of, 12
Quadriceps tendon allografts, 60
Quadriceps tendon autografts, 58–59, 59f

R
Radiculopathy, lumbar, as footdrop cause, 170
Radiography, 29–30, 33, 135
    of knee dislocations, 66, 66t
    of multiple ligament injured knees, 113
    preoperative, in revision surgery patients, 229
    stress, 30, 30f, 229
    of posterolateral knee injuries, 99, 100f
Range-of-motion exercises, postoperative, 122, 210, 212–213, 212t
Rehabilitation, postoperative, 207–216, 239–240
    after multiple ligament knee reconstruction, 122, 209–214, 211t, 2127
    of anterior cruciate ligament injuries, 93
    of medial side knee injuries, 93
    open-chain knee exercises in, 209
        versus closed chain exercises, 207–208
        during months 4 to 6, 211t, 213–214
        during weeks 1 to 6, 210, 211t, 212t
        during weeks 7 to 12, 211t, 212–213
    of posterior cruciate ligament injuries, 93
    of posterolateral knee injuries, 107
Reverse pivot shift test
    contraindication in acutely dislocated knees, 67
    positive, 98
    posterolateral complex injury-related, 28
Revision surgery, in the multiple ligament-injured knee, 227–242
    anterior cruciate-posterior ligament ligament reconstruction in, 232–241
    drill guide system for, 233, 234f
    medial reconstruction in, 237–238
    operative technique, 232–235, 233f, 234f
    posterior tibial and femoral tunnels in, 233–234, 234f, 235
    posterolateral reconstruction in, 235–237, 236f, 237f
    results of, 240
    grafts for, 229, 230f, 232
    hardware removal in, 230, 230f, 231f
    indications for, 228
    operative technique in, 231–232
    preoperative evaluation of, 229
    technical considerations in, 229

S
Sagittal tibial alignment, 187, 187f
Sag sign, 72, 73f
Saphenous vein grafts, interposition, 160f
Schenck classification system, for multiple ligament injured knees, 19, 20t
Sciatic artery, 151
Sciatic nerve, anatomy of, 168
Segond injuries, 21
    radiographic evaluation of, 29, 29f
Shunts, temporary vascular, 159
Skin examination, in open knee dislocations, 97–98
Slocum maneuver, 26–27
Spasms, of popliteal artery, 161, 162f
Spin-out/dial sign, 28
Spin test, 98, 98f
Split biceps tendon transfer, 117–118, 119f
Sports, as knee injury cause, 20, 39–40, 154, 154t
Stability examination, 25
Stocking paresthesia, 171
Strain rate, effect on ligament failure, 40–42, 42f
Stretch injuries, 65
Superficial peroneal nerve, anatomy of, 168, 169f
Sural nerve grafts, 22, 175

T
Tensioning device, 238, 239f
Thrombosis, deep venous, 112
Tibia
    dislocation of, 64
    displacement of, 63
    knee dislocation-associated bruising of, 67f
    proximal, fractures of, 66
Tibial eminence fractures, 72
Tibial external rotation testing, in anesthetized patients, 77
Tibial inlay technique, in revision surgery, 234–235
Tibial nerve examination, pre- and postreduction, 97
Tibial nerve injuries, 169
Tibial plateau fractures
    iatrogenic, 129
    knee dislocation-associated, 22, 66
    radiographic evaluation of, 29
Tibial subluxation, chronic fixed posterior, 193–205
    clinical presentation of, 193–194
    incidence of, 193
    physical examination of, 194–195, 195f
    postoperative care in, 198, 204–205
    radiographic evaluation of, 195–196, 195f, 196f
    treatment options for, 196–197
        amputation, 197
        arthrodesis, 197
        hinge-based reconstruction, 199–204, 199f, 200f, 203f, 204f
        nonoperative treatment, 196–197
        reconstruction, 198
        reduction, 197–198
Tibiofemoral joint, cruciate intact rotatory dislocation of, 38–39, 39f
Tinel's sign, 172, 173, 174
Tolazoline, 161
Total knee arthroplasty
    medial parapatellar approach in, 8
    as popliteal artery injury cause, 154
Tourniquets, 101, 135
Traction injuries, peroneal, 172, 174, 176
Trampoline injuries, 20, 154
Trauma, postreconstruction, 228
Triple-varus knee, 186

V
Valgus malalignment, osteotomy treatment for, 185–186
Valgus motion, role of medial collateral ligament in, 13
Valgus stress testing, 27
    in anesthetized patients, 77
Varus deformity, with lateral thrust, 121–122
Varus malalignment, osteotomy treatment for, 185–186
Varus motion, role of cruciate ligaments in, 13
Varus stress testing, 27
    in anesthetized patients, 77
Vascular examination
    in anesthetized patients, 77
    of knee dislocations, 66, 66t
Vascular injuries
    iatrogenic, 218–219
    knee dislocation-associated, 52, 64–66, 133–134, 134

Vascular injuries (*cont.*)
  in high-velocity dislocations, 217
  in low-velocity dislocations, 217
  in multiple ligament-injured knees, 170
  obesity-related, 217
Vasculature, of the knee, 6
Vastus intermedius muscle, anatomy of, 5
Vastus lateralis muscle, anatomy of, 5
Vastus medialis muscle, anatomy of, 5, 14
Venography
  diagnostic, 112
  indications for, 114
Venous injuries
  knee dislocation-associated, 151–165

W

War, popliteal artery injuries during, 151, 160
Work-related injuries, as knee dislocation cause, 154, 154t